MILADY'S AESTHETICIAN SERIES

Peels and Peeling Agents

MILADY'S AESTHETICIAN SERIES

Peels and Peeling Agents

PAMELA HILL, R.N.

THOMSON

DELMAR LEARNING

Australia Canada Mexico Singapore Spain United Kingdom United States

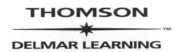

THOMSON

DELMAR LEARNING

Milady's Aesthetician Series: Peels and Peeling Agents
Pamela Hill, RN

President, Milady:
Dawn Gerrain

Director of Editorial:
Sherry Gomoll

Acquisitions Editor:
Brad Hanson

Developmental Editor:
Jessica Burns

Editorial Assistant:
Jessica Burns

Director of Production:
Wendy A. Troeger

Production Editor:
Nina Tucciarelli

Composition:
Cadmus Professional Communications

Director of Marketing:
Wendy Mapstone

Channel Manager:
Sandra Bruce

Cover and Text Design:
Essence of 7

Library of Congress Cataloging-in-Publication Data

Hill, Pamela, RN.
    Peels and peeling agents / Pamela Hill.
        p. ; cm. –(Milady's aesthetician series)
    Includes bibliographical references.
    ISBN 1-4018-8177-7 (pbk.)
    1. Chemical peel. 2. Skin–Surgery. 3. Face–Surgery. 4. Surgery, Plastic.
    [DNLM: 1. Keratolytic Agents. 2. Skin Care–methods. QV 60 H647p 2006] I. Title.
RD520.H55 2006
617.4'770592–dc22

2005015633

NOTICE TO THE READER

Contents

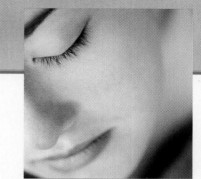

CHAPTER 2

CHAPTER 3

CHAPTER 4

CHAPTER 5

Preface

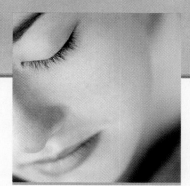

A skilled and knowledgeable clinician who understands and feels comfortable providing chemical peels can achieve a substantial result for the patient. However, unlike microdermabrasion, chemical peels can carry a greater risk of complications and potential scarring. Until now, little valuable information has come to the clinical aesthetician and cosmetic nurse about the concepts of peeling and the normal healing that follows. As the leader of a network of medical skin care clinics, I have heard clinicians beg for more information to expand their knowledge base about peels. For the last 14 years I have spent my days managing medical spas. Part of my job as the president and chief executive officer was the development and oversight of the training programs for our facilities. Needless to say, I have met and trained many clinicians. What I noticed is that my first-rate, curious clinicians (aestheticians and nurses) can never get enough information. They are always looking for more information, improved technology to provide advanced results, a new book, and more and more! Although these questions are obvious signs of good clinicians, they are wrought with peril given that unbiased information is not always available.

This book is intended for persons who are studying to become first-rate clinicians, as well as for clinicians who thirst for more information, expanding on what they already know. That said, this text is written to expand on the basic knowledge of aesthetician training, taking it from a conceptual level to the practical level.

I have researched and written this book so that I could satisfy the hunger that makes a great aesthetician and cosmetic nurse. Chemical peeling has developed into one of the most popular procedures in the skin care industry, but great variation exists in the results, peel solutions, and postcare processes. Research exists that shows remarkable results in the improvement of both the epidermis and the dermis. However, chemical peeling is technique dependent, and success is based in decreasing the variables and the ability to teach your patient all the tricks of the trade. This book takes modern research, facts, and opinions, and shapes them into a start-to-finish model. This model has one fundamental intent: ideal results for both the clinician and the patient.

This *clinical handbook* for chemical peeling is my answer to the chants for more information. The chapters are organized one on top of the other, with *essential, must-have information* on chemical peeling. To this effect, general knowledge is expanded on, and insightful hints and recommendations allow you to optimize your knowledge and achieve the optimal, replicable results that will ensure your success. Each chapter has questions and "Top Ten Tips to Take to the Clinic," which will help you well beyond your training and give you the knowledge that is helpful beyond the classroom. Each specific peel chapter is dedicated to the process from beginning to end. The book was developed to help you learn the basics of chemical peeling while adding information that will allow you, the clinician, to develop, refine, and redefine your skills.

Good luck!

About the Author

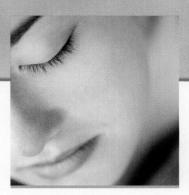

Pamela Hill, RN, CEO, received her diploma from Presbyterian/St. Luke's Hospital and Colorado Women's College. She followed through to practice as a registered nurse for more than 20 years with her initial emphasis in cardiac surgery and then in cosmetic surgery and medical skin care. In 1992, Ms. Hill founded Facial Aesthetics®, a network of medical skin care clinics in association with John A. Grossman, MD Since then, Ms. Hill has been an industry pioneer in the growth and development of the medical spa industry. As the president and chief executive officer of Facial Aesthetics®, Ms. Hill has been a proactive member and pioneer in the evolution of the medical spa model and the integration and union of cosmeceuticals and nonsurgical skin care. In addition to her leadership in the medical spa industry, she has also been actively engaged in the research and development of the successful Pamela Hill Skin Care product line.

Ms. Hill has devoted her passion for nonmedical skin care to the instruction of a higher level of education and skill for those aspiring to be the aestheticians of tomorrow. To further this mission, Ms. Hill founded the Pamela Hill Institute® in 2004. The goal of the Pamela Hill Institute® is to develop a uniform and comprehensive curriculum, as well as resources for aesthetic education, the advancement of cutting-edge technologies, while placing an emphasis on client care and safety for patients, students, and product lines as well.

Reviewers

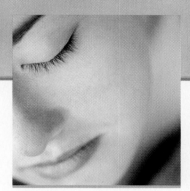

The author and publisher wish to thank the reviewers for their assistance and expertise in producing this text. We are indebted to them.

Darlene Battaiola,
Butte, Massachusetts

Alan Bunting,
Loxahatchee, Florida

Pat Cavenaugh,
Carolina Beach, North Carolina

Sallie Deitz,
Bellingham, Washington

Patricia Heitz,
Albany, New York

Ruth Ann Holloway,
Providence, Utah

Rose Policastro,
Little Ferry, New Jersey

Ellen Thorpe,
Mesa, Arizona

Karen Wackerman,
Phoenix, Arizona

Acknowledgments

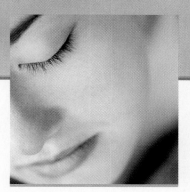

The Medical Aesthetics Series is a group of books that will help clinicians grow to a new level. As the president and chief executive officer of a multi-location medical spa, I know how important this information is to our industry. I would like to acknowledge all of the aestheticians, nurses, and physicians assistants who strive each day to make a better place in our world.

I would also like to acknowledge the love of my life, my husband, John. Always at my side, he has been my best critic, my beacon of light, my teacher, and my best friend without whom this book would not exist.

I would also like to acknowledge the staff at all of my clinics who supported me, taught me, and rallied me on to the goal line. But, there are two individuals at my clinics that stand out. First, Carmela, the aesthetician who took care of the patients represented in this text. Without her help, we would not have achieved our goals. And in the "writing dug-out" was Christian Sterling. He has been with me each day, documenting references, researching, and helping me to stay focused. Without these two very dedicated individuals, this book would never have found completion.

Additional thanks go to everyone at Milady who believed in my message and supported me through this process.

Milady and the author would like to thank the following for contributing to this series:

Larry Hamill Photography, Denver, CO

The owner, Edit Viski-Hanka, and her entire staff at Edit Euro Spa in Denver, CO, for allowing us to use their beautiful location for our photo shoot.

Aesthetic Technologies for graciously allowing the use of the Parisian Peel® Prestige™

Models who participated in the photo shoot:

Jessica Anderson Barbour	Julie O'Toole
Marnie Brooks	Jeffrey Robison
Tina Marie Castillo	Melissa Ryan
Beverley J. Grant	Kathryn Staples
Velma Guss	Christian M. Sterling
Alysa K. Hill	Kavina Trujillo
Patricia Iannacito	Lawrence P. Trujillo, Jr.
Rosalyn Kurpiers	Nina Tucciarelli
Sandra D. Martinez	Karyn Turner
Connee McAllister	Phyllis Walsh
Patricia J. McIntyre	Pamela Whatcott
Polly McKibben	Lisa Williams
Barbara J. Miller	Donna R. Wilson
Susan Nathan	Sandra Vinnik
Janene T. Newell	Edit Viski-Hanka

Illustration credits

Introduction to Peels and Peeling

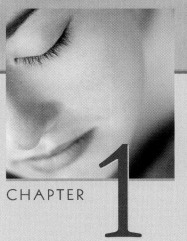

CHAPTER

1

KEY TERMS

5-flourouracil (5-FU)
alpha hydroxy acids
anatomy
Ayurveda
Blue Peel®
carbolic acid
carbon dioxide (CO₂)
    laser
career plan
chemical peeling
chemoexfoliants
Chi (or Qi)
clinic protocols
collagen
continuing educational
    units (CEUs)
cosmeceutical
deep epidermal wounding
dermaplaning
dyschromias
epidermal cells
erbium laser

four humors
glycolic acid
ground substance
Health Insurance Porta-
    bility and Accountabil-
    ity Act (HIPAA)
hepatitis
herpes simplex
Hippocrates
Hippocratic oath
human immunodeficiency
    virus/acquired immu-
    nodeficiency syn-
    drome (HIV/AIDS)
hypopigmentation
Jessner's solution
keratolysis
lymphatic drainage
mission statement
necrosis
nonsurgical aesthetic skin
    care

papillary dermal wounding
partial-thickness injury
peel depth
phenol
physiology
postinflammatory hyper-
    pigmentation
poultices
professional ethics
progressive improvement
    plan (PIP)
pyruvic acid
radio frequency (RF)
reflexology
resorcinol
Retin A®
salicylic acid
technique sensitive
telangiectasia
trichloroacetic acid
yin and yang

LEARNING OBJECTIVES

After completing this chapter you should be able to:

1. Describe the history of peels and peeling.
2. Discuss the value of clinical training for peeling.
3. Discuss variations in licensure regulations and insurance requirements.
4. Name the career options available with peel training.
5. Understand the key points of professional ethics.

1

INTRODUCTION

Lines, wrinkles, and sagging skin were once considered irreversible consequences of the aging process. Prior generations grudgingly accepted their right of passage into the golden years. Some elders wore their lines proudly as a testament to their survival through war, depression, and oppression. Today, the opposite is true. The signs of aging are considered unwarranted and unwanted. As the baby boomers pass into their own golden years, they have been responsible for the creation of a multi-billion dollar industry we call **nonsurgical aesthetic skin care**. In a desire to sustain a youthful appearance, these baby boomers and the generations that follow them have forced our industry to develop products and refine services to meet their needs. Among these services is **chemical peeling.** Chemical peels are exactly as they sound, using agents to peel the outermost layer or layers of skin, allowing newer and healthier skin to present itself. Peels can be an individual procedure or a single step in a multifaceted treatment plan. A large number of different types of peels, as well as different peel depths, have been developed. Some of the deeper peels can cause serious injury, more so than most other treatments that an aesthetician will perform on patients; these are the peels with the greatest amount of success, as well as greatest potential for consequences. Therefore a thorough understanding of chemical peels is vital to your success as an aesthetician.

Chemical peels have an expansive appeal with young and old persons alike. With many positive attributes to recommend it, chemical peels are the preferred treatment for many signs of aging, including **dyschromias** and fine lines. However, these results do not come without risks. Depending on the particular peel, the downtime, as well as the risk of infection and scarring, can be significant.

Progress in medical science and **cosmeceutical** research has made great strides in our ability to treat the skin and generate nonsurgical results. Our society puts a high value on the commodity of youth, and this means looking younger and fit. However, let us start at the beginning with the origins of skin care.

■ EVOLUTION OF SKIN CARE

Beginning with the Chinese, whose appearance and hygiene were considered to be a defining characteristic, skin care has held a place in every culture, including Egyptian, Greek, Roman, Indian, and African, through to the present day. From decorating and celebrating, to masking and concealing, every culture throughout time has placed a value on faces and

---

The four levels of peeling include very superficial, superficial, moderate, and deep.

Chemical peeling is basically an accelerated exfoliation induced by a chemical agent. Superficial peeling agents cause increased slough of the stratum corneum, and deeper peels cause necrosis and inflammation in the epidermis, papillary dermis, or reticular dermis.[1]

nonsurgical aesthetic skin care
Any noninvasive procedure that is intended to improve overall skin health and appearance.

chemical peeling
The use of chemical agents to destroy layers of skin.

dyschromias
Discoloration of the skin.

cosmeceutical
Products that do more than decorate or camouflage but less than prescription drugs would do. The term was originally coined by Dr. Albert Kligman.

how they look. Today, we use a much more scientific and medical approach that not only enhances the appearance of our faces, but also improves it down to the cellular level. Presently, the medical and aesthetic arts continue their convergence. Although the two disciplines seem distant cousins, both are of an ancient origin.

The Chinese were the first to understand medical fundamentals, which are still practiced today. Traditional Chinese medicine dates back over 5000 years to the writings of Fu Xi. His texts, called the *Trigrams*, relied on the theories of **yin and yang**. Yin and yang represent harmony between nature and its daily phenomenon. The Yellow Emperor of the Han Dynasty later wrote of the need for a *positive physician-patient relationship*. The Chinese methods involving **Chi (or Qi)**, the balance of nature and imbalance of illness, are important foundations on which contemporary western medicine was constructed.[2]

In ancient Egypt, materials were commonly used to enhance the skin's appearance. Ancient Egyptians routinely used animal oils, alabaster, and salts to this effect. Some Egyptian women even soaked their skin in sour milk, unaware that the lactic acid was the source of their positive results. In addition, the Egyptians are credited for inventing the process of distillation, which they used to extract oils and other essences for use in both ceremonial and aesthetic contexts.[3]

Simultaneously, physicians in the Greek empire were making medical and aesthetic advancements of their own. **Hippocrates** had named the **four humors** (blood, phlegm, yellow bile, and black bile), the balance of which defined a person's character. Hippocrates also created the **Hippocratic oath**, which is taken still today by physician and which requires that persons in attendance work cohesively (a point that has modern-day relevance for students who are reading this text). Concurrently, the Greeks also used accessories and adornments to enhance their physical appearance, including pigments such as vermillion to enhance facial coloration.

From then on, many other cultures compounded previous knowledge and learned their own techniques in both medicine and aesthetics. The Indian concept of **Ayurveda,** or the science of living, became part of the foundations of Western medicine. In Africa, colorful decorations of the body were offered as gifts to the gods. Different colors and their use in varied combinations reflected equally varied meanings, many of which are still celebrated today. Similarly, Native Americans wore elaborate beads and headdresses for hierarchical and aesthetic purposes. Native Americans also were quite adept in herbal wound healing, a skill they shared with their new neighbors, the European immigrants.

In Europe, the Dark Ages and the frequent bouts with plague and disease were causes for King Henry IV to issue the "Order of the

yin and yang
Concept, originally devised by Fu Xi, that describes the harmony between nature and its daily phenomenon.

Chi (or Qi)
Concept originally theorized by the Yellow Emperor of China's Han Dynasty. According to Chi, nature has a delicate balance and describes illness as an imbalance.

Hippocrates
Greek physician and "father of medicine" who theorized the Hippocratic oath and the four humors.

four humors
Early medical concept originally documented by Hippocrates that states that the character of a man was determined by the specific balance of the four fluids (as he perceived as) running through the body: black bile, yellow bile, blood, and phlegm.

Hippocratic oath
Oath taken by all physicians relative to the practice of medicine and created by Hippocrates.

Ayurveda
Indian theory, dating back to 2500 B.C., known as the *science of living*. Ayurveda defines the essentials that were perceived as being necessary to health.

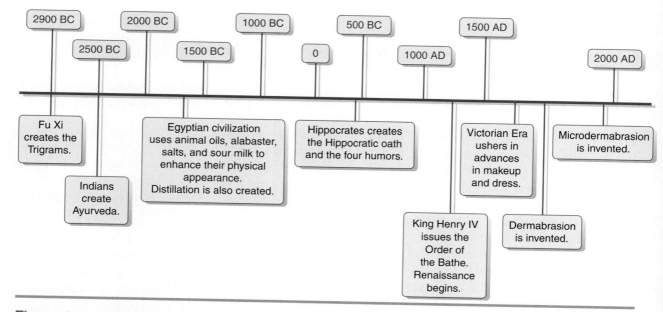

Figure 1–1   Evolution of skin care. This time line depicts the progress of skin care.

chemoexfoliants
The use of chemical agents to exfoliate the stratum corneum.

Bathe,"[4] which required all men and women to bathe frequently. Similar to the Egyptians, Europeans in the Middle Ages used old wine and sour milk for facial rejuvenation. Today, these historical **chemoexfoliants** are known to contain alpha hydroxy acids, which are the active ingredients responsible for the skin exfoliation.[5]

During the Renaissance, amazing breakthroughs in science and technologies of all kinds made medicine more reliable and aesthetics more beautiful. During the Victorian Era, elaborate gowns, headdressings, and makeup made women stand out, at least the wealthy ones (Figure 1–1).

Some of the most remarkable advancements in medicine and aesthetics, however, have been made in the last 25 years. Understanding epidermal cellular migration, dermal collagen content, and advanced wound healing has allowed the development of procedures and products that can truly affect the skin. Notably, however, these advancements created chaos and fragmentation in industries such as the retail product industry, the medical industry, and the spa and skin care industry. Members of the skin health industry are further fragmented into those who treat skin disease and those who treat skin aging, leaving consumers many choices. Combine these choices with the abundance of products and services that claim to fight the effects of aging, and consumers may wonder, "Where do I go and for what?" For all of these reasons and much more, advanced skin care has "gone medical" and is creating a name for itself.

■ HISTORY AND ORIGINS OF PEELS AND PEELING

Chemical peeling has its foundation thousands of years ago in Ancient Egypt. As mentioned, the Egyptians were quite advanced with regard to aesthetics. One of the earliest known treatments involved the application of abrasive tapes composed of alabaster, honey, and sour milk. After removal of the tape, the tightened skin was then abraded with finely ground sand. Later, Greeks developed early facial peeling techniques using various combinations of limestone, mustards, and sulfurs. Early facial peeling techniques also consisted of **poultices** treated with plant and mineral derivatives, sanding techniques, application of various acids, and even burning with fire.[6]

A German dermatologist, Dr. P. G. Unna, ushered in the modern era of chemical peeling in 1882. Unna used **carbolic acid,** derived from coal tar, as a means of peeling. In the early 1900s, **phenol** was discovered to treat acne scarring effectively. Later, phenol was used to treat facial gunpowder wounds during the First World War.

Realizing the efficacy of phenol, Sir Harold Gillies first used chemical peeling in an aesthetic context. Gillies used phenol to remove fine lines under the lower eyelid. For years, the process was replicated and perfected. Later, in 1941, Eller and Wolf suggested combining **resorcinol** paste with phenol and afterwards using carbon dioxide cryotherapy to rejuvenate the face. Soon afterwards, Dr. J. C. Urkov introduced **salicylic acid** as a chemoexfoliant. In the 1960s, Drs. Baker and Gordon developed a phenol-peeling agent, which smoothed deeper furrows, especially around the mouth. Beginning in the 1980s and continuing to the present day, research has continued on phenol and the variables used to create a positive result.[7] In the latter half of the twentieth century, other chemicals, successful for use in aesthetic peeling, made their way into the marketplace. Including, **trichloroacetic acid, Jessner's solution,** and **alpha hydroxy acids.** Formulas, concentrations, and specific techniques were all reviewed, modified, and perfected to ensure safety and efficacy. Today, chemical peels are performed routinely in spas, physicians' offices, and clinics.[8]

poultices
An herb or other substance made into a paste, used to relieve congestion or pain on the skin.

carbolic acid
See phenol.

phenol (carbolic acid)
Highly corrosive acid used in peel solutions that dissolves cells to make room for newer and healthier ones.

resorcinol
Equal parts of hydroquinone and catechol, a peeling agent with similarities to phenol.

salicylic acid
Beta-hydroxy acid, a peeling agent usually reserved for acne treatment.

trichloroacetic acid
Chemical used in peel solutions that dissolve aging cells to make room for newer and healthier ones.

Jessner's solution
Peel solution for the skin that is 14% resorcinol, 14% salicylic acid, and 14% lactic acid in ethanol.

alpha hydroxy acids
Mild organic acids used in cosmeceutical products. AHAs "unglue" cells in the epidermis, allowing keratinocytes to be shed at the stratum granulosum, providing skin with a healthier texture.

partial-thickness injury
A wound that penetrates only the epidermis or the upper layer of the papillary dermis. These wounds tend to heal more quickly and with less risk of scarring.

peel depth
The depth of skin injury by chemical peeling agents.

Retin A®
Topical vitamin A, also known as tretinoin.

5-flourouracil (5-FU)
A chemotherapy agent that is given as a treatment for some types of cancer. Used as a topical peeling agent. Also known as Efudex® when used on the skin.

pyruvic acid
An alpha keto acid that has properties of acids and ketones. Pyruvic acid is a powerful peeling agent.

■ CHEMICAL PEELING

Chemical peels are intended to remove the outermost layers of the skin. To accomplish this task, the chosen peel solution induces a controlled **partial-thickness injury** to the skin. Resulting wound healing processes begin to regenerate necrosed epidermal tissues.[9] When the new skin replaces that which was removed, the skin will be healthier and more youthful in appearance. Depending on their depth, peels will reduce imperfections or damage caused by sunlight exposure, pigmentation irregularities, and fine wrinkles.[10]

Results from chemical peels can be controlled to an extent by the amount of time, concentration, and type of the chemical peel used; pretreatment; the number of treatments; and application technique. These variables determine the **peel depth** (predicting and managing the peel result). Peel depth will be your key to success. Similarly, peel depth will be the source of any complications. Great attention should be paid to peel depths, which will be discussed in greater detail later (Table 1–1).

Separating the Fact from the Fiction

Because of the wide variety of peels, a great deal of misinformation has been given about the processes and after-care results. Many myths exist such as lunchtime peels never scar, peels are easy to do, peels are for every skin type, peels replace facelifts, peels take weeks to heal, peels always leave the skin red, peels always risk hyperpigmentation, peels are really painful, and peels are better (or worse) than other skin procedures. Statements such as these create fiction for the public and an educational challenge for the clinician. To eliminate the fiction, let us talk briefly about the realities of these statements.

Table 1–1   Peeling Agents
Retinoic acid **(Retin A®)**
5-flourouracil (5-FU)
Resorcinol
Salicylic acid (BETA)
Jessner's solution
Alpha hydroxy acids (AHAs)
Trichloroacetic acid (TCA)
Alpha keto acids **(pyruvic acid)**
Phenol

Practitioners of lunchtime peels carved out a niche for themselves in the mid 1990s, and, in reality, these light peels should not scar. However, an exception to the rule can be found. A risk for scarring increases if these peels are used in correlation with **dermaplaning** (BioMedic, circa 1993) or the use of dry ice. Dermaplaning is an exfoliation treatment using a sharp scalpel blade to remove dead layers of skin cells. As such, the stratum corneum is thinned, allowing for a faster penetration of the peel solutions. This procedure in combination with aggressive peeling agents can cause scarring. The use of dry ice as a finishing treatment also weakens the stratum corneum; this too can increase the risk of scarring. The tools that you use need to be handled with respect. Simply because the peel is billed as a light peel does not mean it will not be harmful, if used improperly.

The notion that peels are easy to do is another misconception. Some clinicians and patients believe that the skin is washed and that the peel solution is put on and washed off. In simple terms, this belief is valid, but performing a peel is so much more. The condition of the skin must be considered, as well as the home program and the clinical preparation of the skin, in addition to the technique and skills of the clinician. Peels are not easy to do and require education and practice to ensure a positive outcome.

What about the idea that peels are for every skin type? Well, this assumption is simply not true. The decision to perform a peel depends on the indications that the patient presents and the analysis of the age and type of skin. When a peel is performed on a skin type or for an indication that is inappropriate, not only do you risk a poor result, but also you risk potential complications such as scars or **postinflammatory hyperpigmentation.**

Peels do not replace facelifts. Even the most aggressive of peels (phenol) will not provide the surgical result of a facelift. If your patient has loose and sagging skin, guiding her or him in the right direction—to your physician's office—will be important. Remember, peels are for skin quality; surgery is for skin quantity (i.e., too much skin).

Do peels make the skin red? Well, yes. Reddening is the normal response of the skin when an irritant is applied. Nonetheless, how red and for how long are the important questions. The answers are associated with the specific peel solution applied, the time it was left in place, and the aftercare.

Benefits of Peeling

Every day, our skin is undergoing the normal process of sloughing older dead skin cells. In place of these dead cells, newer cells have traveled up

dermaplaning
The use of a sharp surgical blade to exfoliate the stratum corneum.

postinflammatory hyperpigmentation
Pigment that occurs in response to skin injury.

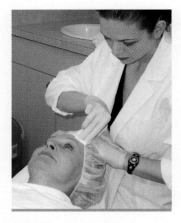

Figure 1–2 Peel treatments are valuable for all skin types.

necrosis
Death of cells when tissue is deprived of blood supply.

collagen
An insoluble protein found in connective tissues. Particularly, type I collagen forms a network in the epidermis, and it is credited with providing skin with its tensile strength and firmness.

ground substance
Consists mainly of glycosaminoglycans (hyaluronic acid, chondroitin sulfate, and dermatan sulfate); involved in maintenance and repair of dermis.

through the layers of skin. These new cells will replace the dead cells and ultimately suffer the same fate. However, as we get older, the time required for the older cells to slough off increases, meaning that the older cells stay in place longer, causing our skin to look dull and aged (Figure 1–2).

Chemical peels accelerate this process in three different ways. First, resurfacing the stratum corneum stimulates epidermal growth, which makes the epidermis thicken. Second, chemical peels cause **necrosis**, or destruction of damaged skin. Ideally, the damaged or dyschromatic skin will be replaced with healthier, normalized tissue by means of the skin's wound healing processes. Finally, deeper peels will induce the production of new **collagen** and **ground substance** within the dermis, which occurs as an inflammatory response to wounding deeper basal layer and papillary dermis tissue. This entire process will be discussed in greater depth later in this text. Given that peeling can cause necrosis, you will want to do as little damage as possible while still stimulating as much new tissue formation as possible. This task is best accomplished with repeated superficial and medium-depth peels.[11]

Peeling versus Other Treatments

The four levels of peeling include very superficial, superficial, moderate, and deep. The peels that are associated with very superficial peeling would include *lunchtime peels, 20% glycolic peels, and herbal designer peels*. Superficial peeling is *30% to 50% glycolic peels, salicylic peels, or Jessner's peels*. Moderate peels are defined as *TCA peels and 70% glycolic peels*. The deep peel category is saved for phenol or pyruvic acid peels (Table 1–2).

Each peel category is related to the associated level of skin injury. For example, very superficial peels are acting only on the stratum corneum, and moderate peels are wounding into the papillary dermis. Additionally, peels require some "downtime" for the patient to peel and heal. Healing is related to peel depth. Some peels can also pose a slightly higher risk of scarring, infection, and postinflammatory hyperpigmentation.

In most cases, the potential risks and the result are directly related to the depth of the peel. Interestingly, however, the repetitive nature of the very superficial to superficial peels creates enough minor injury to stimulate collagen remodeling in the dermis and new collagen formation. For this reason and the minimal healing associated with superficial and very superficial peels, very superficial to superficial peels have become popular with the public. This trend is not to discount the moderate peels, especially TCA, which provides

Table 1–2 Comparison of Treatments

Treatment	What It Does	What It Does Not Do
Trichloroacetic acid (TCA) peels	Flattens scarring Reduces rhytides Corrects photo damage Improves hyperpigmentation	Reduce pore size Eradicate all rhytides Remove **telangiectasia** Remove deep scarring
Jessner's solution and glycolic acid peels	Reduces rhytides Corrects photo damage Improves hyperpigmentation	Reduce pore size Eradicate all rhytides Remove telangiectasia Remove deep scarring
Dermabrasion	Flattens scarring Reduces rhytides Corrects photo damage Improves hyperpigmentation	Reduce pore size Eradicate all rhytides Remove telangiectasia Remove deep scarring
Carbon dioxide CO_2 laser	Removes some acne scarring Removes coarse static rhytides Reduces coarse dynamic rhytids Corrects photo damage Improves hyperpigmentation	Reduce pore size Eradicate all rhytides Remove telangiectasia Remove deep scarring
Erbium laser	Removes some acne scarring Removes coarse static rhytides Reduces coarse dynamic rhytides Corrects photo damage Improves hyperpigmentation	Reduce pore size Eradicate all rhytides Remove telangiectasia Remove deep scarring
Microdermabrasion	Flattens scars Removes hyperpigmentation Reduces fine dynamic rhytides Corrects photo damage Improves hyperpigmentation	Reduce pore size Eradicate all rhytides Remove telangiectasia Remove deep scarring

> The peels that create deep epidermal wounding are considered superficial peels, papillary dermal wounding is created by TCA or 70% glycolic acid, moderate depth peeling.

telangiectasia
Dilation of a group of small blood vessels.

deep epidermal wounding
Injury that reaches deep into the epidermis, as with peeling solutions.

papillary dermal wounding
Any injury to the skin that is sufficient to cause bleeding.

glycolic acid
Alpha hydroxy acid derived from sugar cane. It has a small molecular size that allows for easier penetration into the skin.

Blue Peel®
TCA peel solution that is combined with blue color and acid penetration—slowing or modifying agents.

improvement with usually one peel. The most popular TCA peel is known as the **Blue Peel**® developed by Dr. Zen Obagi. This TCA peel combines a blue dye into the TCA to assist with application and observation of the peel. In recent years, these peels have become well accepted, with few complications.

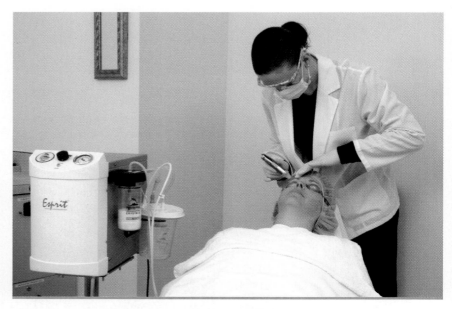

Figure 1–3 Medical microdermabrasion machine using crystals. Photograph courtesy of Aesthetic Technologies®.

> AHAs *melt* epidermal cells and exfoliate the skin. These peels act differently on the skin by causing separation of the layers of the epidermal cells (keratolysis) and then sloughing those *necrotic* cells off.

epidermal cells
Cells found in the outermost layer of skin.

keratolysis
Separation of the skin cells in the epidermis.

carbon dioxide (CO_2) laser
Aggressive type of laser used for skin resurfacing, which vaporizes skin and causes thermal injury, allowing for improved collagen production.

erbium laser
Less-aggressive type of laser that causes less thermal injury while still causing epidermal and papillary dermal injuries.

hypopigmentation
The lack of melanin production.

Microdermabrasion

Chemical peels have many of the same indications as those of microdermabrasion, including light acne scarring, dyschromias, rough texture, and fine lines. Although microdermabrasion has less downtime, and potentially fewer complications, it cannot match chemical peels with regard to collagen stimulation and the number of treatments required for improvement. Patient satisfaction between the two procedures was addressed in a recent study, stating only 1 in 10 patients preferred microdermabrasion treatments over peels (Figure 1–3).[12]

Carbon Dioxide (CO_2) Laser

Resurfacing lasers cause epidermal and papillary dermal injury. Two major types of skin resurfacing lasers have been developed: the **carbon dioxide (CO_2) laser** and the **erbium laser.** The CO_2 laser vaporizes the skin, causing a thermal injury, which, in turn, causes additional improvements in the dermis through collagen formation.

Unfortunately, because of the aggressive nature of CO_2 laser, the skin is at great risk for **hypopigmentation.** The erbium laser causes an epidermal and papillary dermal injury. However, this "lighter" laser does so with little thermal injury. Therefore the result is somewhat less than that of the CO_2 laser resurfacing procedure. The erbium laser also creates a slightly lower risk of hypopigmentation.

Several lasers have been developed that now combine the effects of erbium and CO_2 laser. The benefit of these lasers is the ability to treat, for example, the skin around the eyes with a lighter setting and more aggressively in other areas. These lasers are often used in conjunction with facial surgery such as blepharoplasty and facelift.

Laser treatments can be a preferred treatment to some deeper chemical peels. Because the laser beam is small and easy to manipulate, it allows the physician to treat specific areas intricately. The laser also has the capability to be *turned up or turned down* and thus creates a tailored injury for the problem. No single "hammer" that works best to treat aging skin has been found. In fact, a combination of peeling and laser can provide the best results.

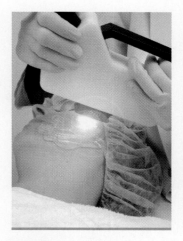

Figure 1–4 Intense pulsed light or Foto Facials® are another treatment for solar damage.

Intense Pulsed Light

Intense pulsed light (IPL) therapy, also known as Foto Facial® or Photo Facial®, is a light treatment. Using a broad spectrum of light energy in a range of wavelengths, IPL therapy supplies high levels of light power in millisecond bursts.[13] This phenomenon treats colors—red and brown. When alternated with peeling treatments, such as glycolic, the skin responds faster, and the result is more dramatic (Figure 1–4).

Radio-Frequency Therapy

Radio-frequency (RF) therapy is the newest "high tech" therapy available today in the medical spa. This therapy, though still new, has been shown to tighten the skin effectively on the lower face and neck. Tightening of the skin, not unlike surgery, does not improve the *quality* of the skin, and therefore a skin program that includes peeling and home therapies is appropriate.

radio frequency
Frequency used with the newest technology for promoting collagen growth.

Facial Surgery

Facial surgery is directed at improving loose skin on the face and neck. The objective of cosmetic facial surgery is *not* to improve the *quality* of the skin. Therefore a program of clinical peels and therapeutic home products are appropriate for an optimal result. Additionally, healing the skin after surgery is helpful if the patient has been on a preoperative skin care program that includes peels and home programs.

■ TRAINING

There is no *getting started* without training. This area is, as they say, "where the rubber meets the road." Because chemical peel treatments are **technique sensitive**, clinicians must understand the processes, concentrations, indications and contraindications, the importance of home products for the skin, and proper management of aftercare, all of which are important factors for success.

The training process for peeling should not be left to the individual clinician to figure out on his or her own. Given that chemical peeling can be risky, the clinician must have the necessary training. (Although state licensure does not generally depend on peel training or theory, the qualified clinician will have advanced training in this area.) This preparation will give the spa the confidence necessary to allow the clinician to provide care to the patient. If the clinician is not trained, the spa must have a trainer available to teach and mentor the new clinician in the use of these chemicals.

Chemical peel training should take place in a dedicated class that addresses theory and hands-on practice. The classroom work should include a review of the **anatomy** and **physiology** of the skin, the basics of wound healing, the indications and contraindications of treatment, and the fundamentals of the at-home skin programs. The course should require familiarity with **clinic protocols** for chemical peels and the variety of available treatments and programs available. Once the student completes the classroom work and has passed the recommended examination, he or she can move to hands-on clinical training.

The review of anatomy and physiology should be specific to the layers of the skin and the response to the application of peel solutions. Additionally, the trainer should be able to tie these responses into wound healing and the anticipated result of the treatment. Obviously, all the conditions that reflect indications and contraindications should be covered. This information may vary by facility and is based on predetermined policy and procedures.

In the clinic, a training program should focus on how to observe for skin injury, wound healing, and the benefits of chemical peeling. The clinician should also be introduced to the specific solutions such as glycolic acid, lactic acid, Jessner's solution, TCA solutions, and phenol solutions. The protocols will differ in each facility as to which peel solutions can be used by aestheticians, which solutions are to be used by nurses, and, finally, which solutions are to be used only by physicians. Once the clinician is introduced to the theories of the solution, the clinical education begins.

technique sensitive
Results of a treatment that depend on the clinician's ability to administer consistent results.

anatomy
The study of the body and how its structures work in relation to one another.

physiology
The study of body function.

clinic protocols
Any set of rules or guidelines established by a clinic to ensure safe practice. These guidelines will vary by location yet are expected to be observed by clinicians working within the individual clinic.

The ability to reproduce a treatment comes with practice, and therefore extra time should be built into this area of the training process. The clinician should not provide chemical peel treatments to patients until he or she has completed a thorough clinical training program. Remember that completion of a training program does not always reflect competency. Therefore skill testing and observation of the clinician are critical for the safety of the patient.

Training Protocols

Training protocols are specific documents that help you understand the processes that are deemed acceptable for training. Protocols address subjects such as who can be trained, how the training takes place, and the necessary test scores to be approved as a skilled clinician. Each clinic should have a protocol to guide its behavior and options for training.

Who can be trained should be addressed in protocols and dictated by the physician. The qualifications of the personnel category (aesthetician versus nurse) should be used to differentiate which peel solutions can be used and why. How the training takes place is also important to differentiate in the policy and procedure. This aspect protects the facility from potential litigation from patients and employees alike. The training outline should be complete and available. Additionally, it should be updated yearly. Finally, evaluating the training process is important for both the clinician and the facility. Everyone wants to be successful, and a meaningful evaluation helps in this process.

Clinical Training Process

In the clinical segment of the training, the clinician should be working one-on-one with the clinic educator or instructor to master the technique of the chemical peels. The clinical training should be directed at three specific processes: the consultative process, the chemical peel technique itself, and the pre- and post-home–care programs. When learning about the consultative process, the clinician should take the specifics learned in the classroom, such as indications and contraindications, and apply them appropriately to specific skin types and clients' complaints. When focusing on the chemical peels techniques, the issues of skin quality, specific peeling solutions, recovery time, and potential complications are addressed. Finally, at home-adjunct therapy for the patient is a critical component of the long-term success of the clinical program (Figure 1–5 on page 15).

Peeling Protocol

Standard Policy and Procedure: Training and Certification for Peels

Date of origination: June 1996

Creator: Pamela Hill, R.N.

Date of review: January 1996

Revisions by: S. Smith M.E.

Date of revisions: Jan. 1997, Jan. 1998, Jan. 1999, Jan. 2000, Jan. 2001, Jan. 2002, Jan. 2003

Policy #: 01-003

Attachments: Policy and procedure document for peels, certificates of completion, written test, clinical test

Title of policy: Training and Certification for Peels

Policy: All clinical staff will be licensed and insured in the state of employment. Certification through the company training program is required before patient care is given.

Purpose: To ensure that all clinical staff employed by the company are properly trained and certified in the techniques, policies, and procedures through the company training programs.

Scope: All clinical personnel

Definition: Clinical aesthetic personnel

Procedure indications: All clinicians seeking certification will be recommended to the training program by their supervisors.

Procedure contraindications: Not applicable

Required paperwork: "Recommendation for Training # PER- 22" signed by the clinician supervisor

Testing if necessary: Score of 80% or greater on the written examination is required before proceeding to clinical training. A score of 90% or greater on the clinical examination is required to treat patients.

Required reading: Articles and technical information provided by the instructor

Classroom training: The training will consist of two classroom days. The curriculum for these days includes a review of anatomy and physiology of the skin, wound healing, principles and techniques of chemical peels, and home-care regimens for chemical peels. A written test will be given at the conclusion of the 2-day classroom course. A score of at least 80% is required to move to the clinical training.

Clinical training: The clinician will be responsible for finding 25 models on whom to practice the chemical peel treatment. These models should have different skin types and different skin problems. Preferably, models have not had any previous skin care or treatments. A full consultation is done, followed by the treatment. The clinician will need to prove competency in consultation skills, in the development of home-care programs, and in the techniques of chemical peeling described in the policy and procedure document. A passing score of 90% is required on the clinical training to be released to treat patients.

Clinician requirements: Licensed professional

Clinician required training: Certificate of completion in a chemical peeling course with a state recognized school or company training program

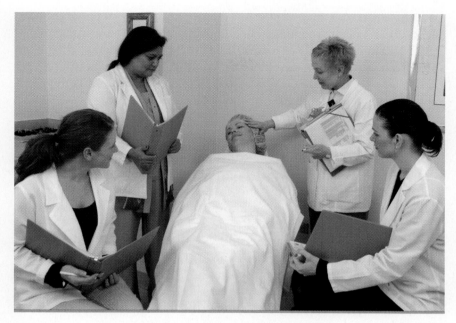

Figure 1–5 Peel treatments are *technique sensitive*. Proper training should always take place before treating patients.

The clinic must require at least 25 *model* patients with varying skin types and clinical concerns to be treated before treatment of *client* patients. A clinical examination is also required to ensure that the clinician understands the application of the chemical peels treatment.

Requirements for Training

A specific document within the clinic protocols called *requirements for training* should be provided. These training requirements are the specific actions that must take place *for the clinician to be placed* into a training program and, after completing the training, to be released to treat patients. Within this document should be an outline of the requirements such as any necessary previous experience, any additional education (college courses for example), a written recommendation by the physician, and the number of years that the clinician must be employed with the company before receiving this type of training. Once all of the qualifications have been met, the criteria to treat patients must be addressed, for example, a passing score on the written examination, treatment of 25 models, or the written permission of the physician. Several important points regarding training requirements bear succinct repetition: clinicians must have a current and valid license in the state in which the clinician is practicing, the physician or clinic manager should recommend the clinician be trained for the procedure, and the clinician must score at least 80% on the theoretic testing and at least 90% on the clinical testing.

Evaluating Clinician Skills

Although written testing is a valuable tool to evaluate the student through the treatment-related educational process, it is not always an accurate indicator of the clinician's true clinical abilities. In other words, a clinician may be adept at performing the chemical peel treatments, but he or she will also need to be reviewed on other aspects of performing in the clinic. A simple checklist for the clinician and the clinical instructor might be useful. This *skill list* should include tasks such as draping the client, patient communication skills, home program evaluation, and the ability to orient to the physical space. These skill sets and those identified in Table 1–3 will help the clinician expand his or her knowledge.

Continuing Education

Continuing education is a professional obligation and privilege. Educational updates can be provided using three methods: an annual recertification process through the clinic, **continuing education units (CEUs)** obtained at meetings, and online study and education. Annual recertification processes within a clinic usually have two phases. The first phase is through self-managed workbook reading and quizzes. These workbooks can be printed or put on your intranet (an efficient way of managing the process). The second phase is the clinical recertification. This recertification is the process by which the clinic educator or physician observes the clinician treating patients. The educator uses a score sheet to evaluate the clinician in all areas of the treatment room, including the actual treatment, cleanliness of the room, professionalism with the client, and so forth. The score on this evaluation must be at least 90%. If the clinician does not achieve a passing score then a problem-solving document called a **progressive improvement plan (PIP)** should be implemented to help the clinician improve his or her treatments.

The next approach to ensuring educational updates is by requiring recognized CEUs. In some states, CEUs are required for licensure renewal. The concept can be translated to the clinic requiring each practicing clinician (aesthetician, registered nurse,

continuing education units (CEUs)
Any certified training or event that is intended to build or add skills.

progressive improvement plan (PIP)
Administrative document intended to record a problem and the actions taken to correct the problem and prevent its reoccurrence.

Table 1–3 Additional Clinician Skills

Clinical Skills	Score 1–10	Recommended Improvements
Communications Skill		
Clarity		
Education		
Sales abilities		
Safety Skills		
Wears protective gear		
Understands machine		
Charting		
Understands the record		
Makes appropriate notes		
Takes pictures		
Products		
Understands product lines		
Professionalism		
Appropriate to patient		
Appropriate to peers		

licensed practical nurse, or physician's assistant) to obtain a certain number of hours each year to maintain employment. CEUs can be obtained at annual meetings of professional organizations. Each year, one or two people can be selected from the clinic to attend the annual meetings. Although expensive, these meetings are usually illuminating and help the clinician stay current on the newest products and services. If clinicians at the clinic cannot attend the meeting, the returning clinician should give a report and provide copies of any relevant literature.

Finally, learning can take place through a variety of web sites on the Internet that are dedicated to education. These sites provide recognized CEUs or simple educational information.

Ongoing education is the most important thing you will do for your career. It is your annuity for increased wages, improved treatment results, and self-improvement.

Ongoing training should be part of a yearly *self-improvement plan*. After you graduate from school, plan to take at least one course a year to learn a new subject that will add depth and power to your resume.

Table 1–4 Career Opportunities	
Medical Office	Plastic surgery
	Dermatology
	Family practice
	Gynecology
	Otolaryngologist (ear, nose, and throat [ENT])
	Dentistry
Spas	Salon spas
	Fitness club spa
	Country club spas
	Holistic spas
	Day spas
Resorts	Destination spas
	Resort/hotel spas
	Cruise ship spas

◾ EMPLOYMENT OPTIONS

Career opportunities abound for the educated and skilled medical aesthetician and cosmetic nurse. Creating a **career plan** for success is the first step to realizing your dream. Many professionals in the area of *self-improvement* recommend identifying the goal and working backward to achieve that goal (Table 1–4).

career plan
Action taken by an individual to set goals and actions taken to ensure that these goals are realized.

Using this technique, identify where you want to be and what you want to be doing in 5 years. Then, create a list of objectives to achieve the goal. For example, if you are currently an aesthetician without medical experience and you would like to be in a medical office as a chemical peel specialist, identify objectives that will allow you to meet the goal. Find out where to gain the training, expertise, and experience that will allow you to be a valued employee in a medical setting. Identify internships or learning situations that will help you perfect your clinical skills. Take communication courses that will help you learn how to communicate with patients, peers, and superiors in a medical setting. Take sales courses that will help you make a contribution to your employer and to yourself. Learn the basics of building a business. Create a professional resume. Practice interviewing skills that will help you get the job.

Marketing yourself to a business will become an important skill in acquiring the right job. Whether you want to land a job in a medical spa, a destination spa, or a holistic spa, the tactics you use to get there will be the same. Remember, just as you are looking for the perfect job, the employer is looking for the perfect employee. Not every opportunity will be a good match for you or the employer, and that is reasonable; understanding the components of a good match will be the key to long-term success. By marketing yourself, you will have a sound understanding of what positions will be a good match for you personally.

Several components of marketing yourself should be addressed, including your values, your integrity, your skills, and your needs. Before looking for a job, a worthwhile activity may be to write out each category. This exercise will help you ask potential employers the right questions, which will assist in your own determination. Then, practice with a friend. Remember, you are interviewing the employer as much as the employer is interviewing you.

Values are defined as "the abstract concepts of what is right, worthwhile or desirable, principles or standards."[14] Ask questions about the business's philosophies and goals (businesses should have both financial and nonfinancial goals). Specifically ask about patient care philosophies. Then, discuss these values with which you can identify. Important values to you may include being on time, following company protocol, providing the quality care to patients, or even volunteering at the local women's shelter. Think twice about taking a position in which your values differ from those of the clinic or employer.

Under the subject of *your value,* you will want to itemize specifics such as the location of your primary education. Some schools have more prestige than others do; build on this if it is possible. Include a list of your advanced education, including college (name, location, degree), advanced aesthetic education classes (with whom and where), and experience in the field in which you are looking to be employed.

Integrity is different from values. Integrity is defined as "uncompromising adherence to moral and ethical principles; *honesty.*"[15] In this category, you will want to ask questions about patient care such as how complications are handled, how unhappy patients are handled, and how fee disputes are managed. Additionally, ask direct questions about the ethical principles of the company. A written philosophy should be available, usually known as the **mission statement.** Then, consider if these ethical principles are similar or the same as your own. They should be.

Your skills are important to an employer, but sometimes the position is not exactly what we want. You may be underqualified or overqualified. You need to assess this aspect with the employer. Ask questions about the specific skills needed, and respond with information about your skills. If you are underqualified but otherwise matched to the position, what training will be available to help you become

mission statement
A written statement of a business's individual philosophy.

qualified? How quickly will that training happen, and who will do the training? Could a pay raise be expected once the training is complete? These are important questions to ask before committing to a position. What you hear at the interview and what comes to pass in a job are not always the same things. Putting some of what would otherwise be a "handshake" deal in writing is in your best interest. This approach eliminates any future misunderstandings or hard feelings. If the employer is unwilling to provide a written agreement, maybe the position is not a match.

Your needs are especially important but not exclusive of the employer's needs. The best situation is when you find a *need match*. List your needs, such as salary (pay rate, pay schedule, commission), benefits, vacation time, sick day policies, hours to be worked, desired job description, and any other important needs you may have. In advance, decide which ones you can compromise and which ones will be "deal breakers." Making this decision in advance prevents you from feeling "sour grapes" if you give in and then regret the decision later.

Once you have your credentials, your resume, and your marketing plan, you are ready to go get the job for which you are uniquely qualified.

License and Insurance

| The clinician must be properly licensed by the state in which he or she plans to be working.

Whether you are an aesthetician, nurse, physician's assistant, or medical assistant, you must be licensed in the state in which you work (Table 1–5). Confirmation of licensure should be provided to the employer and kept in the employee record. Many clinicians like to keep their license hanging in their treatment rooms for all to see. In some states, this posting is a requirement. Unlicensed clinicians should not be working in a medical setting (or at all for that matter), and the license should be obtained before employment begins.

| Before you begin your employment, be sure to contact the state board that recognizes your license and find out what specific implications should be noted when you are working in a medical setting versus a spa setting. Once you have completed this task, the next contact should be made to your insurance agent to ensure that you have the proper coverage for the procedures you will be doing.

Several types of insurance are necessary for a spa business. For the clinician, the most important insurance policy will be the malpractice policy. This insurance policy covers your actions when treating patients. If something goes wrong, this policy will protect you. When working in the medical office, the physician will sometimes have a broad policy under which you will be covered. This practice is also true in the luxury spa. For you, as the individual clinician, getting proper coverage is a fact-finding mission. First, find out from your employer what the status of coverage for your position will be. Second, find a reputable company, and have a consultation with one of the agents. Take the agent's counsel, and then consider a discussion with an attorney to ensure that your best interests are served.

Table 1–5   Sample State Regulations

State	State Requirements
Alabama	Esthetician: 1500 hours Massage therapist: 650 hours
California	Esthetician: 600 hours
Florida	Esthetician: 260 hours Massage therapist: 500 hours
Georgia	No separate licensing requirements
North Dakota	Esthetician: 900 hours Massage therapist: 750 hours
Texas	Esthetician: 600 hours Massage therapist: 250 hours
Utah	Esthetician: 600 hours Master esthetician: 1200 hours Massage therapist: 200 hours
West Virginia	Esthetician: 600 hours Massage therapist: 500 hours

Adding Peel Treatments

Peels, especially repetitive superficial peels, can be among the best treatments to address solar aging, fine lines, and hyperpigmentation. Peel treatments are sometimes overlooked for *high tech* solutions, which is unfortunate because all peels have a proven record of epidermal or dermal improvement and, as such, appearance enhancement for the patient.

Glycolic acid peels in particular can be a beneficial monthly treatment that will, over time, provide a noticeable result for the patient, with very little if any downtime. The patients who opt for more aggressive treatments such as a TCA peel can also achieve a result that is remarkable, with a moderate amount of downtime. However, peels alone do not necessarily provide the best results. Other treatments help enhance the peel treatment and ensure a positive outcome. Included in the *partner* treatments are facials, especially hydrating and exfoliating facials.

Additional considerations to be evaluated when deciding on whether peels fit into your facility menu are the capabilities of the facility, the abilities of the clinicians, and the image that the company wants to portray. These considerations bring us to the concept of whether peels can be done only in the medical office or whether peels are appropriate for the salon setting. Finally, the consideration of liabilities for the clinician and the facility itself should be addressed.

Medical Offices

Busy aesthetic medical offices are always looking for proficient aestheticians and cosmetic nurses. A physician will often be looking for an employee who can multi-task and who can take on additional job responsibilities. Depending on the scope of the practice, you may have an opportunity that will allow you to learn more than simple aesthetics and to expand your skills. Some medical offices are willing to train aestheticians or cosmetic nurses.

Working in a medical office has many rewards, among them prestige, advanced knowledge, complex treatments, and working with other medical professionals. Medical professionals—physicians, nurses, and physician assistants, as well as residents and interns—are unlike any other professional you will meet. The training of these professionals has spanned life and death, and their commitment to their patients is unlike any other commitment to a customer. Mistakes are not tolerated by physicians or nurses, or patients for that matter. This type of environment can be an intense and intimidating place to work, but the payoffs will be worth the effort you put into the job. The ability to make a difference in the life of a patient is among the most meaningful rewards. To learn and become more skilled, to participate, and to bring visible results to patients in need are some of the benefits of working in a medical office. Working in a medical office requires expert skills, willingness to learn, compassion, understanding, and expert professionalism.

The peels that are done in a medical office are more advanced, more aggressive, and, as such, provide a better result compared with peels that are performed in a salon setting. The care of the patient undergoing a peel requires advanced knowledge in skin anatomy and physiology, wound healing, and wound care. The clinician is also expected to know about the different peeling solutions, how they will act on the skin, and the potential outcome. The clinician must have the ability to talk with patients, explain procedures, and work alongside the physician. Acting as a representative for the physician, conveying important information, and providing treatments to the patient will make the clinician a valuable asset to the medical office and to the patient.

Working in a medical office will not always be easy. The challenging aspects of working in a medical office include dealing with the politics (though all offices seem to have politics), being the *low person on the totem pole* (the aesthetician or cosmetic nurse often feels out of the loop and unimportant), adhering to many new rules that seem to have little

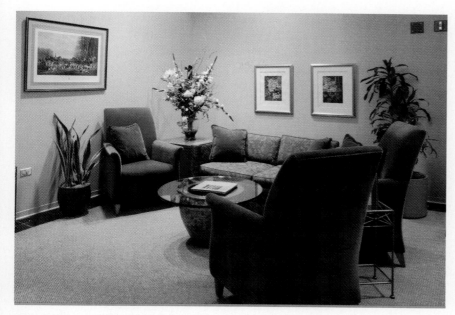

Figure 1–6   Medical spas are comfortable and also have facilities conducive to more technical procedures. They may resemble a physician's office.

or no apparent meaning, learning a new business sector, and building the nonsurgical aesthetic business in isolation. Physicians are often busy performing surgery or seeing patients and do not have the time to dedicate to the growth and development of the aesthetic arm of a business, even though it is important to them. Physicians will be looking to the aesthetician or cosmetic nurse to build the nonsurgical aesthetic side of the business. Understanding all of the potential pitfalls of building a nonsurgical aesthetic business will be important in this situation. Learn how to maneuver through the landmines, and you will find this career rewarding and financially profitable (Figure 1–6).

Salons and Spas

Salons and spas offer a sense of well-being and luxury to the client. As treatments have become more sophisticated and our tools have become more advanced, we have the opportunity to provide our clients treatments that may supplement medical treatments (**lymphatic drainage**) or help to reduce the stress (**reflexology**) from an extraordinarily busy world. Peels can also take place in the spa or salon setting. However, treatment should be appropriate to the setting. That is to say, the peel should be limited in its aggressiveness and the need for potential

lymphatic drainage
Drainage of lymphatic fluids.

reflexology
A system of massage in which certain body parts are massaged in specific areas to influence other body functions favorably.

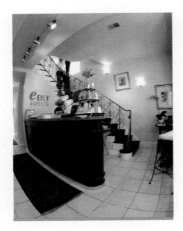

Figure 1–7 Traditional spas offer nonmedicinal treatments in a professional and aesthetically pleasing environment. Traditional spas may be more luxurious and have a retail focus. Photograph courtesy of Edit EuroSpa, Denver, Colorado.

physician oversight. TCA peels or even higher-percentage glycolic peels are simply not appropriate for the spa or salon setting. The salon or spa should consider light rejuvenative peels such as 20% glycolic acid, lactic acid, or designer peels that have less of a potential for complications and fall within the laws of the state. Because peels can be popular, the spa should have protocols in place about the types of peels that can typically be provided. This precaution reduces the liability exposure for both the clinician and the spa.

As the medical spa has become more popular and many aestheticians have the desire to work in the medical spa, other types of spas are looking for qualified and valuable employees. Many different types of spas exist. Among them are salon spas, resort spas, cruise ship spas, day spas, club spas, destination spas, and holistic or mineral bath spas. Each spa has a different focus and requires the aesthetician to understand the advanced treatments he or she will be providing. Especially popular in resort spas and destination spas are body treatments and nutritional counseling. Cruise ship spas are looking for employees with excellent customer service skills, as well as extensive technical skills.

Spa directors expect their employees to be professional, educated, and willing to work hard to build their clientele. Having some experience or education in marketing will give you an opportunity to excel and build your clientele more quickly. As is the case in the medical spa, acquiring advance education and refining techniques is important for the aesthetician to be successful in the specific spa that he or she happens to have interest (Figure 1–7).

Liability Issues for the Clinician

Liability issues for the clinician are an important factor in preparing for a career. Our United States society is far more litigious than ever before. If something goes wrong, the client is always looking for someone to blame, and usually a lawyer will take the case. Whether a case ever comes to settlement or trial, the stress of being blamed will be overwhelming, a situation in which no clinician should be caught.

Clinicians face many potential liability risks. The most common injuries at risk for lawsuits are scarring, burns, product reactions and allergies, infections, and failure to keep information confidential. When speaking specifically of chemical peels, the greatest risks of liability are burns, infection, and scarring.

Burns that are caused by chemical peels can develop into deep wounds and finally into scars. The burns caused by chemical peeling are sadly the result of either a failure to understand the peel solution or a failure to recognize an unusual circumstance. Regardless of the cause, the safeguard is for the clinician to be well qualified. Nonetheless, bad things can happen. Having an understanding of wound healing and wound care is important for the clinician so that he or she can quickly recognize a problem and seek help once a problem is determined.

Scarring is an obvious concern, especially in the medical clinic. No one is exempt from causing a scar, and, as we know, even improperly performed extractions can cause scarring. Although medical aestheticians are more at risk, all aestheticians should be aware that, each day they work, they might cause a scar. With aggressive treatments, the clinician needs to follow protocol carefully and ensure that he or she is skilled in that treatment. As previously stated, being qualified and knowing when to ask for help from the physician is important for the clinician. Knowing when to ask for help is an important skill in and of itself, one that is directed by protocol and experience.

Infection is most commonly the result of a clinician's failure to provide an adequate standard of care. Infections can happen in a variety of ways: failure to properly clean and sterilize implements, including extractors, microdermabrasion tips, makeup brushes, peel brushes, electrodes, tweezers, bowls, reusable masks, or basically anything that touches the skin; failure to wear gloves during treatments (including spa treatments); or failure to understand the sterilization and contamination process. The transmission of **hepatitis C, human immunodeficiency virus/acquired immunodeficiency syndrome (HIV/AIDS),** and **herpes simplex** should be of concern to the clinician.

Regulatory Agencies

The agencies that regulate spas are not federalized but are implemented on a state-by-state basis. Therefore you need to check with the licensing agency in your state to determine any specific requirements related to your job, aside from general licensure. For example, you might need a certificate indicating that you have completed a course on chemical peels to perform the treatment.

Professional Organizations

Our industry is so fractured. Many organizations are trying to accomplish lofty goals for our industry only to be in conflict with another organization with the same goals. Supporting organizations that have our best interests in mind will be important over the coming years for us as we work toward goals to create uniform educational requirements. The most progressive organization is the National Coalition of Esthetic & Related Associations (NCEA), which is an umbrella for the many small organizations in the marketplace. Check with NCEA to find out if a

hepatitis
A condition caused from multiple viruses defined as hepatitis A, B, or C; it is a contagious inflammation of the liver, with possible chronic consequences, particularly with hepatitis C.

human immunodeficiency virus/acquired immunodeficiency syndrome (HIV/AIDS)
Opportunistic infections that are associated with a compromised immune system.

herpes simplex
An infectious disease caused by herpes simplex virus (HSV)-1, characterized by thin-walled vesicles that tend to occur repeatedly in the same place on the skin's surface.

Belonging to a professional organization can be educational and a great place to network. However, finding a good fit is important. The physician with whom you are working usually belongs to a professional organization. If associations for ancillary staff are available, consider these organizations first.

professional ethics
A set of guidelines that should set a framework for professional behavior and responsibilities.

professional organization can be located that meets your individual needs. Meanwhile, if you work for a plastic surgeon, check into the Society of Plastic Surgical Skin Care Specialists; and if you work for a dermatologist, check into the Society of Dermatology Skin Care Specialists.

Professional Code of Ethics

The first question to ask ourselves is, "Why have a code of ethics?"[16] Two types of ethical codes are (1) personal ethics and (2) **professional ethics**. Although these two areas may overlap, each individual document is important. Individually, the personal code of ethics is a document that discusses how you will live your life and what will be your priorities in daily decision making.

A professional code of ethics, on the other hand, should be public and well known to all in our profession, as well as our clients. If we are to be considered as a member of trained service professionals (sometimes referred to as allied health professionals) as are our counterparts in nursing, social work, nutrition, or other areas, we should extend ourselves to the highest level, and this includes professional ethics. Therefore exactly what does a code of ethics need to include? "It should discuss appropriate and inappropriate behavior, it should promote high standards of patient care, it should be used for self evaluation, it should establish a framework for professional behavior and responsibilities, it should identify us and create an image of occupational maturity."[17]

Given all of these criteria, we recognize that creating a code of ethics is not an easy task. Although the National Coalition of Esthetic & Related Associations publishes a code of ethics, creating one in your place of work is a good idea. For codes of ethics to be meaningful, they should be developed by the group that is going to *use* the document. This task may appear overwhelming because the subject matter can be broad and diverse, especially if the group that is writing the code of ethics is large. The focus of the code is based on moral principles. The process should begin by asking certain questions such as, Why have a code of ethics? What is the purpose of our organization? For what purpose will this code be used? For the code to be useful, it must reflect the qualities of the group. This point can be difficult, given that each person within the group has different qualities and moral viewpoints. However, finding a place of compromise will create a useful document. The code of ethics must be broad enough to take into consideration the number of people using it but specific enough to direct behavior. Therefore if the code fails to provide substantive guidance for the organization, then it creates confusion. As for the skin care industry at large and your business specifically, a few tips can be offered (Table 1–6).

Table 1–6 Writing a Professional Code of Ethics

Component	Considerations
Preamble	What is the purpose of the organization?
Statement of intent	What is the purpose of the code itself?
Fundamental principles	What population is affected by your organization? What is your organization's area of expertise?
Fundamental rules	What unethical situations does your organization want to prevent? What are the likely problem situations in which unethical solutions might arise?
Guidelines for the fundamental principles and fundamental rules	How can these unethical situations be prevented? How can you prevent conflicting principles?

NCEA Esthetician Code of Ethics

CLIENT RELATIONSHIPS

- Estheticians* will serve the best interests of their clients at all times and will provide the highest quality service possible.
- Estheticians will maintain client confidentiality and provide clear, honest communication.
- Estheticians will provide clients with clear and realistic goals and outcomes and will not make false claims regarding the potential benefits of the techniques rendered or products recommended.
- Estheticians will adhere to the scope of practice of their profession and refer clients to the appropriate qualified health practitioner when indicated.

SCOPE OF PRACTICE

- Estheticians will offer services only within the scope of practice as defined by the state within which they operate, if required, and in adherence with appropriate federal laws and regulations.
- Estheticians will not use any technique or procedure for which they have not had adequate training and shall represent their education, training, qualifications, and abilities honestly.

Continued

> "A code of ethics is a means of uniquely expressing a group's collective commitment to a specific set of standards of conduct while offering guidance in how to best follow those codes."[18]

NCEA Esthetician Code of Ethics—cont'd

- Estheticians will strictly adhere to all usage instructions and guidelines provided by product and equipment manufacturers, provided those guidelines and instructions are within the scope of practice as defined by the state, if required.

PROFESSIONALISM

- Estheticians will commit themselves to ongoing education and to provide clients and the public with the most accurate information possible.
- Estheticians will dress in attire consistent with professional practice and adhere to the code of conduct of their governing board.

* For the purpose of the NCEA Code of Ethics, the use of the term *Esthetician* applies to all licensed skin care professionals as defined by their state law.

Reprinted with permission from the NCEA.

A Higher Standard of Professionalism

When we work in the medical office, more is expected of us by both the patient and the physician. We are expected to adhere to a higher level of professionalism and customer service than is familiar to us in the spa setting. You must train yourself to refrain from laughing, joking, and loud behavior. Patients may think you are talking or laughing about them. Additionally, this kind of "party" atmosphere does not reflect positively on our image or our profession. In fact, this unprofessional activity may negatively reflect on you in the eyes of the patient. Your ethical conduct should be present in your contact with patients, their charts or records, and your communication with others about the patient. The information you must pass along about the patient to colleagues or others involved in their care should be complete but comply with **Health Insurance Portability and Accountability Act (HIPAA)** regulations (see later discussion). The patient list of the medical spa belongs to the physician, and, according to the laws of HIPAA, the information should never leave the medical office.

Health Insurance Portability and Accountability Act (HIPAA)
A federal regulation that dictates procedural protocols to protect patient privacy.

Client List

Although you may believe that the client you meet and treat *belongs* to you, the reality is this client belongs to the medical spa and physician.

Without the physician's license, you would be unable to extend your services. Therefore, if and when you leave the employ of the clinic, taking a list of patient names and telephone numbers to contact for your next job is inappropriate and unethical. This activity constitutes poor judgment, and if you are a medical professional (registered nurse, physician's assistant), your professional license may be at risk. This behavior will not gain you points in the medical and professional community. If the physician for whom you are going to work asks you to do this, you should be concerned. All you have is your reputation, not only in the eyes of clients, but also in the eyes of physicians and medical community. You may some day require the referral of your current manager or physician or need to work with them on some professional level, such as a committee. Do not embarrass yourself by doing something inappropriate or worse yet illegal.

HIPAA and the Clinician

When working in a medical office, the clinician must understand all of the laws and regulations that affect the practice. Among these rules and laws is the HIPAA. Passed by Congress in 1996 and signed into law in January of 1997, the purpose of this Act is to protect the privacy of patients' health information. Uniform standards are now in effect across the nation identifying how health information changes hands. Health information is protected by stringent rules that apply to information in the chart, on the computer or fax, and by spoken word. Seven categories of the law are of concern: access to medical records, notice of privacy practices, limits on use of personal medical information, prohibition on marketing, stronger state law, confidential communications, and complaints.[19]

Proper Handling of Medical Information

Access to medical records: patients are entitled to have copies of their records and to have access to their medical records.

Notice of privacy practices: medical facilities are required to communicate with patients in writing about how their medical information will be used and what the patient's rights are under the law.

Limits on the use of personal medical information: this section of the law deals with insurance plans and how the patient's information is communicated between insurance companies and medical professionals.

Prohibition on marketing: this area involves restrictions on how the patient's information can be used for marketing purposes.

Continued

Proper Handling of Medical Information—cont'd

Stronger state laws: The national law does not affect stricter state laws. However, all states must abide by the national law.

Confidential communications: Patients can dictate where and how they are contacted.

Complaints: All patients may file a complaint if they believe that their privacy has been violated.

The following are a few basic tips to keep you out of trouble and respect HIPAA laws:

- Do not talk about patients within earshot of other patients (especially at the front desk and near or in the waiting area).
- Do not share information about the patient with others, including the patient's family.
- Do not fax medical records.
- Do not gossip about patients.
- Do not leave charge tickets where other patients can see the name.
- Do not make a computer screen available for the patient to see.
- Do not release information over the telephone.
- Do not release copied information without a signed release by the patient.
- Take only the record for the patient you are treating into the treatment room.
- Chart immediately and file the chart; do not leave charts where others can see them.
- Be an ethical professional, and consider how you would like to be treated.

▶ ›› TOP TEN TIPS TO TAKE TO THE CLINIC

1. Aging baby boomers will be the thrust of your practice, and they can be demanding.
2. Four levels of chemical peels have been developed; know and understand them.
3. The origins of skin care date back over 5000 years. From the beginning of time, people have wanted to improve their appearance.
4. Chemical peels accelerate the rate of cellular turnover and, as such, improve the appearance of the skin.

5. Many organizations for skin care specialists are available; find the right one for you.
6. Know your state regulations before you start to practice.
7. Obtain insurance that covers and protects you.
8. Hold yourself to a higher standard of professionalism.
9. Understand and abide by HIPAA regulations.
10. Respect your physician.

CHAPTER REVIEW QUESTIONS

1. How does peeling fit into today's advanced skin care programs?
2. What basic training is required for a clinician to be deemed competent in administering chemical peels?
3. How should a clinician be evaluated for peeling technique and knowledge?
4. What is the recommended continuing education for a clinician administering chemical peels?
5. What are the licensure requirements for providing chemical peels?
6. Are there professional organizations to which a clinician can belong in which he or she can meet other clinicians providing chemical peels?
7. What is the difference between performing peels in the medical setting and performing peels in the salon setting?
8. What are the principles of a higher code of ethics?
9. What are HIPAA regulations?

CHAPTER REFERENCES

1. Rubin, M. (1995). *Manual of chemical peels: Superficial and medium depth.* Philadelphia: Lippincott, Williams & Wilkins.
2. D'Angelo, J., Dean, P., Dietz, S., Hinds, C., Lees, M., Miller, E., et al. (2003). *Milady's standard: Comprehensive training for estheticians.* Clifton Park, NY: Thomson Delmar Learning.
3. Rubin, M. (1995). *Manual of chemical peels: Superficial and medium depth.* Philadelphia: Lippincott, Williams & Wilkins.
4. D'Angelo, J., Dean, P., Dietz, S., Hinds, C., Lees, M., Miller, E., et al. (2003). *Milady's standard: Comprehensive training for estheticians.* Clifton Park, NY: Thomson Delmar Learning.
5. Kuwahara, R. T. (2001, December 5). *eMedicine: Specialties: Dermatology: Surgical, Chemical Peels* [On line]. Available: http://www.emedicine.com

6. Ancira, M. A. (1998). Chemical peels: An overview. *Plastic Surgical Nursing*, 19, 179.

7. Kuwahara, T. (2001, December 5). *eMedicine: Specialties: Dermatology: Surgical, Chemical Peels* [On line]. Available: http://www.emedicine.com

8. Ancira, M. A. (1998). Chemical peels: An overview. *Plastic Surgical Nursing*, 19, 179.

9. Kuwahara, T. (2001, December 5). *eMedicine: Specialties: Dermatology: Surgical, Chemical Peels* [On line]. Available: http://www.emedicine.com

10. A Board Certified Plastic Surgeon Resource. (2004, April 7). *Chemical peel, find a chemical peel surgeon near you!* [On line]. Available: http://www.aboardcertifiedplasticsurgeon.com

11. Rubin, M. (1995). *Manual of chemical peels: Superficial and medium depth*. Philadelphia: Lippincott, Williams & Wilkins.

12. Omura, A. M. N. E. (2002). *Glycolic peels compared to microdermabrasion: A right-left controlled study trial of efficacy and patient satisfaction* [On line]. Available: www.ncbi.nlm.nih.gov

13. http://www.aesthetic.lumenis.com

14. *Webster's college dictionary*. (1992). New York: Random House.

15. *Webster's college dictionary*. (1992). New York: Random House.

16. MacDonald, C. (2004, March 9). *Why have a code of ethics?* [Online]. Available: http://www.ethicsweb.ca

17. MacDonald, C. (2004, March 9). *Why have a Code of Ethics?* [Online]. Available: http://www.ethicsweb.ca

18. Olson, A. (2004, March 11). *Authoring a code: Observations on process and organization* [Online]. Available: http://www.iit.edu

19. United States Department of Health and Human Services. (2004, March 9). *Fact sheet* [Online]. Available: http://www.hhs.gov.html

BIBLIOGRAPHY

A Board Certified Plastic Surgeon Resource. (2004, April 7). *Chemical peel: Find a chemical peel surgeon near you!* [On line]. Available: http://www.aboardcertifiedplasticsurgeon.com

Ancira, M. A. (1998). Chemical peels: An overview, *Plastic Surgical Nursing*, 19, 179.

Barad, R. (2004, March). *Laser skin resurfacing* [Online]. Available: www.laserexpert.com

Bernard, R. W., Beran, S. J., & Rusin, L. (2000, October). Chemical peels in clinical practice, *Journal of Clinical Plastic Surgery*, 27(4), 71–77.

Birket, W. P. (2000, July). *Ethical codes in action* [Online]. Available: www.ifac.org

Brennan, H. G. (2001, April). Skin care in my practice: The spectrum concept, *North American Journal of Facial and Plastic Surgery*, 9(3), 383–394.

Brody, H. J., Geronemus, R. G., & Faris, P. K. (2003, April). Beauty versus medicine: The non-physician practice of dermatologic surgery. *Journal of Dermatologic Surgery*, 29(4), 319–324.

Callen, J. P., Paller, A. S., Greer, K. E., & Swinyer, L. J. (2000). *Color atlas of dermatology* (2nd ed.). Philadelphia: W. B. Saunders.

D'Angelo, J., Dean, P., Dietz, S., Hinds, C., Lees, M., Miller, E., et al. (2003). *Milady's standard: Comprehensive training for estheticians.* Thomson Delmar Learning.

Deitz, S. (2004). *Milady's the clinical esthetician.* Thomson Delmar Learning.

Freeman, S. (May, 2001). Chemical peels, *North American Journal of Facial and Plastic Surgery*, 9(2), 257–266.

Gerson, J. (2004). *Milady's standard: Fundamentals for estheticians* (9th ed.). Thomson Delmar Learning.

Goldberg, G. (2004, January 15). *Chemical peels* [Online]. Available: www.pimaderm.com/chemical peels.htm

Guttman, C. (2002, August). Histologic studies: Chemical peels: Not just superficial. *Cosmetic Surgery Times* [Online]. Available: http://www.cosmeticsurgerytimes

Hinds, A. (2003, August). *Not convinced yet? Aestheticians turn the tide, washing in new opportunities* [Online]. Available: www.cosmetic-surgerytimes.com http://www.aesthetic.lumenis.com

Koch, R. J., & Hanasono, N. M. (2001, August). Chemical peels, *North American Journal of Facial and Plastic Surgery*, 9(3), 377–382 .

Kuwahara, R. T. (2001, December 5). *eMedicine: Specialties: Dermatology: Surgical, Chemical Peels* [On line]. Available: http://www.emedicine.com

Lee, W. R., Shen, S. C., Kuo-Hsien, W., Hu, C. H., & Fang, J. Y. (2003, November). Lasers and chemical peels enhance and control topical delivery of vitamin C, *Journal of Investigative Dermatology*, 121(5), 1118–1125.

MacDonald, C. (2004, March). *Guidance for writing a code of ethics* [Online]. Available: www.ethicsweb.ca

Olson, A. (2004, March). *Authoring a code: Observations on process and organization* [Online]. Available: www.iit.edu

Omura, A. M. N. E. (2002). *Glycolic peels compared to microdermabrasion: A right-left controlled study trial of efficacy and patient satisfaction* [On line]. Available: www.ncbi.nlm.nih.gov

Palmer, G. D. (2001, October). Regarding the study on chemical peels on acne, *Journal of Dermatological Surgery*, 27(10), 914.

Pilla, L. (2002, October). *Medical spas: Where medicine and luxury meet in the middle* [Online]. Available: www.skinandaging.com

Poulos, S. (2004, March). *Erbium laser skin resurfacing* [Online]. Available: www.poulosmd.com

Prague Aesthetic Surgery. (2004, March). *CO_2 Laser & erbium laser: Skin smoothing & non-invasive facial rejuvenation* [Online]. Available: www.aesthetia.com

Rubin, M. (1995). *Manual of chemical peels: Superficial and medium depth*. Philadelphia: Lippincott, Williams & Wilkins.

Shim, E. K., Barnette, D., Hughes, K., & Greenway, H. G. (2001, June). Chemical peels: A clinical and histopathologic study, *Journal of Dermatologic Surgery*, 27(6), 524–530.

United States Department of Health and Human Services. (2004, March 9). *Fact sheet*. [Online] Available: http://www.hhs.gov

Webster's college dictionary. (1992). Random House.

Whitaker, E. (2003, December 2). *Chemical peels* [Online]. Available: www.emedicine.com

Anatomy and Physiology of Aging and Solar Damaged Skin

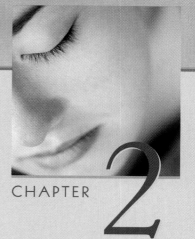

CHAPTER 2

KEY TERMS

adipose cells
aging
albinism
atrophic
avascular
basal cell carcinoma (BCC)
ceramides
cholesterol
dermal-epidermal junction
dermis
desmosomes
elastin
epidermis
extrinsic aging
fatty acids
filaggrin
generalized posttraumatic
    dyschromias
glycosaminoglycans
    (GAGs)

hemochromatosis
hyperpigmentation
hypodermis
hypopigmentation
integumentary system
intrinsic aging
keratinization
keratinocyte
lamellar granules
lamellar ichthyosis
Langerhans cells
lichen simplex chronicus
lipids
melanin
melanocytes
melanoma
melasma
melasma gravidarum
natural moisturizing factor
    (NMF)

normal aging
organelles
papillae
postmitotic cells
rete-pegs
reticula
reticular dermis
senescence
skin turgor
squamous cell
    carcinoma (SCC)
stem cells
stratum basale
stratum corneum
subcutaneous
transepidermal water loss
    (TEWL)
vitiligo

LEARNING OBJECTIVES

After completing this chapter you should be able to:

1. Know each layer of the skin.
2. Identify the functions particular to each layer of skin.
3. Describe the difference between intrinsic and extrinsic aging.
4. Describe transepidermal water loss.
5. Understand the constituents of natural moisturizing factor.

35

INTRODUCTION

integumentary system
The skin and its appendages (nails, hair, sweat glands, and oil glands).

As clinicians in the field of dermal techniques, we must be familiar with the skin, its layers, and the cells within them. Your deeper understanding of skin structure and function will help you be a better clinician. In turn, this knowledge will provide your client improved results and safer care.

The skin and its appendages—nails, hair, nerve endings, sweat, and oil glands—comprise the integumentary system, sometimes referred to as "integument." Skin not only keeps our bodies and its various components intact, but it is also, and equally important, our most immediate contact with our environment. Our skin senses vital information about the world in which we live; therefore it ensures our survival.

Although seemingly uniform and simple in its presentation and purpose, the skin is far more complex and variant than meets the eye. It changes in thickness and in sensitivity based on the areas of the body. Parts of the skin develop (in utero) from brain tissues and remain attached to the brain through nerves that conduct pleasure as well as pain.[2] Although not all of the sensations we feel are pleasurable, they are all *purposeful*. If we could not *feel* cold air, we would freeze to death. If we could not *sense* a cut, we could bleed to death. The sensations we feel are, in turn, sent to our brains for processing and translation. The skin overall possesses most of the nerve endings that transmit vital information about our environment to the brain. Relatively few nerve endings are found on our posterior sides; however, in *lips, fingers,* and *genitals,* they are abundant.

Similarly, because the skin is our outermost organ, it also serves as a unique identifier, which we see and use to associate and differentiate one person from another. Being the psychosocial creatures we are, we have put great emphasis on how others perceive the way we appear. The way we dress, decorate, and posture ourselves conveys gender, age, strength, and most noticeably, attractiveness.

Healthy skin has become synonymous with youth and beauty in our society. For this reason, we strive to preserve and maintain healthy skin as best we can. To the chagrin of most of us, the means to halt the aging process is not currently available. For most of us, this understanding may seem a little late. The good news is that not all damage is irreversible. The marketplace is driving the demand for more effective and useful products and services, and science is stepping up to the challenge.

For persons who are committed to undoing the damage, and turning over a new leaf, hope can be found. As skin care professionals, you will be able to offer a host of effective treatment programs that will help slow the clock down and reverse the previous damage (Figure 2–1). To this avail, a basic understanding of the skin and the functions of aging are the logical starting point (Table 2–1 on page 38).

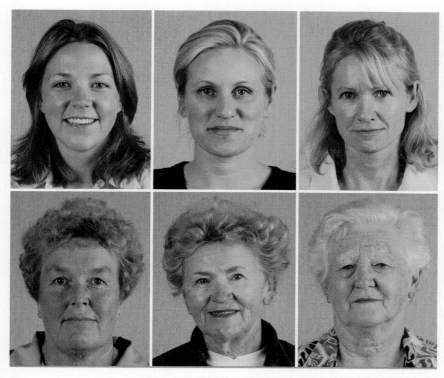

Figure 2–1 Aging through the years is predictable and presents itself in lines, wrinkles, and loose skin.

The outermost layer of the skin is the epidermis. It shields us from the environment, potential injury, bacteria, pollution, and most everything else that wants to get in. The lower layer of the skin, called the dermis, is the support, providing the epidermis with strength and stability. Beneath the dermis is subcutaneous fat, called the hypodermis. The hypodermis acts as a thermal barrier and mechanical cushion, with varying thickness from person to person and at different places on the body.

■ LAYERS OF THE SKIN

The skin is composed of two main layers: the epidermis and the dermis. The epidermis is the top layer. It is tough and, because of its exposure, is constantly being worn down and replaced.[3] This layer contains no blood vessels or nerves and is vital in preventing loss of moisture from the body. The dermis, or deeper layer of the skin, and the subcutaneous fat beneath it, lend strength and elasticity to the skin. Within both layers of skin are sublayers with cells that perform specific functions.

If you look at a microscopic slice of skin, it will appear as though some objects, such as hair follicles, project from the dermis through the epidermis. This is not really the case. The epidermis *encases* these objects and projects down into the dermis beneath it.

Let us drill down into the skin from above.

epidermis
Outermost, avascular, protective layer of skin.

dermis
The second layer of skin, which is responsible for attaching the skin to the body.

subcutaneous
Beneath the skin.

hypodermis
A layer of subcutaneous fat and connective tissue lying beneath the epidermis.

Table 2–1   Facts About Aging Skin[4]

- Changes in the skin inevitably happen as years pass.
- A natural order of life is that matter changes as it ages.
- Skin is not immune to the law of gravity.
- Collagen and elastin production slows down a dramatic 65% between the ages of 20 and 80 years.
- The thickness of the skin decreases a staggering 6% every 10 years.
- 90% of the visible signs of aging are caused by sunlight exposure.
- TWENTIES: wrinkles first appear around eyes and lips.
- THIRTIES: skin becomes less resilient as elastin declines, allowing gravity to begin to have its way.
- FORTIES: as elasticity begins to diminish, skin loses its memory and becomes less able to snap back. Repetitive movements such as frowns and squinting, as well as cigarette smoking, form the first permanent wrinkles.
- FIFTIES: normal aging changes become more apparent; gravity is certainly a factor. Gravity combines with the decrease in collagen and elastin, causing skin and muscle to sag. Gravity also causes the tip of the nose to droop and the ears to elongate.
- SIXTIES: hormonal activities have ceased to be a problem, and, as such, the skin is loose and sagging. If the skin has not been protected, lines, wrinkles, and dark spots develop.
- SEVENTIES: increased thinning of the skin and loss of collagen in the dermis occur. Additional wrinkles, lines, and sagging develop.

Epidermis and Aging

The epidermis is the top layer, the outer skin, the skin that we see. This layer is avascular (without blood vessels), impermeable to water, physically tough, and dry at the surface to impede the growth of microorganisms (Table 2–2).

Within the epidermis are tiny pockets that house sweat glands and pilosebaceous glands.[5] Contrasting the dermis, the epidermis is often very thin, having a thickness of approximately 0.12 mm, but this can vary dramatically over the body.[6] This layer is thickest on the palms of the hands and soles of the feet and thinnest on the eyelids.

Unlike other cellular components of the body such as nerves, epidermal cells are born, they die, and are ultimately replaced by new ones. Hence the epidermis is continually replacing itself. When the epidermis is injured or diseased, its replacement speeds up in response; this factor is important to us as clinicians. In short, the epidermis is our self-replicating defense against everything outside of us.

The epidermis is further divided into five *sublayers* (Figure 2–2). These sublayers are characterized by *stages* of hardening, maturation,

avascular
Lacking in blood vessels and thus having a poor blood supply.

Table 2–2 Layers of the Epidermis and Their Functions

Layer	Function
Stratum corneum	Outermost layer of skin characterized by the death and ultimate sloughing of the aged keratinocyte
Stratum lucidum	This thin, clear band ("lucidum" means *clear* or *bright*) of closely packed cells is most prominent in areas of thick skin and may be absent in other areas[7]
Stratum granulosum	Similar to the other sublayers of the epidermis, this layer signals transition of the cells within it.[8] In this layer, the keratin loses the nucleus and organelles, becoming flat, before moving farther up into the stratum corneum. In effect, these granules write the death warrant of the cell because as the granules grow in size, the nucleus—the power generator of the cell—disintegrates and dies.[9]
Stratum spinosum (stratum germinativum)	Stratum spinosum means *spiny layer*. Cells in this sublayer are intertwined with desmosomes. Lamellar granules are also found here. These granules control lipids that migrate to the stratum corneum and become another component of NMF.
Stratum basale (basal layer)	The *basal layer*; it anchors the epidermis to the dermis. This layer contains germinal cells, cells of regeneration, for all sublayers of the epidermis.

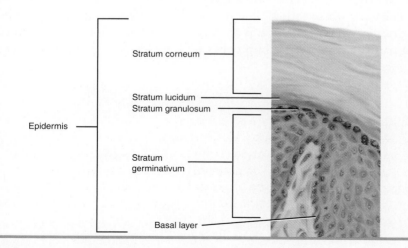

Figure 2–2 The epidermis has five sublayers: the stratum corneum, the stratum lucidum, the stratum granulosum, the stratum germinativum (stratum spinosum), and the basal layer (stratum basale).

keratinocyte
Any cell in the skin, hair, or nails that produces keratin.

stratum basale
The lowest layer of the epidermis. The stratum basale (basal layer) houses germinal cells and regenerating cells for all layers of the epidermis.

stratum corneum
The superficial sublayer of the epidermis; this layer varies in thickness over the body.

natural moisturizing factor (NMF)
A compound found only in the top of skin that gives cells their ability to bind with water.

filaggrin
Synthesizes lipids (fats) that are thought to serve as "intercellular cement," an important component of NMF.

and eventual death in the migration of their major cell type, the keratinocyte.[10]

Each month, these cells migrate from the bottom layer (stratum basale or basal layer) of the epidermis and travel upward until they arrive at the outermost layer (stratum corneum). Each cell begins as a healthy plump cell with a fully functioning nucleus. However, as the cells near the summit, they shrivel and flatten out. [11]

The stratum corneum is the *top* or superficial layer of the epidermis, and it varies in thickness. It can be thin on the upper arm and thick on the soles, palms, and other areas of chronic friction. This is the area where cells complete their journey, soon to transition to death, at which time they are eventually sloughed off.

Although it is drier than lower skin layers, the stratum corneum contains a compound called natural moisturizing factor (NMF). NMF helps keep the skin soft and moisturized, even in dry climates.[12] NMF is composed of amino acids and filaggrin, water-soluble chemicals capable of absorbing large quantities of water. The presence of NMF in the stratum corneum is critical for soft and flexible skin. Although NMF is contained only in the uppermost layer of the skin, its existence is made possible by ingredients provided by deeper structures.[13]

NMF gives the cells of the stratum corneum their ability to bind with water. NMF is found only in the stratum corneum, and it is solely responsible for the regulation of water in the very superficial layers of the stratum corneum. Not surprisingly, the presence of NMF is diminished by age and excessive exposure to soap. This factor is the key to understanding the phenomenon of dry skin.

Worth noting, NMF and TEWL have nothing to do with water loss associated with sweating. The notion that drinking water will improve hydration levels of the skin is a common misconception. This is simply not true. Drinking water improves the water level inside the body but is

transepidermal water loss (TEWL)
The process by which our bodies constantly lose water via evaporation.

Preventing Excessive Water Loss

As long as we are not submerged, our bodies constantly lose water via evaporation through our skin. This gentle process is called transepidermal water loss (TEWL),[14] and we are totally unaware of it. In the normal epidermis, the water content decreases the closer we get to the surface. Water makes up to 70% to 75% of the weight of layers beneath but only 10% to 15% of the weight of the stratum corneum. When too much water evaporates, not only our skin, but also our bodies suffer ill effects. Preventing excessive water loss is important both to the skin itself and to the body as a whole.

used up there. The best way to rehydrate the skin is by applying a topical moisturizer.

Below the stratum corneum is the stratum lucidum. This thin, clear band ("lucidum" means *clear* or *bright*) of closely packed cells is most prominent in areas of thick skin and may be absent in other areas.[15]

Similar to the other sublayers of the epidermis, the stratum granulosum signals transition of the cells within it.[16] In this layer, the keratin loses the nucleus and organelles, becoming flat, before moving farther up into the stratum corneum. This layer is called the stratum granulosum because of the granules that now appear in the cells. In effect, these granules write the death warrant of the cell because, as the granules grow in size, the nucleus—the power generator of the cell—disintegrates and dies.[17]

Stratum spinosum means *spiny layer*. Cells in this sublayer are intertwined with tiny structures called desmosomes. Under the microscope, desmosomes resemble hair combed with an eggbeater, which is why this part is often called the *prickly-cell* layer. The hairlike desmosomes permit materials to move around them in the intercellular space (the spaces between cells). Lamellar granules are also found here. These granules control lipids that migrate to the stratum corneum and become another component of NMF.

In this first leg of the journey, keratinocytes depart the basal layer and show the first signs of keratinization. Here also, we find lamellar granules, organelles that deliver fats to the stratum corneum. These granules contain the lipids and other components such as cholesterol, fatty acids, ceramides, and enzymes necessary to produce NMF. Once these granules reach the stratum corneum, they release their contents and cause the production of NMF to occur.

The basement of the epidermis is appropriately called the basal layer, or stratum basale. It anchors the epidermis to the dermis. This layer contains germinal cells, cells of regeneration, for all sublayers of the epidermis. Here, stem cells produce two types of cells. Basal cells remain in the basal layer, creating a solid skin foundation, and keratinocytes begin their upward migration to the stratum corneum.

The basal layer houses several types of basal cells, including stem cells, amplifying cells, and postmitotic cells. In part, the stratum basale creates its own stability, and, in part, it initiates the cell migration and maturation toward the more superficial layers. The cells of the basal layer form the "basement" of the epidermis, attaching to the dermis below and the spiny layer above. This layer generates the epidermal cellular process.

The epidermis has much to do with how our skin presents the signs of aging. Healthier, happier people are sometimes called *radiant*.

organelles
A specific location within the cell.

desmosomes
Small hairlike structures in the spiny layer of the epidermis.

lamellar granules
Control lipids that produce NMF.

keratinization
The process keratin cells go through as they move up to the stratum corneum layer.

lipids
Fat or fatlike substances that are descriptive not chemical.

cholesterol
A precursor to most steroid hormones; a single molecule is called alcohol.

fatty acids
One of many molecules that are long chains of lipid-carboxylic acid found in fats and oils.

ceramides
A class of lipids that do not contain glycerol cholesterol.

stem cells
Unspecialized cells that give rise to a specific specialized cell.

postmitotic cells
Cells that have completed mitotic division.

Table 2–3 Layers of the Dermis and the Functions

Layer	Function
Papillary dermis	Papillary dermis, the most superficial layer of the dermis, is the first skin layer to contain capillary blood vessels, small nerves, and lymphatic vessels. This sublayer also houses GAGs.
Reticular dermis	Reticular dermis is located beneath papillary dermis and rests on the thick pad of fat known as subcutaneous tissue. Here lies the real anchor of the skin.

melanocytes
A group of cells (in the epidermis) that produces the pigment melanin.

reticula
A netlike formation or structure; a network.

elastin
Connective tissue proteins.

dermal-epidermal junction
The superficial side of the dermis, connected to the epidermis.

On its superficial side, the dermis holds the epidermis at the dermal-epidermal junction (DEJ). On its distal side, the dermis attaches to subcutaneous tissue.

Actually, this description is equally a reference to healthy, functioning skin given that it is about disposition. As we get older, the radiance begins to fade. Translucent skin gives way to opaque, grayer skin, which can more easily reveal the effects of prolonged environmental exposure. Pigment-containing melanocytes decrease in quantity but increase in size. This change allows brown spots to appear in sunlight-exposed areas.[18] As if that were not bad enough, the upward migration of the keratinocyte slows over time. Consequentially, the mature cells that comprise the stratum corneum must lay in wait for their replacement well beyond their means. The older we get, the longer the skin cell's lifespan becomes. In effect, our skin (outwardly) appears even more lackluster and dull. These older, necrotized cells must be removed for younger, healthier looking cells to come to the forefront. Accomplishing as much is what makes many treatments successful, including chemical peels.

Dermis and Aging

The dermis resides below the epidermis and provides the vital function of attaching skin to body (Table 2–3).

The dermis is crisscrossed with three types of fibers that lend strength and elasticity. These fibers—reticula, collagen, and elastin—form a network that creates stability for the skin. Type I collagen runs throughout the dermis and is responsible for its tensile strength and for providing skin its youthful appearance of tightness, firmness, and fullness.[19] The combined strength of these tissues anchors the epidermis above to the subcutaneous tissue below.

Epidermal appendages such as sweat glands and hair follicles are embedded in the dermis and serve as the end point for blood vessels and nerves.[20]

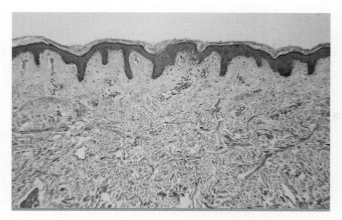

Figure 2–3 The dermis has two layers: the papillary dermis and the reticular dermis.

The dermis, which varies but is approximately 2 mm thick, is further subdivided into the papillary and reticular layers.[21] This subdivision is based on differences in collagen texture.[22] The papillary dermis, the most superficial layer of the dermis, is the first skin layer to contain capillary blood vessels, small nerves, and lymphatic vessels (Figure 2–3).

Because the papillary dermis contains blood vessels and blood vessels provide temperature changes when they constrict or dilate, the papillary dermis is specifically responsible for thermoregulation of the body. In addition to its *holding* properties, the papillary dermis has another important function in regulating the appearance of the skin's surface because this sublayer houses glycosaminoglycans (GAGs). GAGs are a variety of "chains" made of polysaccharide, a type of complex carbohydrate. Attracted almost fanatically to water, GAGs are presumably capable of binding up to 1000 times their weight in water.[26] This moisture-attracting property makes GAGs one of the most important components in our study of the skin. Many histologic studies of the skin show a decrease in the number of GAGs with age.[27]

The reticular dermis is located beneath the papillary dermis and rests on the thick pad of fat known as subcutaneous tissue, which represents the real anchor of the skin.

Within the reticular dermis are structures called rete-pegs. These *pegs* extend up into the epidermis (and similar structures extend from above down into the dermis) to hold the dermis to the epidermis. These structures are responsible for holding the epidermis and dermis together

glycosaminoglycans (GAGs)
Polysaccharide chains, most prominent in the dermis that bind with water, smoothing and softening the surface from below.

reticular dermis
The sublayer of the dermis that connects the dermis to the epidermis and is home to the skin's appendages (nails, hair, and glands).

rete-pegs
Anatomic features that hold the dermis and epidermis together.

papillae
Projections of any kind; in the skin, papillae hold the dermis and the epidermis together.

Collagen in the papillary dermis is finely textured[23] and contains projections called papillae that fit the dermis to the epidermis.[24] We are accustomed to using these uniquely individual ridged patterns in foot- and fingerprinting.[25]

Collagen in this layer (reticular means *similar to a network*) is larger and more coarsely textured.[28] In the example of a cow's skin after *tanning*, the cow's dermis makes the leather.[29]

skin turgor
The flexibility of the skin.

adipose cells
Fat cells.

to create *the skin*. Capillary networks run through rete-pegs as tiny elevators, bringing nutrients to the epidermis. Widened vessels in the rete-pegs cause *broken capillaries*. People with transparent or very light skin may flush or blush, causing a dilation of the capillaries in the rete-pegs.

Even though it is situated below the epidermis, the dermis also suffers some catastrophic changes with the passage of time. Collagen and elastin weaken, and the skin begins to lose tensile strength and skin turgor.[30] In turn, lines of expression deepen. The dermal-epidermal junction flattens and begins to undergo atrophy. Meanwhile, the quantity of blood vessel decreases. This decrease in vascularity causes the hair, nails, and other appendages to appear gray and dull; the appendages can also become weaker through the process of aging. Whereas young skin is translucent and can retain moisture easily, older skin can no longer retain moisture as it was once able to do. As a result, skin becomes drier and flakier.[31] As a result of the dermal aging process and the degradation of the dermal layer, the skin has impaired healing abilities as we grow older. This process sounds dismal. Although we cannot turn back the hands of time, we can stimulate the dermal layer to continue to produce collagen and encourage increases in vascularity. Some of the improvement in the dermal layer will come with exercise, and other improvements will come with skin treatments. Let us read on to find out more.

Hypodermis or Subcutaneous Tissue

Under the reticular dermis lies the hypodermis, or subcutaneous fat (Figure 2–4). The hypodermis is made up of clumps of fat-filled cells called adipose cells. This area is the *cushion layer* of the skin and helps protect internal organs from trauma; it also acts as an insulator, conserving body heat.[32]

The attachment of subcutaneous tissue to reticular dermis is not tight or rigid. Rather, it is loose, allowing the skin a degree of shifting movement over muscle and skeletal structures. The subcutaneous tissue is crisscrossed with connective tissue to fibers and layers interspersed with fat to hold it together. When pockets of fat accumulate between the connective tissue bands beyond the ability of the connective tissue to hold it smooth, the appearance is called *cellulite* or *orange-peel* skin. Because women generally have thinner skin and less rigid connective tissue bands than do men, *cellulite* is generally more apparent in women. Cellulite is also more likely to appear in certain areas of the body as well, such as the hips, thighs, and buttocks.

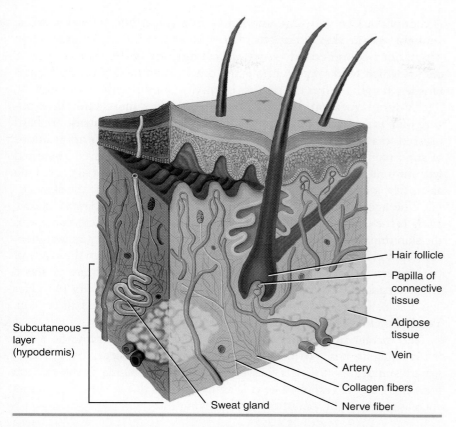

Hair follicle

Papilla of connective tissue

Adipose tissue

Vein

Artery

Collagen fibers

Nerve fiber

Sweat gland

Subcutaneous layer (hypodermis)

Figure 2–4 Beneath the reticular dermis lies the hypodermis, or subcutaneous fat.

■ AGING SKIN

As children, we take our soft, pliable, quickly healing integument for granted. We play outside, frolic in any available water, and roam hills, valleys, and flats. Additionally, during this time, our skin is absorbing the effects of this *trauma*. The effects are not all bad, but they are certainly cumulative, and every bit of *exposure* has its consequences.

Realistically, we cannot completely avoid sunlight; in fact, most of our sunlight exposure is normal (everyday exposure). In an earlier time, people of wealth, good breeding, and leisure valued a pale, tanless complexion. In the late twentieth century, sun-bronzed skin took on its sexy aura of vigor and well being. This appearance connoted the ability to spend leisure time on beaches, golf courses, and tennis courts. Within boundaries, sunlight exposure is not all bad; in fact, we need the sun.

Although we can get some vitamin D from plant and animal sources, sunlight on our skin is responsible for up to 90% of the vitamin D on which our bodies depend.[33] In tight conjunction with calcium, neither one of which works well without the other, vitamin D gives our bones tensile strength,[34] thus the process of enriching milk with vitamin D.

Without question, however, many people get more sunlight exposure than is necessary for bone health. People who work outside are hard pressed to avoid the effects of weather, even with generous applications of sunscreen. Even if the sunlight never reaches us, we are bombarded with tiny molecular renegades (radiation) that do their damage. As long as we live, we cannot completely avoid damage and aging to the skin.

The aging process is both complex and yet simple. Simply stated, aging is the degradation of the dermis and epidermis over time that leaves the skin thin, lacking elasticity, wrinkled, and speckled with pigmentation. A reduction in skin turgor occurs.[35] Loss of adhesion between the layers of the epidermis, as well as between the epidermis and dermis, creates a greater tendency for injury and more visible effects of gravity (wrinkles and folds). Decreases in filaggrin and NMF mean dry and flaky skin. Wound healing slows from decrements in Langerhans cells.[36]

To further understand the process of aging, we employ the terms intrinsic aging and extrinsic aging. Intrinsic aging occurs by virtue of genetics and gravity—it is unavoidable. Extrinsic aging is the portion for which we are responsible; it is aging attributable to external factors such as the sunlight, pollution, and smoking.

Intrinsic Aging

Aging is a "process of gradual and spontaneous change, resulting in maturation through childhood, puberty, and young adulthood and then decline through middle and late age."[37] Senescence, on the other hand, is the "process by which cell division, growth, and function is lost over time ultimately leading to an incompatibility with life."[38] The idea of *successful* aging implies growing old without debilitating diseases that eventually end in death. Intrinsic aging is the process of normal aging that is related to our genetic code. Some people age differently than others do; this fact we know. Some people grow old quickly, with diseases such as *diabetes* or *heart disease*, while others remain healthier and younger than their chronologic age. Baby boomers in particular are insistent that they live longer, healthier lives. Longevity and the rate of intrinsic aging have not only to do with how healthy we are, but also how we look. However, because genetics play a noteworthy role in the aging process, part of its individual effects is out of our hands. The longer we live, the more likely we will face our mother or father in the mirror one

Langerhans cells
Cells that are intimately involved in the immune response of skin.

intrinsic aging
Changes that would occur over time without the effects of any environmental factors.

extrinsic aging
Changes that are brought on by the effects of the environment and our choices relating to them, specifically sunlight exposure.

aging
The universal experience of change associated with the passage of time.

senescence
Growing old; aging.

normal aging
Intrinsic aging.

day. Intrinsic aging happens over time and regardless of resistance (Figure 2–5). Clients seen for problems such as deep smile lines or more typically vertical upper lip lines will report that either their mother or father has the same aging phenomenon. Some of the hallmarks of aging are pigmented lesions, dry skin, or thinning skin, although the skin generally does not become extraordinarily thin until the eighth decade.[39] Although most of intrinsic aging is out of our control, it does not mean that we should throw up our hands and consider it a lost cause. Advanced skin-care techniques, among them chemical peels and sophisticated home-care regimes, can blunt the onset of the inevitable.

Extrinsic Aging

Degradation of collagen is the result of exposure to environmental hazards such as wind, severe temperature changes, sunlight, smoking, and pollution. This exposure to the elements creates free radicals that hasten the aging process and increase the potential for skin cancers. The process of extrinsic aging is different histologically and physiologically compared with intrinsic aging.[40] However, as clinicians, we do not generally differentiate the aging process for our patients. The appearance of extrinsic aging, however, is easily identified and is present in all humans because it is cumulative and begins in childhood. The evidence is usually quite strong in persons over the age of 60 and is presented as wrinkling, pigmentation, telangiectasias, and rough textures. The extreme, of course, are skin cancers. Although basal cell carcinomas are the most common, more serious squamous cell and melanoma cancers are on the rise. Recent statistics tell the story of decades of sun worship. The American Cancer Society tells us that, as of this writing, over one million cases of skin cancer have been diagnosed yearly. Most of these cases are considered sunlight related. Of the one million diagnosed cases each year, over 55,000 of these cancers will be melanoma! Of the persons diagnosed with melanoma, nearly 10,000 will die!

To the clinician, extrinsic aging may appear as the type of aging over which we have complete control. For instance, we can protect our skin from extrinsic aging by using sun-block or avoiding extremes of hot and cold temperature. Simply being outside, unprotected, will age the skin faster. However, blaming the sun for all of our aging symptoms is easy. Although a large percentage of extrinsic aging is sunlight related, other insults play a role. For example, cigarette smoking, extreme temperatures (especially cold), and living in polluted environments are addition factors. Not surprisingly, the sunlight-protected sights (abdominal skin or breast skin) are less aged and atrophic than is exposed skin. This phenomenon makes for a useful educational tool when working with patients to explain the effects of the sunlight and environment.

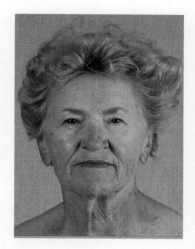

Figure 2–5   Persons who have had limited or restricted access to sunlight will exhibit primarily intrinsic aging. This woman is in her 70s.

atrophic
To undergo deterioration.

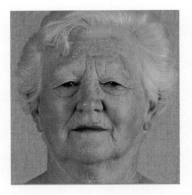

Figure 2–6 Yesterday's tan will eventually present as tomorrow's extrinsic aging. This woman is also in her 70s.

melanin
The cells that produce color in the skin.

hyperpigmentation
The overproduction of melanin.

hypopigmentation
The lack of melanin production.

melasma
An overproduction of melanin.

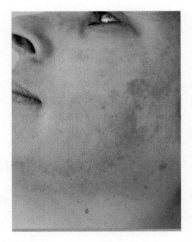

Figure 2–7 Melasma presents as dark spot or areas on the face and neck.

Although chemical peels are effective in treating solar damage specifically and extrinsic aging in general, the most important task for the clinician is educating the client. All clients should be reminded of potential injuries to the skin that occur with extreme or prolonged exposure to the sunlight, wind, temperature extremes, and pollution (Figure 2–6).

Pigmentary Disorders

As we know, the pigment of the skin is directly related to the production of melanin, from the melanocytes. Melanin production can increase or decrease beyond normal, creating a change in the skin color. The overproduction of melanin, or hyperpigmentation, is related to several phenomena, for example, postinflammatory hyperpigmentation, solar damage, pregnancy, some types of drug use, and dermatologic disease processes. The problem of hypopigmentation is often associated with the disease known as vitiligo but can also occur as a result of injury (Table 2–4).

Hyperpigmentation

Hyperpigmentation results from the increased deposition of melanin, which causes the skin to become darker in patches. It is one of the most common problems seen in the medical spa. This irregular patchy pigmentation has origins in solar exposure, pregnancy, medications, birth control, and dermatologic skin diseases. Hyperpigmentation can be frustrating yet is a simple problem to solve.

Hyperpigmentation can also result from aggressive or mismanaged peeling, microdermabrasion, or intense pulsed-light therapy (Foto Facial™), that is, any procedure in which the skin is overstimulated or injured. Hyperpigmentation is especially common in darker skin types. These skin types should be treated with care both in the clinic and at home to avoid hyperpigmentation.

The treatment for hyperpigmentation varies depending on the probable cause. In general, a bleaching cream of prescription strength is necessary: hydroquinone 4%+ and, of course, sunscreen. Some patients will be under the misguided assumption that using the bleaching cream will be enough to solve the problem. The patient needs to be educated to understand the need for sunscreen, because without sunscreen, the hydroquinone is likely to have little, if any, effects.

Melasma

Melasma is an overproduction of melanin and is a problem normally found in women (Figure 2–7). It is generally associated with pregnancy or the use of birth control pills, although 10% of the population affected

Table 2–4   Descriptions of Pigment

Skin Pigment Disorders Present in the Medical Spa Environment

Melanin	Pigment that protects skin from ultraviolet damage
Melanocytes	The type of cell that produces the pigment melanin
Albinism	An inherited skin dyschromia that is a lack of pigment; people with albinism typically have light skin, white or pale yellow hair, and blue or light-gray eyes
Hypopigmentation	A form of skin dyschromia that results from a lacking production of melanin from melanocytes
Hyperpigmentation	A skin dyschromia that occurs as a result of an overproduction and over deposits of melanin
Lichen simplex chronicus	A skin disorder with severe itching that causes thick, dark patches of skin to develop
Vitiligo	A skin disorder that creates smooth depigmented white spots on the skin
Lamellar ichthyosis (also known as fish scale disease)	An inherited skin disorder that is characterized by darkened, scaly, dry patches of skin
Melasma gravidarum (also known as mask of pregnancy or chloasma)	A dark, masklike discoloration that covers the cheeks and bridge of the nose; caused by an over-production of melanin
Hemochromatosis (also known as hemosiderosis)	A form of dyschromia characterized by a buildup of pigments not ordinarily found in such abundance to cause darkening
Generalized posttraumatic dyschromias	Patchy pigment loss at or near the sight of an insult, for example, a burn or an infection

albinism
Inherited skin dyschromia which is characterized by a lack of pigment.

lichen simplex chronicus
Itching papules; also known as Vidal's disease.

vitiligo
Smooth depigmentation white spots on the skin.

lamellar ichthyosis
An inherited skin disorder with scaly, dry patches of skin; also known as fish scale disease.

hemochromatosis
Dyschromia characterized by a buildup of pigments; known as hemosiderosis.

generalized post-traumatic dyschromias
A hyperpigmentation caused by an insult.

melasma gravidarum
An increase in melanin production caused by pregnancy, also known as the mask of pregnancy.

are men.[41] Although many researchers speculate as to the specific physiologic cause that triggers the overproduction of melanin, the true cause is as yet unknown. We know that many women are affected during pregnancy and when using birth control pills, causing us to postulate the hormonal relationship to melanin. We call this melasma gravidarum. Unprotected sunlight exposure will also contribute melasma, as will overirritation of the skin (Fitzpatrick IV, V, and VI) and skin injuries such as picking at acne cysts.

> Over time, skin that is consistently exposed or has extreme exposure to the environment may develop skin cancers.

SKIN CANCERS

Moles and lesions that appear suspicious or concern you should be examined by the physician. This protocol should be part of the policy and procedures at your spa. Take photographs of these particular moles or lesions. Make notes regarding the length of time the lesion or mole has been present, if it is changing, and any other pertinent information. Moles or lesions for which you should be looking include melanomas, basal cell carcinomas, and squamous cell carcinomas. When the physician examines the patient, a copy of the physician's report should be added to the patient's skin-care record. If a biopsy or lesion removal is done, file a copy of that pathology report in the skin-care chart.

Basal Cell Carcinomas

basal cell carcinoma (BCC)
A slow-growing tumor that generally does not metastasize. It is the most common form of skin cancer, which usually occurs in regions of repeated sunburn.

A basal cell carcinoma (BCC) is the most common skin cancer, often found in areas of repeated sunburns and sunlight exposure. A BCC is a slow-growing tumor and generally does not metastasize (spread to other areas). A basal cell carcinoma can, however, cause extensive disfigurement if left untreated or treated ineffectually. In the United States, the incidence of BCC annually is nearly 900,000 million—550,000 men and 350,000 women.[42] BCCs are divided into six subtypes: nodular, pigmented, superficial, micronodular, cystic, and morpheaform. Each subset has its own distinct features. The most common appearance of BCC is as a pearly nodule. It can exhibit some but not necessarily all of the following features: bleeding, crusting, and a small center depression (Figure 2–8).

Squamous Cell Carcinomas

squamous cell carcinoma (SCC)
A malignant cancer of the epithelial cells.

melanoma
The most serious form of skin cancer.

A squamous cell carcinoma (SCC) is the second most common skin cancer, with over 200,000 cases diagnosed annually.[43] Unlike BCC, SCC can sometimes metastasize if left untreated. As with BCC, chronic sunlight exposure seems to be the main precursor to SCC, although SCCs have been found in areas without sunlight exposure, such as the mucous membranes of the mouth. Areas such as the inside of the mouth have usually been exposed to frequent and persistent sores, such as leukoplakia. On a rare occasion, SCC will spring up in an area of healthy skin. The hypothesis is that SCC may be passed genetically (Figure 2–9).

Melanomas

Melanoma is the most dangerous of all skin cancers. Melanoma will metastasize and cause death, if left untreated. You must always be alert

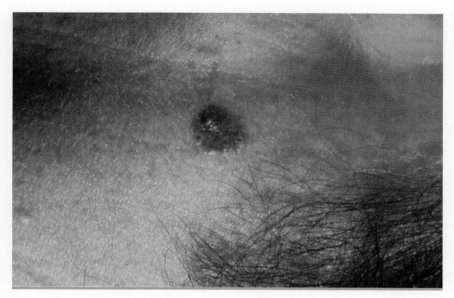

Figure 2–8   Basal cell carcinomas result from chronic sun exposure.

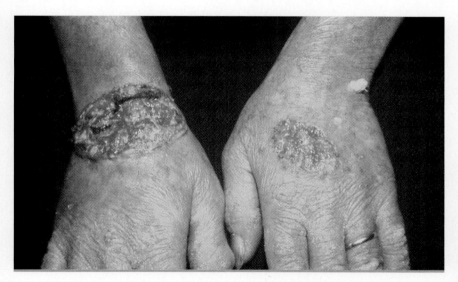

Figure 2–9   Squamous cell carcinomas from chronic sun exposure and irritation.

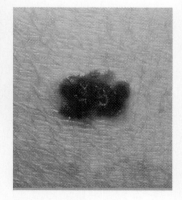

Figure 2–10   A melanoma carcinoma from chronic and intense sun exposure.

to the potential for melanoma. Melanoma is an irregularly shaped and colored mole, most commonly occurring on the back of the legs and trunk. People who have had one to two significant sunburns are at risk for melanoma (Figure 2–10). Because these moles are not primarily located on the face, the clinician must be an *investigator,* asking the client about moles that are new or have changed. You can never be too careful when you suspect a melanoma. Always refer this client to your physician. You might save a life. Remember the ABCDs of skin cancer.

ABCDs of Cancer

Asymmetry—Growth that, when divided in half, has two mismatched halves.

Border irregularity—Ragged or uneven edges that are blurred and poorly defined.

Color—Uneven black, brown, and tan coloring; other colors, like red, white, and blue, can also be interspersed in the growth; any change in the color of the preexisting mole or lesion.

Diameter—Any growth larger than the top of a pencil eraser, which is approximately 6 millimeters in diameter; any unusual or sudden increase in size should also be checked.

▶ ▷ ▷ TOP TEN TIPS TO TAKE TO THE CLINIC

1. Understanding the physiology of the skin will help you be a better clinician.
2. If you understand how the skin ages, you will be better suited to educate your patients.
3. The stratum corneum contains NMF, a critical component to the hydration of the skin.
4. Know the different types of skin cancers and how they appear.
5. Consult with patients about the benefits of sunscreen.
6. Understand the different types of aging.
7. Understand the different layers of the skin and their functions.
8. Know how the skin ages and how it presents on the surface of the skin.
9. Glycosaminoglycans represent an important part of the ground substance.
10. Most people would prefer a younger appearance.

CHAPTER REVIEW QUESTIONS

1. What are the two principle aging processes?
2. What are the two main layers of the skin?
3. How is the skin affected by the sunlight?
4. What are the skin cancers that are induced by the sun?

5. What are GAGs?
6. What is NMF?
7. Why is TEWL important?
8. Define intrinsic aging.
9. Define extrinsic aging.

CHAPTER REFERENCES

1. Burchill, J. (1999). In Moore, E. (Ed.) *Quotation finder*. p. 69. Harper Collins: Glasgow, Scotland.
2. Gray, J. (1997). *The world of skin care* [On line]. P & G Skin Care and Research Center. Available: www.pg.com
3. Gray, J. (1997). *The world of skin care* [On line]. P & G Skin Care and Research Center. Available: www.pg.com
4. Arbonne International. (2004, June 8). *The wiser way: Facts about the aging process* [On line]. Available: www.thewiserway.com
5. King, D. (2003, November 14). *Introduction to skin histology* [On line]. Available: http://www.siumed.edu
6. Spense, A. P. (2004, February 22). *Basic human anatomy* (3rd ed.) [On line]. Available: http://www.sawyerproducts.com
7. King, D. (2003, November 14). *Introduction to skin histology* [On line]. Available: http://www.siumed.edu
8. King, D. (2003, November 14). *Introduction to skin histology* [On line]. Available: http://www.siumed.edu
9. Spense, A. P. (2004, February 22). *Basic human anatomy* (3rd ed.) [On line]. Available: http://www.sawyerproducts.com
10. King, D. (2003, November 14). *Introduction to skin histology* [On line]. Available: http://www.siumed.edu
11. Lowe, N., & Sellar, P. (1999). *Skin secrets: The medical facts versus the beauty fiction*. New York: Collins & Brown.
12. Baumann, L. (2002). *Cosmetic dermatology practices and principles*. New York: McGraw Hill.
13. King, D. (2003, November 14). *Introduction to skin histology* [On line]. Available: http://www.siumed.edu
14. Baumann, L. (2002). *Cosmetic dermatology practices and principles*. New York: McGraw Hill.
15. King, D. (2003, November 14). *Introduction to skin histology* [On line]. Available: http://www.siumed.edu
16. King, D. (2003, November 14). *Introduction to skin histology*. [On line]. Available: http://www.siumed.edu
17. Spense, A. P. (2004, February 22). *Basic human anatomy* (3rd ed.) [On line]. Available: http://www.sawyerproducts.com

18. Gray, J. (1997). *The world of skin care* [On line]. P & G Skin Care and Research Center. Available: www.pg.com

19. Baumann, L. (2002). *Cosmetic dermatology practices and principles.* New York: McGraw Hill.

20. King, D. (2003, November 14). *Introduction to skin histology* [On line]. Available: http://www.siumed.edu

21. Spense, A. P. (2004, February 22). *Basic human anatomy* (3rd ed.) [On line]. Available: http://www.sawyerproducts.com

22. King, D. (2003, November 14). *Introduction to skin histology* [On line]. Available: http://www.siumed.edu

23. King, D. (2003, November 14). *Introduction to skin histology* [On line]. Available: http://www.siumed.edu

24. Nemours Foundation. (2004). *Skin, hair, and nails* [On line]. Available: http://kidshealth.org

25. Spense, A. P. (2004, February 22). *Basic human anatomy* (3rd ed.) [On line]. Available: http://www.sawyerproducts.com

26. Obagi, Z. (2000). *Skin health restoration and rejuvenation.* New York: Springer-Verlag New York.

27. Baumann, L. (2002). *Cosmetic dermatology practices and principles.* New York: McGraw Hill.

28. King, D. (2003, November 14). *Introduction to skin histology* [On line]. Available: http://www.siumed.edu

29. Spense, A. P. (2004, February 22). *Basic human anatomy* (3rd ed.) [On line]. Available: http://www.sawyerproducts.com

30. Brannon, H. (2005, May 5). *What causes wrinkles* [On line]. Available: http://dermatology.about.com

31. Gray, J. (1997). *The world of skin care* [On line]. P & G Skin Care and Research Center. Available: www.pg.com

32. Nemours Foundation. (2004). *Skin, hair, and nails* [On line]. Available: http://kidshealth.org

33. Falkenbach, A. (2000). Muscle strength and vitamin D (letter), *Archives of Physical and Medical Rehabilitation*, 81, 241.

34. Rao, D. S. (1999). Perspective on assessment of vitamin D nutrition. *Journal of Clinical Densitometry*, 2(4), 457–464.

35. Obagi, Z. (2000). *Skin health restoration and rejuvenation.* New York: Springer-Verlag New York.

36. Bisaccia, E., & Scarborough, D. (2002). *The Columbia manual of dermatologic cosmetic surgery.* New York: McGraw Hill.

37. Merck Pharmaceuticals Company. (2004, May 15). *The Merck manual of geriatrics, Section 1: The basics of geriatric care* [On line]. Available: http://www.merck.com

38. Merck Pharmaceuticals Company. (2004, May 15). *The Merck manual of geriatrics, Section 1: The basics of geriatric care* [On line]. Available: http://www.merck.com
39. Venna, S. S., & Gilchrest, B. (2002, February). *Skin aging and photoaging* [On line]. Available: www.skinandaging.com
40. Merck Pharmaceuticals Company. (2004, May 15). *The Merck manual of geriatrics, Section 1: The basics of geriatric care* [On line]. Available: http://www.merck.com
41. American Academy of Dermatology. (2004 January 14). *Rosacea. Public resources* [On line]. Available: http://www.aad.org
42. Revis, D. R. Jr. (2001, July). *Skin grafts, split thickness* [On line]. Available: www.emedicine.com
43. The Skin Cancer Foundation. (2004). *About squamous cell* [On line]. Available: www.skincancer.org

BIBLIOGRAPHY

American Academy of Dermatology. (2004 January 14). *Rosacea. Public resources* [On line]. Available: http://www.aad.org

American Society of Plastic Surgeons. (2002). Quick facts on cosmetic and reconstructive Quick facts on cosmetic and reconstructive plastic surgery trends plastic surgery trends [On line]. Available: http://www.plasticsurgery.org

Baumann, L. (2002). *Cosmetic dermatology practices and principles.* McGraw Hill.

Bisaccia, E., & Scarborough, D. (2002). *The Columbia manual of dermatologic cosmetic surgery.* McGraw Hill.

Blitzner, A., Binder, W. J., Boyd, J. B., & Carruthers, A. (Eds.). (2000). *Management of facial lines and wrinkles.* Philadelphia: Lippincott, Williams & Wilkins.

Brody, H. J. (1997). *Chemical peeling and resurfacing* (2nd ed.). Mosby.

Elsner, P., & Maibach, H. L. (Eds.). (2000). *Cosmeceuticals: Drugs vs. cosmetics.* New York: Marcel Dekker.

eMedicine.com, Inc. (2004). *Hair growth* [On line]. Available: http://www.emedicine.com

Falkenbach, A. (2000). Muscle strength and vitamin D (letter). *Archives of Physical and Medical Rehabilitation, 81,* 241.

Ganong, W. F. (1989). *Initiation of impulses in sense organs. Review of medical physiology* (14th ed.). Appleton & Lange.

Gray, J. (1997). *The world of skin care* [On line]. P & G Skin Care and Research Center. Available: www.pg.com

King, D. (2003, November 14). *Introduction to skin histology* [On line]. Available: http://www.siumed.edu

Lowe., N., & Sellar, P. (1999). *Skin secrets: The medical facts versus the beauty fiction.* New York: Collins & Brown.

Merck & Company. (2001). Resource library [On line]. Available: http://www.mercksource.com

Moore, E. (Ed.). (1999). *Quotation finder.* Harper Collins: Glasgow, Scotland.

Moschella, S., Pillsbury, D., & Hurley, H. (1975). *Dermatology* (Vol. 1). W. B. Saunders.

Nemours Foundation. (2004 February 25). *Kid's health for parents. Impetigo* [On line]. Available: http://www.kidshealth.org

Nova. (2000, November). *Surviving Denali* [On line]. Available: http://www.pbs.org

Obagi, Z. (2000). *Skin health restoration and rejuvenation.* New York: Springer-Verlag New York.

Oneskin.com. (December 8, 2003). *Anatomy of the skin* [On line]. Available: www.oneskin.com

Owens, S. (February 11, 2004). *Photobiology of the skin* [On line]. Available: www.consumerbeware.com

Parsad, D., Sunil, D., & Kanwar, A. J. (2003, October 23). Quality of life in patients with vitiligo, *Journal of Health and Quality of Life Outcomes,* 1(1), 58.

Rao, D. S. (1999). Perspective on assessment of vitamin D nutrition. *Journal of Clinical Densitometry,* 2(4), 457–464.

Revis, D. R. Jr. (2001, July). *Skin grafts, split thickness* [On line]. Available: www.emedicine.com

Shea, C., & Prieto, V. G. (2003, October 13). *Merkel cell carcinoma* [On line]. Available: http://www.emedicine.com

Spense, A. P. (2004, February 22). *Basic human anatomy* (3rd ed.) [On line]. Available: http://www.sawyerproducts.com

Students of Elert, G. (Ed.). (2001). *Temperature of a healthy human (skin temperature)* [On line]. Available: http://www.hypertextbook.com

The Skin Cancer Foundation. (2004). *About squamous cell* [On line]. Available: www.skincancer.org

Thomas, M. P. H. C. L. (Ed.). (1997). *Taber's cyclopedic medical dictionary* (Vol. 18). Philadelphia: F. A. Davis.

University of Iowa Healthcare. (March 15, 2004). *Fluid replacement* [On line]. Available: www.uihealthcare.com

Venna, S. S., & Gilchrest, B. (2002, February). *Skin aging and photoaging* [On line]. Available: www.skinandaging.com

Healing Peeled Skin

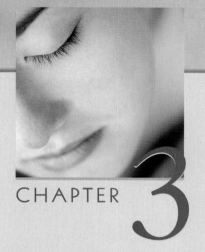

CHAPTER 3

KEY TERMS

acute
anagen
apocrine sweat glands
appendages
arrector pili muscle
atrophic scars
basophils
carbohydrates
catagen
chronic
cornified
diabetes
discoid lupus
drug-induced lupus
eccrine sweat glands
eosinophils

epithelialization
epithelium
full-thickness wounds
granulocytes
hypertrophic scar
inflammatory phase
insult
ischemia
keloid scars
leukocytes
lupus
lymphocyte
macrophages
malnutrition
necrosis

neutrophils
pilosebaceous unit
proliferative phase
protein
Raynaud's phenomenon
reepithelialization
remodeling phase
scar
sebaceous glands
systemic lupus
telogen
vasoconstriction
wound
wound healing

LEARNING OBJECTIVES

After completing this chapter you should be able to:

1. Identify the different types of wounds.
2. Explain the different stages associated with the healing process.
3. List the medications that interfere with wound healing.
4. Discuss smoking and wound healing.
5. Discuss scarring.

57

INTRODUCTION

The way skin heals itself is a multifactorial, multistage, and multilevel marvel that is easy to take for granted. Although we seldom give it a thought, wound healing is a complex subject, with details that only a scientist or pathologist can fully understand or enjoy. However, for the clinician, it is valuable to have a thorough understanding of the different types of wounds and the processes they undergo to repair themselves.

Fundamentally, a **wound** is "a disruption of normal anatomical structure which results from **pathologic** processes beginning internally or externally to the involved organ."[1] **Wound healing** is "the restoration of tissue continuity after injury."[2] Therefore, when an injury or an **insult** affects tissue (most often the skin), it becomes inconsistent with the uninjured tissue nearby. For example, suppose you cut your leg. The contact with the sharp object is the insulting event, and the specific area that has sustained the cut is the wound. The wound is open and can become red and painful. The wounded area is damaged and hence inconsistent with the normal tissue that had not come in contact with the offending source. In this chapter, we will examine the phases that this and most wounds will undergo to repair themselves in hopes of becoming consistent once again.

Wound healing basically traces three physiologic stages or phases: (1) inflammatory, (2) proliferative, and (3) remodeling or maturation. Although each stage has distinctive cellular events, they often work concurrently (overlapping) at times. A good analogy would be to consider wound healing as if it were a symphony composed of several movements. Although each movement has a theme of its own, overlaps exist and, indeed, a return to previous themes throughout the musical composition. Just as we can describe a symphony as separate movements,[3] we can describe the phases of wound healing as separate functions, working toward one goal: tissue continuity.

wound
A disruption of normal tissue that results from pathologic processes, beginning internally or externally to the involved organ.

wound healing
The restoration of tissue continuity following injury or trauma.

insult
An injury or a trauma that causes an inconsistency in tissue.

Phases of Wound Healing[4]

Inflammatory phase: Blood and tissue cells secrete substances to create inflammation, which helps overcome pathogens.

Proliferative phase: Scab and scar tissue build to protect and induce healing; remaining skin cells divide and produce new cells.

Remodeling phase: Scar tissue that was formed during healing is broken down; new skin begins to blend in.

Insult

In the previous example, we used the illustration of a cut or laceration. This type of wound is just one of many types of injuries, or insults, that can cause injury to tissue. Several types of wounds have been identified, and each one is characterized by the type of damage that has been sustained as a result of the insult. Similarly, these different injuries have differing degrees of severity and variations in the specific phases that the tissue will undergo to repair itself. Additionally similar, multiple injuries sustained during one event will have consequences for one another (Table 3–1).

Inflammatory Phase

Within hours of any skin injury, the first phase of wound healing, the **inflammatory phase**, has already begun, *regardless* of the type of wound. Early inflammatory wounds are red, warm, and swollen; the patient feels pain. Blood flow and fluid increase at the site, and cells contained in both blood and skin are rapidly recruited in this first defense. The motive behind the inflammation is to seek and destroy

inflammatory phase
The early wound-healing phase during which blood and fluid collect and substances begin to fight infection and promote healing.

Table 3–1   Types of Wounds

Types of Wound	Description	Example
Contused (or subcutaneous) wound	Injury to tissue below the skin; skin is unbroken	Bruise, broken bones
Puncture wound	Injury caused by a sharp or pointed object, usually collapsed inward; deep-tissue wounding (possibly penetrating additional organ tissues)	Stab wound, gunshot wound
Laceration	Unclean wound with jagged edges; can be of varying depths	Cut with a can or piece of metal
Incision	Clean cut caused by a sharp instrument	Surgical wound
Burn	Tissue injury caused by excessive heat or acids; damage varies, depending on insulting agent	Thermal, chemical

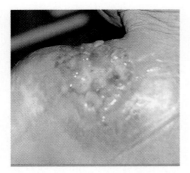

Figure 3–1 The inflammatory stage of healing.

leukocytes
White blood cells without granules involved in immune response; these include lymphocytes and monocytes.

neutrophils
The most common type of white blood cells that kill bacteria and discourage infection.

lymphocytes
White blood cells involved in the body's immune system; their numbers increase in the presence of infection.

macrophages
Part of the immune system in the skin; these cells are scavengers that clear debris in tissue injury.

granulocytes
White blood cells involved in immune response; these include neutrophils, eosinophils, and basophils.

eosinophils
Granulocyte blood cell characterized by multiple-shaped nuclei, present in full-thickness wounds.

basophils
A type of white blood cell.

opportunistic pathogens that may find a vulnerable security lapse in the body's armor. The area is swarmed by an array of substances that deactivate bacteria, activate growth factors, and otherwise participate in the healing process (Figure 3–1).

If the injury penetrates the epidermis, damage to blood vessels activates substances to control bleeding as well.[5] Blood coagulates and platelets aggregate to form a clot on which inflammatory cells and fibroblasts accumulate.[6]

White blood cells (**leukocytes**) are specifically involved in immunity. With regard to healing, each leukocyte has a specific and vital function. **Neutrophils** are among the first healing cells on the scene, scavenging the wound for bacteria and devitalized cells and releasing oxygen free radicals that kill bacteria.[7] Neutrophils usually reach the site of injury within 6 hours and are at full throttle by 24 hours, protecting against infection. Neutrophils that die in the wound release enzymes that dissolve unwanted cells. This activity produces a familiar substance called pus.[8] **Lymphocytes**, white blood cells that are also intimately involved in the immune process, arrive approximately 72 hours later and produce antibodies to combat invaders (Table 3–2).

The blood mostly acts as a delivery device. However, the blood does not act singularly in the process. Tissues are themselves supplied with their own inner first-aid kits. They will activate internal **macrophages**

Table 3–2 Blood and Tissue Cells Involved in Healing

Blood cells: white blood cells, are infection fighters[9] and are composed of two types: with granules (**granulocytes**) and without granules, called leukocytes (*leuko-* is Greek, meaning lacking color).

Granulocytes	Leukocytes
Neutrophils	Lymphocytes
Eosinophils	Monocytes
Basophils	
Tissue cells	

Macrophages: cells in connective tissue that digest by-products of both defense and normal degeneration. They are found in high concentrations in different parts of the body.

Langerhans cells: macrophage cells in epidermis that perform surveillance for the immune system

to the wound. A macrophage[10] is a cell stationed in connective tissue that actually has a limited, ameba-like ability to move itself around inflamed areas as it seeks suspicious substances to engulf.[11] Macrophages secrete various growth factors. Their deficiency has been shown to result in defective healing. Additionally, microphages play an important role in the transition from inflammatory to proliferative phase. Similarly, Langerhans cells, macrophages specific to the epidermis, busily ingest old cells, abnormal cells, and unneeded cellular debris.

Proliferative Phase

Approximately 5 days after injury occurs, the second phase of wound healing begins: the **proliferative phase**.[12] By definition, the name means the phase that builds on or compounds. Granulation tissue, so called because of its granular appearance, is composed of fibrin, cellular components, and blood vessels. Their sheer bulk enables *reepithelialization*—or replacement of protective epithelial tissue—over the old wound site (Figure 3–2).

Collagen, which is prevalent in the dermis, is also a major component of the connective tissue that wraps wounds. For the next 6 weeks, collagen will continue to wrap the wound and act as a surrogate until the wound healing is complete. As collagen increases in the wound, so does its tensile strength,[13] thus becoming even less prone to reopening.

Healing of a wound begins not only from edges, but also from within any appendages lying within it that were not destroyed by whatever caused the wound. The appendages are rooted in the dermis and yet are enveloped by pockets of epithelial tissue extending back up to the epidermis. Wounds not deep enough to remove the pockets with them enable reepithelialization to proceed from remaining pockets.

To this avail, appendages are important to healing. Skin that has a greater density of appendages, such as the face, will tend to heal much more rapidly than will areas with fewer similar structures, such as the palmer and planter regions.

Remodeling Phase

From 1 to 6 weeks after the injury and in conjunction with the proliferative phase, collagen formation occurs at a furious pace. During this time, collagen is distributed in a microscopically haphazard pattern, similar to a box of matches spilled on the floor. In the **remodeling phase** that follows, collagen becomes more organized (Figure 3–3).

As type I collagen is gradually replaced by type III, tensile strength increases. In particular wounds, this process may take as long as 1 to 2 years. This characteristic is why plastic surgeons may tell their patients

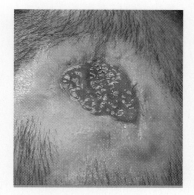

Figure 3–2 The proliferative stage of healing.

proliferative phase
The phase of wound healing during which replacement of protective epithelial tissue occurs over the old wound site.

remodeling phase
Phase of wound healing during which collagen is assembled to replace skin.

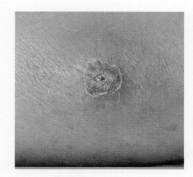

Figure 3–3 The remodeling stage of healing.

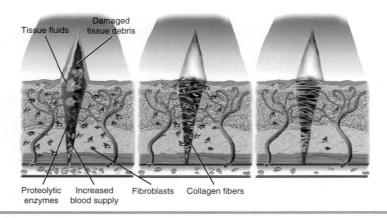

Tissue fluids   Damaged tissue debris

Proteolytic enzymes   Increased blood supply   Fibroblasts   Collagen fibers

Figure 3–4   Illustration of wound healing.

The Nature of Collagen

Although the word collagen is no stranger to this text, the time has come to get a better picture of it. As a major constituent of connective tissue, collagen is the most abundant protein in the body. Connective tissue includes skin, bone, ligaments, and cartilage. Collagen can, in fact, be considered the glue that holds the body's connective tissue together.[14] Because it contributes to a wide range of structures from brain to cornea, constituents of collagen vary, and at least 30 distinct types of collagen inhabit the human body. The most abundant in connective tissue form fibers that assemble themselves into networks capable of supporting more extensive structures; these are labeled type I through type V.[15] These fiber-forming collagens will be our primarily concern.

that the scars from tummy tucks or face lifts take at least 6 months to 1 year to resolve, soften, flatten, and decolorize. During this same period, scars may widen and thicken.

Understanding the broad principles of wound healing—particularly as they apply to skin—and gaining the ability to apply this knowledge skillfully will ensure that your patients have the best possible outcome (Figure 3–4).

▪ TYPES OF WOUNDS

As part of achieving a practical knowledge of chemical peeling, we need to address the concept of wounds to include the unintended possibility

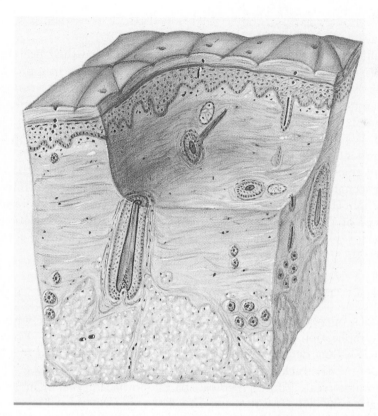

Figure 3–5   Full-thickness wounds are so called because they extend into the lower papillary and reticular dermis.

that a deeper wound might occur. We define the depth of a wound as either partial thickness or full thickness.

Another definition and category that you need to know when considering wounds is *temporal* (i.e., time related, or how long they have been in the area). The descriptors are **acute** and **chronic**. Acute wounds are those of recent (or even emergent) occurrence. Chronic wounds are those that occurred days, weeks, or months before. Chronic wounds might include conditions such as bedsores and leg ulcers or virtually any injury that has not healed in an extended period. (These injuries will not be discussed in this text.)

Full-Thickness Wounds

When wounds penetrate the dermis beneath a certain *threshold level,* wounds tend to heal more slowly and with scarring.[16] These insults are called **full-thickness wounds** (Figure 3–5). The resultant scar tissue is

acute
Having a rapid onset with a short but severe course.

chronic
A disease or occurrence showing little or no change over a long period.

full-thickness wounds
Wounds that penetrate to a specific depth in the papillary dermis or upper reticular dermis. These wounds are associated with slower healing, and scarring will usually develop.

composed of a variety of the original skin tissue; it is neither as strong nor as aesthetically pleasing as the original.

Full-thickness wounds are deeper, and the fact that their healing is far more involved and time consuming makes sense. In this process, dead or dying cells are delineated and destroyed, precursors to collagen form, and eventually, collagen is created, the wound itself shrinks by contraction, and **reepithelialization** eventually occurs across the wound. We will discuss more about the process of wound healing in this environment later.

Full-thickness wounds in the medical spa can result from the following scenarios: (1) microdermabrasion, chemical peel, laser or intense pulsed light (IPL) treatments that become infected; (2) overly aggressive instances of peels and laser therapy; (3) ischemic necrosis (deficient blood supply) from dermal fillers (Zyderm® collagen, and so forth); (4) sclerotherapy; (5) deep hyfrecation; and (6) shave excision.

Partial-Thickness Wounds

Depth of wound appears to have a *threshold level* above which, without other complications, they heal quickly and without scarring.[17] Epidermal and shallow dermal injuries that tend to heal without scarring are known as partial-thickness wounds (Figure 3–6).

Wounds created in the medical spa are not lacerations or incisions penetrating the skin, and they are intended to be only partial-thickness wounds. These wounds do, however, often involve broad surface areas of the face or body. They result from treatments such as microdermabrasion, peels (glycolic acid, trichloracetic acid [TCA], phenol), carbon dioxide (CO_2) and erbium lasers, IPL (also called Foto Facial®or Photo Facial®) treatments, and laser hair removal. These wounds heal quickly, usually within a week. They are superficial enough that only the process of reepithelialization is required (Figure 3–7).

Importance of Appendages

If one of the skin's main functions is to act as a barrier against intruding substances, how, then, do lotions that we apply *soak in?* The primary answer is the **appendages**.

Appendages are defined as smaller parts to a greater part. For the skin, they include the **pilosebaceous unit** (hair follicle and accompanying **sebaceous glands** and **arrector pili muscle**), sweat glands, and nails.[18] Appendages originate in the uppermost layer of the skin (the epidermis) and extend into the lower layer, the dermis.

External substances such as skin creams, ointments, and salves can enter the skin through the appendages of the hair and sweat glands,

---

reepithelialization
The replacement of protective epithelial tissue.

appendages
Any anatomic structure that is associated with a larger structure. For the skin, its appendages include hair, glands, and pores.

pilosebaceous unit
Hair follicle and accompanying sebaceous glands and arrector pili muscle.

sebaceous glands
Small glands, usually located next to hair follicles in the dermis, that release fatty liquids onto the hair follicle to soften hair and skin.

arrector pili muscle
Located at the hair follicle, the arrector pili muscle contracts when we are cold and creates piloerection (goose bumps).

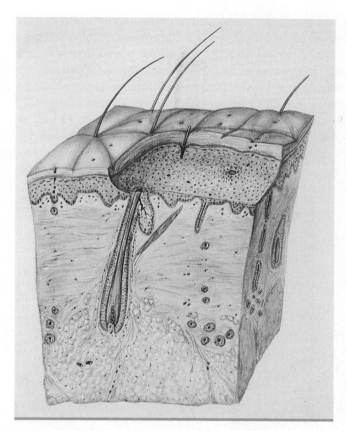

Figure 3–6   Partial-thickness wound.

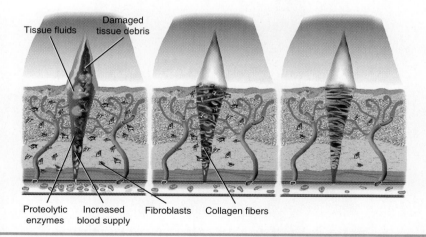

Figure 3–7   Wound healing is a multilevel marvel that is amazing and necessary to our survival.

cornified
Hardening or thickening of the skin.

eccrine sweat glands
The smaller of the two sweat glands that reside all over the body.

apocrine sweat glands
The larger of the two sweat glands that are housed in axillary (under the arm), pubic, and perianal areas.

through the intercellular spaces between the **cornified** cells, or smaller molecules can pass through cells at the surface of the skin (Figure 3–8).

You can think of sweat glands as simple tubes. They are vital for regulating body temperature. Because of the composition of what they carry to the surface, sweat glands also influence water balance and ions.

Ordinary **eccrine sweat glands** are located over most of the body, and large **apocrine sweat glands** are concentrated in axillary (underarm), pubic, and perianal areas.[19] The latter glands develop at puberty.[20] Although sweat from the apocrine glands is initially odorless, it can mix with bacteria on the skin and acquire an odor.

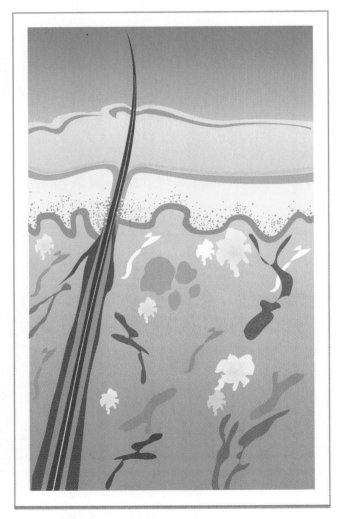

Figure 3–8 An aesthetician must understand how the skin accepts products topically.

Normal, healthy adults secrete approximately 1 pint of sweat per day and more with physical activity.[21] Because of daily loss of water, everyone needs to replace actively water lost inside the body, regardless of their activity level, though the more active you are, the more water needs to be replaced. As much as 4 cups of water can be lost during hard exercise. To avoid dehydration, water should be consumed regularly throughout the day and more before, during, and after exercise. When a person has become thirsty, they are already dehydrated; therefore consuming fluids is important, regardless of thirst. Symptoms of dehydration include dizziness, disorientation, and clumsiness.[22]

Hair is a type of modified skin. It grows everywhere on a person's body except the palmer and planter regions of hands and feet. Hair is most dense on the head, neck, and shoulder regions where the numbers can be from 300 to 900/cm^2. Conversely, approximately 100/cm^2 can be found on the torso and limbs.[23] Hair follicles are tubular. They protrude deep into the skin to develop and nourish the hair. The hair follicle contains epidermal cells, and the hair itself is keratin. Hair follicles have several distinct anatomic components, including the *bulb, root,* and *papilla.*

The hair follicle, gland, nerve, and muscle comprise the pilosebaceous unit. Hair follicles are associated with sebaceous glands (small masses of cells and fat associated with hair follicles), which lubricate the hair; nerve endings, which detect motion of the hair shaft and control piloerection (goose bumps); and smooth muscle, which actually creates the goose bumps[24] (Figure 3–9). The sebaceous glands that are most active reside on the face, chest, and back.

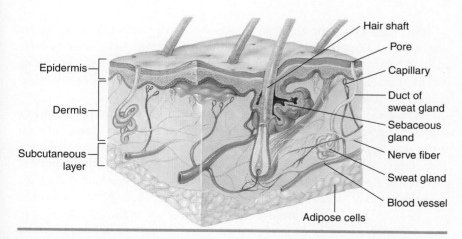

Epidermis
Dermis
Subcutaneous layer
Hair shaft
Pore
Capillary
Duct of sweat gland
Sebaceous gland
Nerve fiber
Sweat gland
Blood vessel
Adipose cells

Figure 3–9 The skin's appendages include the pilosebaceous unit (hair follicle, accompanying sebaceous glands, and arrector pili muscle) and sweat glands.

The Importance of Skin Appendages

The skin's appendages are important in healing, especially superficial healing and protection of the skin. When the skin is superficially injured over a limited surface, it can grow back quickly because of epithelial cells remaining in deeper hair follicles and sweat glands. This feature is important to understand when we begin to discuss wound healing and our care of the client after aggressive treatments.

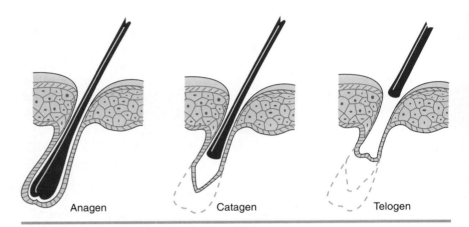

Anagen   Catagen   Telogen

Figure 3–10 All hair goes through three distinct phases in the course of their life cycle: the anagen phase, a catagen phase (transitional), and a telogen phase (resting).

anagen
The growth phase of the hair follicle.

catagen
The transitional phase of the hair follicle.

telogen
The resting phase of the hair follicle.

All hair goes through an **anagen** phase (growth), a **catagen** phase (transitional), and a **telogen** phase (resting)—the hair grows, resides for a while, and then falls out.[25] This growth cycle varies in different parts of the body (Figure 3–10). For instance, the entire cycle takes 4 months for eyelashes and 3 to 4 years for scalp.

As we will discuss, this process of division, growth, and maturation somewhat resembles that of the skin's top layer. In both cases, cells go through a process of hardening and then sloughing (shedding). However, when cells at the bottom of the hair follicle slough, they create a column of keratinized (hardened, "horny") cells. This hair grows up through the shaft and extends through the follicle. Hair growth is a complex process, but understanding this process is key to the success of hair removal with lasers or light. Lasers are known to be effective only on hairs in the growth (anagen) phase.

■ WOUND HEALING COMPROMISED

Not surprisingly, the process of skin healing slows down in older adults. Diminished collagen production thins the skin and slows the inflammatory response to injury. Less collagen will not noticeably affect the healing of an acute partial-thickness wound, however; it is more profound in healing chronic full-thickness wounds. When a client has more than one health problem (e.g., breast cancer, diabetes), healing of even an acute partial-thickness wound is likely to be noticeably compromised.

Aside from older adults and persons with chronic health problems, several other important issues must be considered when assessing a patient for treatment. Among the issues that can possibly affect wound healing and consequently the end result are medications, smoking, and nutrition.

Medications that a patient is taking often have far-reaching consequences unrelated to the disease the medication is ostensibly curing. These consequences, commonly referred to as side effects, are important for the clinician to know before any chemical peeling treatments can begin.

We only have to watch the news or read the newspaper to know how bad smoking is for us. The effects of cigarette smoke include lung disease, heart disease, stroke, and giving birth to low birth weight babies.[26] Additionally, smoking causes **vasoconstriction** (narrowing of the blood vessels).[27] This result is especially significant at the capillary level where the blood oxygen is necessary for wound healing. Patients who smoke are at risk for slow delayed healing and possible infections.

Not enough can be said about proper nutrition. The components of a good diet help improve and accelerate the healing process. Your patient should have a diet high in protein, vitamins, and minerals, which are necessary for healing when the skin is in a compromised state. Supplements, although controversial as a daily addition to the diet, should always be taken during healing.

The clinician and the patient can overcome problems by being proactive, and this begins with the clinician. First, take a complete health history to evaluate whether the client is a candidate for treatment. If a patient is a candidate for treatment but has some bad habits—is a smoker or has poor nutritional intake—you can educate the client regarding these potential problems right away. Then, having cleared the client for treatment, consider which treatments have the highest probability of success.

vasoconstriction
Narrowing of the blood vessels.

Medications

Many medications promote wound healing, and, as suspected, others may compromise the process. Among these latter medications are chemotherapy agents, oral corticosteroids, and Accutane.

Chemotherapeutic agents are drugs used to treat cancers. The process of these agents is usually to alter the DNA of the cancer cell, preventing its reproduction. However, other chemotherapeutic agents destroy the cell structures that are required for reproduction. Unfortunately, these agents do not differentiate between "good" cells and "bad" cells, and all rapidly dividing cells are affected. Therefore any patient who is taking chemotherapeutic agents should be handled carefully and generally are not candidates for peels because their ability to heal is compromised. Check with your clinic physician before treating these patients.

Corticosteroids are hormones that are produced by the adrenal glands.[28] As drugs, corticosteroids are synthetically produced and are usually used as an antiinflammatory agent. Corticosteroids are commonly used for the treatment of asthma, Crohn's disease, or eczema. They are sometimes used, for example, when a patient has an extreme allergic reaction or if excessive swelling from a peel occurs. The most common corticosteroid is Prednisone®. Oral corticosteroids can be dangerous if the dose is decreased too fast. This drug also has serious side effects, among them a potential for slower healing of the skin.

Accutane is a familiar drug to the skin care specialist. Accutane is used to treat recalcitrant nodular acne. The process of action is to decrease the sebum production. Understanding the function of the appendages in healing, the skin care specialist now appreciates why Accutane interferes with the healing process.

Patients who are taking the previously mentioned drugs are not candidates for peeling, and their care should be discussed with the clinic physician for the proper steps to achieve clinical results.

Smoking

The question of delayed wound healing associated with cigarette smoking was proved in laboratory animals in the 1970s.[29] During this time, reports of complications associated with smoking and wound healing began to surface. Since then, a clear correlation between smoking and wound healing has been made. The more patients smoke, and the longer they have had the habit, the greater the potential will be for complications. Even if patients quit smoking before the surgery and during the initial recovery phase, if smoking is resumed before complete healing takes place, complications are likely to occur. The reason? Simply stated, smoking constricts the blood vessels, which reduces the amount of oxygen that reaches the healing tissues. Additional discoveries indicate that the smoking thickens the blood and obstructs collagen formation in the healing wound.[30] We should also comment at this time that the cessation of smoking in favor of a nicotine gum or patch is of no value as it relates to healing. Given that the offending element in the healing process is nicotine, it will be absorbed through the skin or gastrointestinal tract and will have the same effect as if it were being inhaled. So do not be fooled. The nicotine has to go away completely for the healing process to progress unaffected.

Therefore exactly why is this information important for the clinician who provides glycolic or Jessner peels? The question is an important one. Every peel has the opportunity to create a dermal injury and, consequently, a wound and eventually a **scar**. Although this complication is potentially unlikely, it is possible, and the clinician needs to be alert at all times for the possibility. If this unlikely event does occur, knowing what to do and how to heal the wound quickly will decrease the opportunity for scarring and long-term effects with the patient.

Nutrition

Our society has a tendency to consider good nutrition as a preventative measure against disease. Nonetheless, nutrition is equally significant with regard to our capacity for rapid and effective wound-healing capacities. What we eat supplies the building blocks for tissue repair. If the basic elements are not supplied through the food we choose to eat, the healing process is impaired, and the amount of impairment can be serious. This fact is simple yet easily dismissed.

Malnutrition occurs in every corner of the world, not simply in third-world countries; and it need have nothing to do with economics. In the medical spa, you may witness malnutrition in anorexics, bulimics, addicts, senior citizens, and people with cancer or chronic illness.

As the body attempts to heal from an injury, proper nutrition plays a pivotal role. Under most circumstances, and certainly in the case of an epidermal wound, the healthy body should easily be effective in wound healing. Conversely, the presence of malnutrition or diseases such as **diabetes** that impairs circulation can seriously impair wound healing.

To decipher what constitutes good nutrition, let us examine some familiar components of a healthy diet so we can understand the role they play in wound healing.

Protein is made up of amino acids. Although it may seem redundant, our bodies break down proteins into amino acids before rebuilding these amino acids into proteins. This process is crucial for tissue repair.

scar
A mark left in the skin or on an internal organ that is the result of deep tissue trauma. Scars are a result of injury, disease, or medical procedures.

malnutrition
The result of any condition that causes a lack of nutritional substances for the body to use and distribute.

diabetes
Many different types; the most familiar is that which is associated with the rise and fall of blood sugars and the associated complications therein.

protein
A class of complex compounds that are synthesized by all living creatures. Proteins are broken down into amino acids for use, including the rebuilding of tissue.

Tissue repair is an ongoing process in our bodies, even in the absence of wounds. Simply shedding our hair and skin cells requires the repair properties of protein.[31]

Amino acids, the components of proteins, are categorized as essential and nonessential. Essential amino acids must be obtained from the food we eat; we cannot make them on our own.[32] If we do not ingest essential amino acids (of which there are nine), our bodies cannot build protein. Protein is easily obtained primarily through meats, cheese, and eggs. Nonessential amino acids are found in our food; they also occur naturally within our bodies.

Carbohydrates provide sugars, which are easily broken down for use as an energy source. This fuel is either stored away for later consumption or used immediately, which helps spare protein for its ongoing role in building tissue.[33] Carbohydrates that are common in plant cell walls bring with them a bounty of other nutrients with which to feed and heal our bodies.[34] Whole grains (e.g., wheat, barley, nuts) take longer to digest and keep us feeling satisfied longer.

Vitamins are found in everything we eat in varying degrees and can also be made within our bodies. Vitamins are defined as organic dietary components that are required for life, health, and growth. Unlike protein, fats, and minerals, vitamins do not supply energy.[35]

One vitamin that is synonymous with good health is vitamin C. Our bodies do not manufacture vitamin C,[36] meaning that we need to consume it in our diets. Being water soluble, vitamin C remains only briefly in our bodies; thus we need to take it regularly.

During its brief tenure inside our bodies, vitamin C is quite active and in demand. Just one of its critical tasks is to assist in making collagen. Collagen is required for blood vessels to function optimally, that is, to transport blood. Scurvy, the disease caused by vitamin C deficiency, not only slows wound healing because of poor collagen production, but also one half of scurvy fatalities result from burst blood vessels.[37,38]

carbohydrates
One of a group of chemical substances (including sugars) that contain only carbon, hydrogen, and oxygen. Common in fruits, grains, and nuts, carbohydrates are thought to be the most common chemical compounds on earth.

Key nutritional components to the healing process include protein, vitamins, major and trace minerals, proteins, and carbohydrates—all substances easily obtained in our culture. One more essential component of good nutrition is water, the "forgotten nutrient."

Major Minerals	Minor Minerals
Calcium	Iron
Phosphorus,	Zinc
Magnesium	Iodine
Sodium	Copper
Potassium	Manganese
Chloride	Selenium
	Chromium
	Molybdenum

Vitamin B complex contains a spectrum of water-soluble vitamins that are essential to many aspects of health, including the fabrication of new tissue.[39] When scattered filaments of collagen *assemble themselves* into organized networks, they are assisted in that assembly by vitamin B. Vitamin B_6, pyridoxine, is involved in immune function, and vitamin B_{12} is vital for blood formation.[40]

Vitamin A, a fat-soluble vitamin, helps cells reproduce normally, and cell reproduction is heightened following injury.[42] Animal studies have shown that vitamin E diminishes adhesions from surgical wounds, but *provided in massive amounts, vitamin E can actually impair healing.*[43] Vitamin K, another fat-soluble vitamin, assists the blood in clotting, a useful attribute in the presence of any bleeding wound.

Minerals participate in nearly every process that is necessary for living and in several that are integral to healing.[44] The major minerals, such as calcium, are present in your body in the greatest quantities. Trace minerals, such as zinc, are required in much smaller amounts.

Of these minerals, several stand out regarding wound healing. Calcium plays a role in blood clotting, zinc is involved with enzymes that participate in wound healing, and copper helps synthesize protein, which, of course, is necessary to repair tissue.[45]

The issue of whether to supplement with vitamins and minerals is complex, highly individualized, and largely beyond the scope of this text. However, a few pointers can be provided. Vitamins C and B complex are necessary for healing, and supplementing them for the purpose of healing is scientifically documented and generally accepted. However, the value of supplementing with fat-soluble vitamins to assist with healing of minor injuries in people who are not deficient in these vitamins remains unclear.[46] Occasions will certainly occur when the supplement of vitamin A may be recommended, for example, as a topical ointment for skin injuries in persons taking oral corticosteroids. However, fat-soluble vitamins taken orally and in excess can be toxic; therefore under no circumstances would taking them in higher-than-recommended quantities be a good idea.

In taking any supplement, be it vitamin or mineral, balance must be maintained because these nutrients can work for or against each other in the body. Taking too much of one—or taking one at the wrong time vis-à-vis another one—might interfere with your body's ability to absorb that or other nutrients.[47]

All of this information can be overwhelming, and we are not nutritionists, nor should we imply to our patients that we are educated in this specialty. Nevertheless, the clinician should be generally familiar with this information and able to guide the patient through nutritional

> Water-soluble vitamins such as vitamins C and B complex are easily absorbed. Fat-soluble vitamins, such as vitamins A, D, E, and K, are poorly absorbed in the absence of bile and require intake of some dietary fat for their absorption.[41] They can also be toxic if taken in very large doses; thus attending to recommended daily requirements is well recommended.

questions, especially those specific to healing. The clinician must always be aware that a wound can occur from a peel treatment. Knowing this information ensures quick and appropriate action that improves the chances of a complication free recovery.

Illness and Disease

As we have previously discussed, acute illness and chronic diseases can compromise the wound-healing process. Diseases that the clinician may encounter in the medical spa include diabetes, cancer, and autoimmune diseases such as lupus. Other diseases that should be considered are those of the blood vessels that cause ischemia of the skin, such as Raynaud's phenomenon.

The most commonly considered disease associated with healing delays is diabetes. Diabetes is a disease of the pancreas, specifically the islet cells of the pancreas. In diabetes, the pancreas is not secreting enough insulin to balance the glucose in the bloodstream. Diabetes is divided into two types: type I and type II. Type I is usually found in younger people, children, and adolescents, and type II is usually found in individuals who are aging but can happen in children as well.

Cancers of any kind compromise the body's immune system. The treatment of cancer usually includes the administration of chemotherapy agents or radiation therapy, or both. These treatments often wreak havoc with the immune system, creating healing problems and the increased opportunity for infections.

Lupus is a common autoimmune disease in women. Several different types of lupus have been identified, including discoid lupus, systemic lupus, and drug-induced lupus.[48] Lupus is a chronic disease that can affect different parts of the body. In this autoimmune disease, the body loses its ability to identify the difference between normal tissue and foreign body substances such as bacteria or viruses. The body's antibodies attack all cells and tissues, including the body's good cells and tissue; hence the description *autoimmune* disease.

Diseases of the blood vessels, such as Raynaud's phenomenon, are rare. However, the clinician should still have a general understanding of the disease. This disorder affects the capillaries, specifically those that nourish the skin. During an attack, or vasospasm, the skin will turn white and then blue as the capillaries contract and then release. The hands or feet are the most common areas to be affected, but the face, neck, and chest can also be affected.

As we know, clinicians have a responsibility to ensure the safety of their patients and guide them to a superior outcome. Although the peels the clinician may be doing are usually superficial, the opportunities for

lupus
An autoimmune disease that is a chronic, progressive, ulcerating skin disease.

ischemia
A localized restriction of blood flow usually caused by an obstruction of normal circulation.

Raynaud's phenomenon
A chronic peripheral vascular disease.

discoid lupus
Cyclic breakouts and remissions of a scaly red rash.

systemic lupus
Chronic disease of connective tissue, which results in injury to various affected tissue, identified by butterfly mask over the nose.

drug-induced lupus
Growing old; aging eccrine glands.

complications always exist. When these complications occur, they can be made worse by an illness or disease process. Therefore the clinician must be aware of the patient's health.

▪ NORMAL SCARRING

It may sound strange, but *normal scarring* exists. Scarring, as we now know, is the end point of the full-thickness wound-healing process, and normal scarring is the result of uncomplicated healing of such a wound. Normal scar tissue is decolorized and flat, nearly unrecognizable from the rest of the skin. When a wound is treated effectively, most scars will fade into unobtrusive components of skin surface (Figure 3–11).

Events that Lead to Normal Scarring

Recall the three-step process of wound healing. If this process occurs without complication in a dermal injury, a normal scar results.

In the simplest of terms, when dealing with injuries of the skin— absent complicating factors such as infection—the type, size, cause, location, and especially *depth* of injury will determine whether a scar results. In general, injuries that penetrate only the epidermis will heal without a resulting scar. The epidermis is one of the infrequent body organs (also including gastrointestinal-tract **epithelium**, tracheobronchial epithelium, liver parenchyma, bone, and smooth muscle) that can regenerate itself. Therefore, after a superficial injury (what we termed a partial-thickness wound), the epidermis simply re-forms in the defect. This process is called **epithelialization**. Within 24 hours, basal layer cells in injured healthy skin begin to multiply or proliferate and stream across the denuded surface to recreate an intact epidermal layer.

The dermis layer of the skin, beneath the epidermis, presents another story because it cannot regenerate itself. Nevertheless, wounds that penetrate the epidermis and *only the upper part* of the dermis will also often heal without scar formation.

That statement may appear contradictory, but the singular anatomy of the epidermis and dermis enables it. Within the dermis are hair follicles, oil glands, and sweat glands. These appendages, you recall, originate in the epidermis. From that origin, they penetrate down into the dermis while remaining enveloped in epidermal cells.

When a wound involves only the upper part of the dermis, without scraping out these appendages, epithelial cells pocketing these appendages will proliferate and stream out of these structures to form a new intact epidermis. With this kind of wound, still considered a partial-thickness wound, no true scar formation takes place, although additional

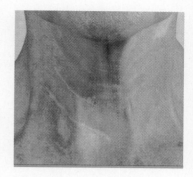

Figure 3–11 Normal scarring is the skin's best attempt to replicate the continuous tissue that is being replaced.

epithelium
Membranous tissue covering internal organs and lining skin appendages.

epithelialization
The growth of new skin over a wound.

collagen is stimulated to form in the dermis. This additional collagen will tend to tighten the skin and is, in part, the reason that we perform procedures that stimulate collagen: microdermabrasion, deeper dermabrasion, chemical peels, and laser resurfacing.

However, generally speaking, dermal injuries will produce scars. When the dermis itself is completely penetrated or disrupted, even by hairline cuts from surgical scalpel or laser beam, the dermis cannot regenerate and instead heals by the formation of *nonspecific connective tissue*—otherwise known as scarring—in what we termed a full-thickness wound. Scars need not be obvious. All things being equal, if the gap between the edges of the wound is very narrow, an excellent scar— an unobtrusive one—should be all that remains.

Abnormal Scarring

Wound healing requires the human body to undergo, in a timely and organized fashion, a multitude of events. When the healing process does not follow the normal drill, failures in healing occur.

Sometimes the fault for these failures lies with the bearers. Many clients do not have the patience for scar resolution; they often want something done to remove a freshly created or still-healing scar, which, of course, is not possible. Clients also like to treat scars themselves. I have seen patients use a variety of tactics on scars to try to resolve them, including nail files, glycolic acid, and vitamin E oil. None of these approaches provide favorable outcomes. Vitamin E is the most popular choice of home therapy. Unfortunately, evidence indicates that vitamin E oil has little or no benefit, and of persons who do use the product, approximately 33% develop dermatitis.[49]

The risk of abnormal scarring is much increased when healing of a deep skin wound is overextended, usually over *three weeks* or longer.[50] Various conditions can prolong healing. Skin that has been burned may be slow to heal. A chronically inflamed earring piercing invites formation of an abnormal scar.

Failures in the process of normal wound healing are called **keloid scars**, **hypertrophic scars**, and **atrophic scars**.

keloid scars
Scar formation in which tissue response is excessive in relation to normal tissue repair.

hypertrophic scar
Overly developed scar tissue that rises above the skin level, often overfed by an abundance of capillaries. These scars usually regress over time.

atrophic scars
Flat, small, round, and generally inverted scars. Usually seen in acne or as chickenpox scarring.

Causes of Longer Healing Times	
▸ Local infection	▸ Smoking
▸ Inadequate wound closure	▸ Malnutrition or chronic disease
▸ Presence of a foreign body	▸ Advanced age
▸ Certain medications	

Keloids

Keloid scars are defined by their growth outside the area of injury. They are seen most commonly on the earlobe, shoulders, chest, and back—areas that may be subjected to excessive skin tension—and usually accompany the healing of a deep skin wound.[51] Keloid scars can form as long as 1 year after the original **insult** (Figure 3–12).

The word keloid means "crab claw," and it describes the way lesions extend, sometimes resembling a starburst, from scar into normal tissue.[52] The excessive development of both hypertrophic and keloid scars occurs only in humans, strangely enough, and in between 5% and 15% of human wounds. Why keloid scars develop is not fully understood. However, some researchers hypothesize that, for some reason, during the proliferation phase, fibroblasts, which form connective tissue, orchestrate an overabundance of collagen fibers.

Keloids are more commonly found in people with darker pigmentation; African-American, Hispanic, and Asian races are more susceptible.[53] Fifteen percent of African-American and Hispanic populations report having keloids.

Keloid scars are difficult to treat. Although most attempts at treatment are frustrating, because the scar can be so unsightly, many patients are willing to try nearly anything to improve their appearance. Treatment options range from shriveling the scar with steroids, to compressing it manually, to removing it surgically.[54] Some physicians prefer to use silicone gel sheeting in combination with other treatments. Multipronged approaches may improve chances of success.

Hypertrophic Scarring

A hypertrophic scar is excessive scar tissue that rises above the skin level yet, unlike keloids, stays within the confines of the original lesion or injury.[55] Hypertrophic scars are often overfed by an abundance of capillaries (Figure 3–13). Additionally, in contrast to keloids, hypertrophic scars usually regress or resolve over time.[56]

When hypertrophic scars are surgically removed, patients may improve. Hypertrophic scarring will also respond to steroid injections and silicon gel–sheeting applications.

If complications in healing a dermal wound occur, the scar can look worse than is expected, or an avoidable scar can develop in a partial-injury wound.

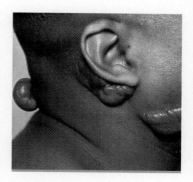

Figure 3–12 Keloid Scarring is abnormal healing that extends beyond the boundaries of the insult.

insult
An injury or a trauma that causes an inconsistency in tissue.

Keloids and to a lesser extent hypertrophic scars seem to run in families. Although men and women are equally affected, women are more likely to seek treatment.

Hypertrophic scarring crosses ethnic barriers and has been reported to be as high as 68% after surgical procedures or injury.[57] Given this high incidence and a general lack of understanding of the difference between keloid and hypertrophic scars, many clients mistake hypertrophic scars for keloids.

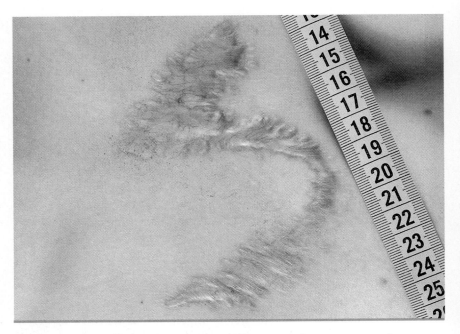

Figure 3–13   Red in color and raised hypertrophic scars are often confused with keloid scars.

Events that Lead to Scarring from a Peel

Now you know that several factors put the patient at risk for scarring in a deep-peel situation or in either a superficial or a moderate peel with complications. To review, conditions that increase the potential for scarring include failure to use a pretreatment program, heredity, and skin type. Once the skin is peeled, three conditions in which scars are likely to develop occur when no scars were anticipated: infection, tissue ischemia, and picking.

Before we discuss the topics of infection, tissue ischemia, and picking, let us briefly review the conditions that may increase the potentials for scarring.

Pretreatment programs are among the most important regimes in which your patients will participate under your care. The benefits of a pretreatment program have been extolled by many physicians and clinicians alike, but let us review them. Pretreatment programs even out the landscape of the skin, especially the stratum corneum. In doing so, the peel application will have an even and more effective *take up* and, as such, will produce a better result. Retin A$^®$ in particular is a must when pretreating patients for peel procedures. Clients who are not treated with

Retin A® will simply not benefit from peels as much as will those who use Retin A®. Pretreatment programs also stimulate the basal layer to increase the keratinocytes and, as such, improve the healing process for the skin during the healing phase of the peel. Finally, the proper home-care program will improve the skin and *boost* the results of the peel.

Heredity and skin type are always a concern for the skin-care professional who is a specialist in peeling techniques. A history of scars, a skin type prone to postinflammatory hyperpigmentation, and skin that is unresponsive to peeling in the past should be noted by the specialist. These potential problems should compel the clinician to select another treatment for this patient. Given the many options in the medical spa these days, pushing the patient into a treatment that has a risk of unfavorable response makes no sense at all.

Infection

Bacteria will always find a wound. Staphylococcus and Streptococcus live on the skin's surface, and when an opening in the skin occurs, these bacteria rarely decline the invitation. Generally, the body controls these invaders. Infection occurs when bacteria in the wound overwhelm the body's defense systems. Many different types of bacteria are in the environment, and they can cause many different types of infection. Infections cause wounds to heal more slowly and, if left unattended, to scar more significantly. Infection can go so far as to cause tissue **necrosis**, the actual death of tissue. Patients must be urged to avoid underestimating the damage potential of infection.

necrosis
Death of cells, when tissue is deprived of blood supply.

Tissue Ischemia

Tissue ischemia is a local shortage of blood supply. Several factors can lead to this deficiency, including infection, smoking, and poor patient health. The most common complication in the medical spa is smoking, as we now know. The client must understand that smoking can and does slow the healing process through tissue ischemia. Small capillaries near the skin are significantly affected by smoking. Smoking causes constriction of these small capillaries, decreasing in the oxygen content of the blood. When blood does not fully serve a wound, the healing process is crippled.

Picking

When a client picks at a wound, it has a greater tendency to scar. You know this to be true from childhood. When you picked at scrapes and cuts, they took longer to heal and left deeper scars. When picking caused the wound to bleed again, the scab would need to re-form, and the healing process would be delayed. We also know this fact to be true from our experiences with acne. Picking disrupts the healing process and causes the cellular repair to begin again and again.

Conclusion

Scar is the terrifying "S" word. Every clinician working in the aesthetic medical spa is terrified of creating a scar, and with good reason. Clients hate scars and, in reality, scars should not be a part of the clinician's eventual outcome. Interviews of people who had never undergone any type of medical skin care revealed the number one reason they had avoided skin care at medical spas was for fear of scars.

Whenever the clinician believes the treatment that he or she has given may have the potential to scar, the clinic's physician should be notified immediately. We now know that avoiding scars can be possible. Keeping in mind our knowledge of anatomy and physiology and the principles of wound healing, the treatments we give our clients will leave them safe and beautiful.

In the end, however, client compliance to posttreatment home instructions may be as important as the clinical care itself.

> ▶ ⟩⟩ **TOP TEN TIPS TO TAKE TO THE CLINIC**

1. Know the wound-healing process.
2. Know the different types of wounds.
3. Recognize processes to improve healing.
4. Understand the different types of scars.
5. Understand complications that may lead to scarring.
6. Smoking and wound healing do not mix.
7. Know that different areas of the body heal differently.
8. Nutrition is important to healing.
9. Counsel patients who pick their skin that doing so may result in a scar.
10. Choose patients carefully; those with diseases may not heal as well as you might think.

CHAPTER REVIEW QUESTIONS

1. What are the three phases of wound healing?
2. How are the three phases of wound healing important?
3. Do all three phases of wound healing occur in epidermal injury?

4. What is an acute wound?
5. How is an acute wound different from a chronic wound?
6. What is a full-thickness wound?
7. What is a partial-thickness wound?
8. How does protein affect the healing process?
9. Which vitamins help the healing process and how?
10. What are scars?
11. What are the three abnormal scars?
12. What events lead to abnormal scarring?

CHAPTER REFERENCES

1. Lazarus, G. S., Cooper, D. M., Knighton, D. R., et al. (1994). Definitions and guidelines for assessment of wounds and evaluation of healing. *Archives of Dermatology*, 130, 489–493.
2. Goepel, J. R. (1996). Responses to cellular injury. In Underwood, J. C. E. (Ed.). *General and systemic pathology* (2nd ed., pp. 121–122). London, UK: Churchill Livingstone.
3. Norman, R., & Bock, M. (2003, March). *Understanding wound management* [On line]. Available: www.skinandaging.com
4. eMedicine.com, Inc. (2004). *Wound healing, skin* [On line]. Available: http://www.emedicine.com
5. eMedicine.com, Inc. (2004). *Wound healing, growth factors* [On line]. Available: http://www.emedicine.com
6. Huang, N. F., Zac-Varghese, S., & Luke, S. (2003). *Apoptosis in skin wound healing* [On line]. Medscape. Available: http://www.medscape.com
7. eMedicine.com, Inc. (2004). Wound healing, growth factors [On line]. Available: http://www.emedicine.com
8. Thomas, C. L. (Ed.). (1997). *Taber's cyclopedic medical dictionary*. Philadelphia: F. A. Davis.
9. Kimball, J. W. (2003). *Blood* [On line]. Available: http://users.rcn.com
10. Thomas, C. L. (Ed.). (1997). *Taber's cyclopedic medical dictionary*. Philadelphia: F. A. Davis.
11. Thomas, C. L. (Ed.). (1997). *Taber's cyclopedic medical dictionary*. Philadelphia: F. A. Davis.
12. Clark, R. A. F. (1993). Basics of cutaneous wound repair. *Journal of Dermatologic Surgery and Oncology*, 19, 693–706.
13. Sholar, A., & Stadelmann, W. (2003). *Wound healing, chronic wounds, Section 4* [On line]. eMedicine.com, Inc. Available: http://www.emedicine.com

14. Thomas, C. L. (Ed.). (1997). *Taber's cyclopedic medical dictionary*. Philadelphia: F. A. Davis.

15. Daresbury Imaging Group. (2005, May). *Collagen* [On line]. Available: http://detserv1.dl.ac.uk

16. Rutledge, B. J. (2004, Jan-Feb). *Modeling dermal scars below and above the threshold* [On line]. Cosmetic Surgery Times. Available: http://www.findarticles.com

17. Rutledge, B. J. (2004, Jan-Feb). *Modeling dermal scars below and above the threshold* [On line]. Cosmetic Surgery Times. Available: http://www.findarticles.com

18. Gray, J. (1997). *The world of skin care* [On line]. P & G Skin Care and Research Center. Available: www.pg.com

19. Gray, J. (1997). *The world of skin care* [On line]. P & G Skin Care and Research Center. Available: www.pg.com

20. Nemours Foundation. (2004). *Skin, hair, and nails* [On line]. Available: http://kidshealth.org

21. Nemours Foundation. (2004). *Skin, hair, and nails* [On line]. Available: http://kidshealth.org

22. University of Iowa Healthcare. (2004, March 15). *Fluid replacement* [On line]. Available: www.uihealthcare.com

23. Elsner, P., & Maibach, H. L. (Eds.). (2000). *Cosmeceuticals: Drugs vs. cosmetics*. New York: Marcel Dekker.

24. Gray, J. (1997). *The world of skin care* [On line]. P & G Skin Care and Research Center. Available: www.pg.com

25. eMedicine.com, Inc. (2004). *Hair growth* [On line]. Available: http://www.emedicine.com

26. Martin, T. (2004, June 10). Cigarette smoking and cancer [On line]. Available: http://quitsmoking.about.com

27. Thomas, C. L. (Ed.). (1997). *Taber's cyclopedic medical dictionary*. Philadelphia: F. A. Davis.

28. Medline Plus, (2005, May). *Corticosteroids (Rectal)* [On line]http://www.nlm.nih.gov

29. Brody, J. E. (1996). *Women's health digest* [On line]. Available: http://geocities.com

30. Brody, J. E. (1996). *Women's health digest* [On line]. Available: http://geocities.com

31. Ganong, W. F. (1989). *Energy balance, metabolism, & nutrition. Review of medical physiology* (14th ed.). Norwalk, CT: Appleton & Lange.

32. Ganong, W. F. (1989). *Energy balance, metabolism, & nutrition. Review of medical physiology* (14th ed.). Norwalk, CT: Appleton & Lange.

33. Quinn, B. (2003). *Nutrition and wound healing: What's the connection?* [On line]. Nutrition. Thomson-Wadsworth. Available: http://www.wadsworth.com

34. Ganong, W. F. (1989). *Energy balance, metabolism, & nutrition. Review of medical physiology* (14th ed.). Norwalk, CT: Appleton & Lange.

35. Ganong, W. F. (1989). *Energy balance, metabolism, & nutrition. Review of medical physiology* (14th ed.). Norwalk, CT: Appleton & Lange.

36. Wooldridge, M. (1993). *Linus Pauling lectures on vitamin C and heart disease* [On line]. Available: http://www.lbl.gov

37. Bender, D. A. (2003). *Vitamins and minerals. Introduction to nutrition and metabolism* (3rd ed.). London: Taylor & Francis.

38. Wooldridge, M. (1993). *Linus Pauling lectures on vitamin C and heart disease* [On line]. Available: http://www.lbl.gov

39. Quinn, B. (2003). *Nutrition and wound healing: What's the connection?* [On line]. Nutrition. Thomson-Wadsworth. Available: http://www.wadsworth.com

40. Mead Johnson & Company. (2003). *Vitamins, minerals, and water* [On line]. Available: http://www.meadjohnson.com

41. Ganong, W. F. (1989). *Energy balance, metabolism, & nutrition. Review of medical physiology* (14th ed.). Norwalk, CT: Appleton & Lange.

42. Quinn, B. (2003). *Nutrition and wound healing: What's the connection?* [On line]. Nutrition. Thomson-Wadsworth. Available: http://www.wadsworth.com

43. Healthnotes, Inc. (2002). *Wound healing* [On line]. Available: www.mycustompak.com

44. Mead Johnson & Company. (2003). *Vitamins, minerals, and water* [On line]. Available: http://www.meadjohnson.com

45. Mead Johnson & Company. (2003). *Vitamins, minerals, and water* [On line]. Available: http://www.meadjohnson.com

46. Healthnotes, Inc. (2002). *Wound healing* [On line]. Available: www.mycustompak.com

47. Mead Johnson & Company. (2003). *Vitamins, minerals, and water* [On line]. Available: http://www.meadjohnson.com

48. Lupus Foundation of America. (2004, June 10). *Types of lupus* [Online]. Available: www.lupus.org

49. Bisaccia, E., & Scarborough, D. (2002). *The Columbia manual of dermatologic cosmetic surgery*. New York: McGraw Hill.

50. eMedicine.com, Inc. (2004). *Wound healing, keloids* [On line]. Available: http://www.emedicine.com

51. eMedicine.com, Inc. (2004). *Wound healing, keloids* [On line]. Available: http://www.emedicine.com

52. eMedicine.com, Inc. (2004). *Wound healing, keloids* [On line]. Available: http://www.emedicine.com

53. eMedicine.com, Inc. (2004). *Wound healing, keloids* [On line]. Available: http://www.emedicine.com

54. eMedicine.com, Inc. (2004). *Wound healing, keloids* [On line]. Available: http://www.emedicine.com

55. Clinics in Plastic Surgery. (2000, October). *Response to tissue injury.* Philadelphia: W. B. Saunders.

56. eMedicine.com, Inc. (2004). *Wound healing, keloids* [On line]. Available: http://www.emedicine.com

57. Clinics in Plastic Surgery. (2000, October). *Response to tissue injury.* Philadelphia: W. B. Saunders.

BIBLIOGRAPHY

American Society of Plastic Surgeons. (2004, February 24). *Everyday wounds: Wound healing* [On line]. Available: www.plasticsurgery.org

American Society of Plastic Surgeons. (2004, February 24). *Everyday wounds: Wound healing* [On line]. Available: www.plasticsurgery.org

Analyst, The. (2004, January 31). *Poor/slow wound healing* [On line]. Available: www.diagnose-me

Baumann, L. (2002). *Cosmetic dermatology practices and principles.* New York: McGraw Hill.

Bender, D. A. (2003). *Vitamins and minerals. Introduction to nutrition and metabolism* (3rd ed.). London: Taylor & Francis.

Bisaccia, E., & Scarborough, D. (2002). *The Columbia manual of dermatologic cosmetic surgery.* New York: McGraw Hill.

Blitzner, A., Binder, W. J., Boyd, J. B., & Carruthers, A. (Eds.). (2000). *Management of facial lines and wrinkles.* Philadelphia: Lippincott, Williams & Wilkins.

Brody, H. J. (1997). *Chemical peeling and resurfacing* (2nd ed.). St. Louis: Mosby.

Brody, J. E., (2003, July 21). *Smoker's face*—an evident reason to quit [On line]. Available: www.geocities.com

Childress, B. B., & Stechmiller, J. K. (2002, July). Role of nitric acid in wound healing, *Journal of Biological Research Nursing,* 4(1), 5–15.

Clark, R. A. F. (1993). Basics of cutaneous wound repair. *Journal of Dermatologic Surgery and Oncology,* 19, 693–706.

Clinical Reviews. (2003, September). *Why does smoking slow wound healing?* [On line]. Available: www.findarticles.com

Clinics in Plastic Surgery. (2000, October). *Response to tissue injury.* Philadelphia: W. B. Saunders.

Coleman, W. P., & Lawrence, N. (Eds.). (1998). *Skin resurfacing.* Baltimore: Williams and Wilkins.

Cumberbach, M., Dearman, R., Griffiths, C., & Kimber, I. (July, 2003). *Epidermal Langerhans cell migration and sensitisation to chemical allergens* [On line]. Available: www.blackwell-synergy.com

D'Angelo, J., Dean, P., Dietz, S., Hinds, C., Lees, M., Miller, E., et al. (2003). *Milady's standard: Comprehensive training for estheticians.* Clifton Park, NY: Thomson Delmar Learning.

Daresbury Imaging Group. (2005, May). *Collagen* [On line]. Available: http://detserv1.dl.ac.uk

Demling, R., & DeSanti, L. (2000). The stress response to injury and infection: Role of nutritional support. *Journal of Wounds*, 12(1), 3–14.

Elsner, P., & Maibach, H. L. (Eds.). (2000). *Cosmeceuticals: Drugs vs. cosmetics.* New York: Marcel Dekker.

eMedicine.com, Inc. (2004). *Hair growth* [On line]. Available: http://www.emedicine.com

eMedicine.com, Inc. (2004). *Wound healing, growth factors* [On line]. Available: http://www.emedicine.com

eMedicine.com, Inc. (2004). *Wound healing, keloids* [On line]. Available: http://www.emedicine.com

eMedicine.com, Inc. (2004). *Wound healing, skin* [On line]. Available: http://www.emedicine.com

Falkenbach, A. (2000). Muscle strength and vitamin D (letter). *Archives of Physical and Medical Rehabilitation*, 81, 241.

Ganong, W. F. (1989). *Energy balance, metabolism, & nutrition. Review of medical physiology* (14th ed.). Norwalk, CT: Appleton & Lange.

Gerstein, A., Phillips, T. J., Rogers, G. S., & Gilchrest, B. A. (1993, October). Wound healing and aging. *Dermatology Clinics*, 11(4), 749–757.

Goepel, J. R. (1996). Responses to cellular injury. In Underwood, J. C. E. (Ed.). *General and systemic pathology* (2nd ed., pp. 121–122). London: Churchill Livingstone.

Gray, J. (1997). *The world of skin care* [On line]. P & G Skin Care and Research Center. Available: www.pg.com

Guirini, J., & Rich, J. (2001, November). *Unlocking the secrets of growth factors. Skin and aging* [On line]. Available: http://www.skinandaging.com

Hamilton, K. (1995, November). Wound healing and nutrition—a review. *Journal of the Australian College of Nutritional & Environmental Medicine*, 14(2): 15.

Healthnotes, Inc. (2002). *Wound healing* [On line]. Available: www.mycustompak.com

Huang, N. F., Zac-Varghese, S., Luke, S. (2003). *Apoptosis in skin wound healing* [On line]. Medscape. Available: http://www.medscape.com

Hubbs, L. (2002, August). Treating complications caused by non-physicians. *Skin & Aging*, 10(8), 57–61.

Kimball, J. W. (2003). *Blood* [On line]. Available: http://users.rcn.com

King, D. (2003, November 14). *Introduction to skin histology* [On line]. Available: http://www.siumed.edu

Lazarus, G. S., Cooper, D. M., Knighton, D. R. Margolis, D. J., Pecoraro, R. E., Rodeheaver, G., et al. (1994). Definitions and guidelines for assessment of wounds and evaluation of healing. *Archives of Dermatology*, 130, 489–493.

Lupus Foundation of America. (2004, June 10). *Types of lupus* [On line]. Available: http://www.lupus.org

Mann, J., & Truswell, S. (Eds.). (2002). *The essentials of human nutrition* (2nd ed.). New York: Oxford University Press.

Martin, T., (2004, June 10). *Cigarette smoking and cancer* [On line]. Available: http://quitsmoking.about.com

Mead Johnson & Company. (2003). *Vitamins, minerals, and water* [On line]. Available: http://www.meadjohnson.com

Moschella, S., Pillsbury, D., & Hurley, H. (1975). *Dermatology* (Vol. 1). Philadelphia: W. B. Saunders.

National Heart, Lung, and Blood Institute. (2004, June 10). *Facts about Raynaud's phenomenon* [On line]. Available: www.nhlbi.nih.gov

Nemours Foundation. (2004, February 25). *Kid's health for parents. Impetigo* [On line]. Available: http://www.kidshealth.org

Newsome, Jr., R. E., Langston, K., & Wang, A. (2003, April 23). *Wound healing, keloids.* [On line]. Available: www.emedicine.com

Norman, R., & Bock, M. (2003, March). *Understanding wound management* [On line]. Available: www.skinandaging.com

Oneskin.com. (2003, December 8). *Anatomy of the skin* [On line]. Available: www.oneskin.com

Parks, J., & Pierce, M. (2002, May). *Effectively treating ethnic skin* [On line]. Available: www.skinandaging.com

Quinn, B. (2003). *Nutrition and wound healing: What's the connection?* [On line]. Nutrition. Thomson-Wadsworth. Available: http://www.wadsworth.com

Rao, D. S. (1999). Perspective on assessment of vitamin D nutrition, *Journal of Clinical Densitometry*, 2(4), 457–464.

Repinski, K. (2003, May). *The best scar treatments. Fitness magazine.*

Reynolds, T. M. (2001, January). The future of nutrition and wound healing, *Journal of Tissue Viability*, 11(1); 5–13.

Roche.com. (2004, January 15). *Accutane product information* [On line]. Available: www.rocheusa.com

Romano, J. J. (2003). *Scar treatment, therapy, and removal* [On line]. Available: http://www.jromano.com

Romo, III, T., (2003, November 18). *Skin wound healing* [On line]. Available: www.emedicine.com

Rubin, M. (1995). *Manual of chemical peels: Superficial and medium depth*. Philadelphia: Lippincott, Williams & Wilkins.

Rutledge, B. J. (2004, Jan-Feb). *Modeling dermal scars below and above the threshold* [On line]. Cosmetic Surgery Times. Available: http://www.findarticles.com

Schardt, D. (2003, Jul-Aug). *The skin game. Nutrition action healthletter* [On line]. Available: http://www.findarticles.com

Sholar, A., & Stadelmann, W. (2003, May 23). *Wound healing, chronic wounds* [On line]. Available: http://www.emedicine.com

Tang, A., Amagai, M., Granger, L., Stanley, J., & Uddy, M. (1993, January). *Adhesion of epidermal Langerhans cells to keratinocytes mediated by e-cadherin* [On line]. Available: www.nature.com

Thomas, C. L. (Ed.). (1997). *Taber's cyclopedic medical dictionary* (Vol. 18). Philadelphia: F. A. Davis Company.

Thomas, D. R. (2001). Age-related changes in wound healing. (2001). *Journal of Drugs and Aging*, 18(8), 607–620.

University of Iowa Healthcare. (2004, March 15). *Fluid replacement* [On line]. Available: www.uihealthcare.com

University of Maryland Medicine. (2003, May 14). *Dermatology health guide: Candidiasis (yeast infection)* [On line]. Available: http://www.umm.edu

University of Maryland Medicine. (2003, May 14). *Dermatology health guide: Cellulitis* [On line]. Available: http://www.umm.edu

University of Maryland Medicine. (2003 May 14). *Dermatology health guide: Fungal infections of the skin* [On line]. Available: http://www.umm.edu

University of Maryland Medicine. (2003, May 14). *Dermatology health guide: Folliculitis, boils, and carbuncles* [On line]. Available: http://www.umm.edu

University of Maryland Medicine. (2004, February 25). *Dermatology health guide: Skin infections* [On line]. Available: http://www.umm.edu

WebMD. (2004, June 10). *Diabetes 'basics'* [On line]. Available: http://my.webmd.com

Wooldridge, M. (1993). *Linus Pauling lectures on vitamin C and heart disease* [On line]. Available: http://www.lbl.gov

Fundamentals of Skin Care

CHAPTER 4

KEY TERMS

acetic acid
acid mantel
acidic
alkaline
alpha hydroxy acids
anthranilates
antimicrobials
ascorbyl palmitate
azelaic acid
benzophenone
camphors
cinnamates
citric acid
cocamidopropyl betaine
d-alpha tocopherol
detergents
dibenzoylmethanes
diethanolamine (DEA)
Eldopaque®
emollients
erythema

ester
free radicals
gel solution
humectant
hydroquinone
isohexadecane
kojic acid
lactic acid
l-ascorbic acid
magnesium ascorbyl
  phosphate
malic acid
Melaquin®
moisturizers
neutral
nicotinamide
para-aminobenzoic acid
  (PABA)
Parsol 1789®
pH (potential of hydrogen)
photodamage

preservatives
Renova®
Retin A®
retinol
retinyl palmitate
salicylates
selenium
sodium lauryl isethionate
sodium lauryl sulfate
sun protection factor
  (SPF)
sunscreens
surfactants
tartaric acid
titanium dioxide
tyrosine
ubiquinone
vitamin B
vitamin C
vitamin E
zinc oxide

LEARNING OBJECTIVES

After completing this chapter you should be able to:

1. Discuss the importance of cosmeceuticals.
2. Identify the importance of moisturizers and cleansers.
3. Describe the use and importance of vitamin C.
4. Discuss the use and importance of sunscreens.
5. Discuss the use and importance of hydroquinone.
6. Discuss the use and importance of retinoids.

INTRODUCTION

Although the focus of this text is chemical peels, the treatment does not happen in isolation. A good treatment program is represented by three components: the pretreatment plan, the clinical treatment, and the aftercare plan. The products used in the at-home segment (pretreatment and posttreatment) of the peel program include cosmeceuticals, quality **sunscreens**, **moisturizers**, and cleansers, as well as the prescription products. As a skin care professional, you already have knowledge in the principles and value of quality sunscreens; and although cleansers and moisturizers seem elementary subjects, they really will influence the success or failure of a program more so than we may have originally understood. Prescriptions are necessities in a medical skin program, and this concept may be new to you. Finally, cosmeceuticals are a type of product that you should understand and know how to represent to your client. This chapter will address medical skin care, products that are absolutely necessary to assist in the desired result of the procedure, and products that will make a noticeable difference if improperly selected.

sunscreens

Any agent that protects the skin from harmful ultraviolet A and B (UVA, UVB) light. In turn, sunscreen helps protect skin from photodamage, including skin cancers, dyschromias, and so forth. Sunscreens block rays by either physical or chemical means.

moisturizers

An agent that replenishes moisture to the skin.

▪ COSMECEUTICALS

The United States Food and Drug Administration (FDA) was created in 1938 to review products and to keep the citizens of our country safe. The product review fell into two categories: the drug category and the cosmetic category. Cosmetics, according to the FDA, are "intended for beautifying and promoting attractiveness."[1] A drug, on the other hand, is defined as a "substance used in the diagnosis, cure, treatment, or prevention of disease, *intended to affect the structure and function of the body.*"[2] Dr. Albert Kligman, a professor emeritus at the University of Pennsylvania's school of dermatology, thought that the two definitions were not black and white. He theorized that drugs and cosmetics overlapped quite a bit. According to Dr. Kligman, it is not the ingredients in the product, but the claims made by the product's manufacturer that differentiate drugs from cosmetics.

In 1980, at a meeting of the Society of Cosmetic Chemists, Kligman introduced a thought-provoking question. "Were there any ingredients that we apply to the skin that *do not* affect its structure?" The idea and the subsequent term, *cosmeceutical,* caused discussion and polarization that continues today. Kligman intended the term to include products that do more than decorate or camouflage but less than a drug would do.[3] To prove his point—that all ingredients penetrate the skin—Kligman did a small yet meaningful experiment. He applied wet cotton to the skin and used a dressing to hold it in place. By the end of the second day, the water had begun to cause an inflammatory response in the dermis. Thus even water can penetrate the skin, making an argument that even the most basic of elements can change the surface of the skin, hence the term *cosmeceuticals.*

The FDA has not updated the cosmetic or drug categories, and the agency has no intention of making changes in the near future. Although this position is a good thing for cosmetic companies and their products, it does leave room for interpretation as to what constitutes drugs and what constitutes cosmetics. The FDA does not recognize *cosmeceuticals;* however, skin care professionals must be aware of the term and what it means. Many interpretations have been offered. If we were to be purists about both the definition and the potential of products on the skin, we would identify all skin-care products as cosmeceuticals because we know that even a moisturizer will change the barrier effect of the skin. The ways in which products are *used* define the new reality. In many ways, national economics drives the unwillingness of the FDA to change the current laws, as defined in 1938. Thank goodness. Think of the chaos that would certainly follow if such significant changes were implemented. Imagine the uproar if body lotion, for example, were to be reclassified as a drug.

Also beneficial would be to further categorize *more active* products versus those *less active* products, such as cleansers and moisturizers. By using the term cosmeceuticals, we can differentiate products and create a sense of value for both the clinician and the client. Among the products that should be classified in this category are **alpha hydroxy acids** (AHAs), **vitamin C**, and **retinol**. The aforementioned products are not prescriptions but do have scientifically known impact on the skin and its layers.

Using Cosmeceuticals

Cosmeceuticals are found in salons, on cable shopping networks, and on retail shelves in varying percentages and **pH (potential of hydrogen)**, making their use (and result) somewhat unpredictable for the average consumer. These places have less of an opportunity to provide the information necessary to help the client learn to use the product properly. Providing cosmeceuticals to the public is a responsibility. Educating the staff, educating the client, and conscientious and ethical marketing are key points to the success of cosmeceuticals in the spa.

Education is an ongoing responsibility of the spa. New employees should be well educated about the product that is available to sell. In turn, employees should be capable of educating clients, recognizing problems, and anticipating results. *Product updates* should be given to the entire staff on a regular basis to remind all employees, front (receptionists) and back (clinical), of the benefits of the products they are selling. In a perfect

> If we were to be purists about both the definition and the potential of products on the skin, we would identify all skin-care products as cosmeceuticals because we know that even a moisturizer will change the barrier effect of the skin.

alpha hydroxy acids
Mild organic acids used in cosmeceutical products. AHAs "unglue" cells in the epidermis, allowing keratinocytes to be shed at the stratum granulosum, providing skin with a healthier texture.

vitamin C
An antioxidant that is a necessary factor for the formation of collagen in connective tissue and maintenance of integrity of intercellular cement.

retinol
A vitamin-A derivative that must first convert to retinoic acid before it can be useful to the skin.

pH (potential of hydrogen)
The scale by which a material is characterized as being acidic (pH less than 7.0), alkaline (greater than 7.0), or neutral (7.0).

world, a manual exists that lists all of the products the spa carries. This manual would provide ingredients, benefits, and features, in effect, everything you need to know about each product. When a new product is introduced, an education meeting would be assembled, everyone would be oriented, and a *product handout* would be provided for each employee.

As we have discussed, the product category is defined by the intended use of the product. Marketing should not be misleading, and should stay within the category. Therefore using words such as *appears to* or *will seem to* are important marketing terms as to not overstep the bounds of the FDA definitions.

Medical Office and Cosmeceuticals

In the medical world of skin care, cosmeceuticals are a staple in the product cabinet. The ingredients are well recognized by clinicians and patients as *active* but not *medicinal*. Choosing the cosmeceutical products and product lines for a business is a daunting task. Many available product lines have been developed directed specifically at medical offices. The basic products that should be in the cosmeceutical armamentarium of the medical office include active cleansers, moisturizers, and vitamin C.

Try to stock at least three cleansers, one with glycolic acid, for normal and combination skin, one with salicylic acid, for oily and acne-prone skin, and one that is void of active ingredients. When considering the treatment products, have a broad selection, including glycolic acids in varying percentages and vehicles (creams, solutions, serums), lactic acids in varying percentages and vehicles, and a salicylic acid toner. When evaluating vitamin C, carry two types of vitamin C (one in an *l*-ascorbic form and one in a **magnesium ascorbyl phosphate** or **ascorbyl palmitate** form). Finally, moisturizers need to contain antioxidants, usually green tea, **selenium**, or **vitamin E**.

Salon/Spa and Cosmeceuticals

The spa world has access to cosmeceuticals, just as does the medical spa, but the vendors may be different. The spa has an increased responsibility to be mindful of these products and dispense them carefully. The public may perceive that the products they purchase from the spa are weaker than those from the medical office, but this is simply not true. Furthermore, the client may believe that, because the products are not those found in the medical setting, he or she will not be at risk for potential complications. Again, this presumption is simply not true. Because the luxury spa may not have a physician on staff, choosing products that are higher in pH than the ones found in the medical spa will

---

The importance of cosmeceuticals in a medical plan cannot go unmentioned. Their effect on the skin is unlike the prescriptions available, but when combined, their sum is greater than the individual parts.

magnesium ascorbyl phosphate
An ester that converts to vitamin C on the skin.

ascorbyl palmitate
A fat-soluble form of ascorbic acid.

selenium
A chemical agent resembling sulfur that helps protect the skin from solar-induced skin cancers.

vitamin E
An antioxidant that has been shown to inactivate free radicals. However, the exact mechanism of function is unknown.

be necessary. This practice is simply common sense to protect the spa from liabilities. The product line chosen by the salon or spa should include the same basic components as the medical spa: cleansers, AHAs, vitamin C, and "power" moisturizers (Table 4–1).

▪ CLEANSERS

A good cleanser will have an immediate, noticeable effect on the skin. However, not all cleansers are created equal. So, what makes a "good" cleanser? Let us start at the beginning with pH, which defines any good cleanser or soap.

A basic rule of thumb is that the more **alkaline** (pH higher than 7.0) a product is, the more drying it will be to the skin. Because the normal pH of the skin is between 4.5 and 6.5,[4] using a more alkaline cleanser or body soap is likely to make the skin feel tight and dry. A moisturizing bar such as Dove®, which contains **sodium lauryl isethionate**, will have a pH of 5 to 7 (Table 4–2).

alkaline
Any substance that has a pH greater than 7.0.

sodium lauryl isethionate
Similar to sodium lauryl sulfate but not as irritating. Additionally, it is less effective as an emulsifier.

Table 4–1   Inventory of Cosmeceutical Products for the Medical Spa and Luxury Spa

- Cleansers, with AHAs
- AHAs, glycolic and lactic
- Salicylic acids
- Vitamin C
- "Power" moisturizers

Table 4–2   Common Hand and Bath Soaps[5]

Soap	pH
Camay®	9.5
Dial®	9.5
Dove®	7.0
Irish Spring®	9.5
Ivory®	9.5
Lever 2000®	9.0
Palmolive®	10.0
Zest®	10.0

acidic
Any substance that has a pH less than 7.0.

detergents
A synthetic cleansing agent that acts as a wetting agent and emulsifier.

surfactants
A surface-active agent that lowers surface tension.

antimicrobials
An agent that halts or prevents the development of microorganisms.

emollients
A product that has a softening or soothing effect on the skin.

humectants
Moisturizing agents.

preservatives
An agent used to prevent spoilage.

sodium lauryl sulfate
A common ingredient in household detergents and soaps most commonly used as an emulsifier.

cocamidopropyl betaine
A foaming agent used in shampoos and cleansers.

diethanolamine (DEA)
An emulsifier or foaming agent.

isohexadecane
A highly emollient cleansing agent.

We can feel comfortable making the general statement that over-the-counter (OTC) soaps are more alkaline and that cleansers are more acidic.

The dry, tight feeling that soap leaves is not an indication of cleanliness but rather a stripping of the acid mantle of the stratum corneum. This is a point of education with your patients, especially the patient who is prone to oily skin or acne.

The second important component of cleansers is the actual ability to cleanse the skin. Cleansing is made possible by a variety of substances, including **detergents, surfactants, antimicrobials, emollients,** moisturizers, **humectants,** and **preservatives.** Examples of common ingredients found in cleansers are **sodium lauryl sulfate** and **cocamidopropyl betaine,** as well as **diethanolamine (DEA)** and **isohexadecane.** These ingredients remove oils, dirt, and makeup and have been used for many years without complications to humans. We know these ingredients work and that they are safe for use around the eyes and mouth.

The choice of a cleanser for your client is based on the two important facts we have just covered: pH and the ability to cleanse. However, one cleanser is not right for all skin types or conditions; thus the clinician must evaluate the skin and choose a cleanser carefully. For example, oily skin requires salicylic acid in the cleanser, and dry skin needs to be cleansed gently, without AHAs. By making a careful evaluation of the patient's skin type and skin condition, you can select the appropriate cleansing product (Table 4–3).

Patient Education for Cleansers

Most individuals are aware of how to use cleansers and moisturizers. However, even the simplest task can sometimes be overwhelming when starting a new program. Therefore explain how to use each product, beginning with the cleanser (Table 4–4 on page 96).

Cleansers should be used with the fingertips: massaged into a wet face, splashed off, and patted dry. Washcloths, sponges, and facial chamois have several drawbacks and are not recommended. First, these items can harbor bacteria and cause breakouts. Second, washcloths often do not rinse clean of the laundry detergent. This fact can be verified by the suds or film of suds in the sink when the washcloth is filled with water before use. When using a washcloth under these circumstances, you are adding detergent (laundry detergent) to the facial cleanser.

If the client insists on using washcloths, chamois, or sponges, teaching the client how to clean the "implement" after each use is important.

Table 4–3 Common Cleansers and Moisturizers in the Medical Office

Manufacturer	Product	pH
Hymed®	Liquid soap	5.81
	Facial cleanser	4.51
	Super hydrating lotion	5.55–6.6
La Roche®	Purifying cleanser	5.25–5.8
	Hydroactive emulsion	5.5–6.5
Jan Marini®	Glycolic cleanser	3.25
	Biocleanser	5.0
	All moisturizers	neutral
Niadyne®	Facial cleanser	6.99
	Moisturizer	7.3
Skinceuticals®	Normal to dry cleanser	4–6
	Oily and combination cleanser	4–6
	Moisturizer	7.1–7.7
IS Clinical®	All skin cleanser	6.0–6.2
	Moisturizer	6.5
Dermalogica®	Cleanser	4.5–5.5
	Moisturizer	4.5–5.5
Neostrada®	Cleanser	4.0
	Antibacterial cleanser	4.0
	Daily moisturizers	8–15
MD Formulations®	Oily and combination cleanser	3.8
	Dry and normal cleanser	3.8
Murad®	Refreshing cleanser	5.5–6.1
	Clarifying cleanser	3.8-4.5

acid mantel
A thin coating on the stratum corneum that is intended to protect the skin from infection. It has a pH of 4.0 to 6.5.

neutral
A pH of 7.0.

The acid mantel is a thin coating on the stratum corneum that measures 4.0 to 6.5 pH. The purpose of this acid cover or mantel is to protect the skin from bacteria and fungal infections. A constant disruption in the acid mantel can cause the skin to be at risk for infection. This action is important as we select moisturizers and cleansers that avoid putting the skin at risk. Most *soaps* are alkaline. Up to 36 hours is required for the skin to recover from a cleansing with an alkaline cleanser. The products we select for our clients should be neutral or slightly acid based to keep the skin from excess dryness and risk of infection.

If possible, these implements should be considered single-use items. Once finished with the facial-cleansing routine, the sponge, washcloth, or chamois should be tossed into the washing machine. That said, disposable sponges are a wise recommendation. If the sponge is disposable, throw it away after use. Do not try to get more than one application out of it. Finally, if a client chooses to use a facial cleansing implement, the tendency is to pull harder, push harder, and generally be rougher on the skin than one would be with using just the fingertips (Figure 4–1).

Table 4–4   Cleansers for Specific Skin Types

Skin Type	Cleanser
Normal	Mild cleanser should contain isohexadecane
Oily	Cleanser should contain salicylic acid
Dry	Cleanser should contain moisturizers such as glycerin or lactic acid
Combination	Cleanser should contain glycolic acid
Sensitive	Cleanser should contain moisturizers such as glycerin but no AHAs

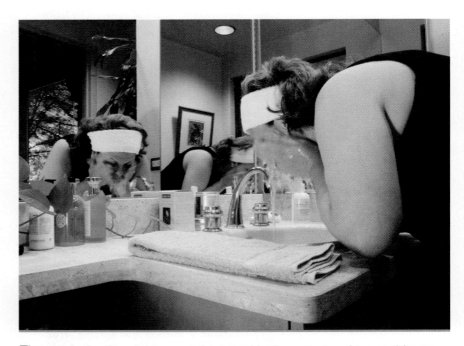

Figure 4–1   Good skin care is important for the patient seeking peel therapy.

Exfoliation

Exfoliation is an important part of the cleansing routine, especially when using cosmeceuticals and prescriptions. Products such as AHAs and **Retin A**® (tretinoin) have a tendency to slough the skin and compact the stratum corneum. The result of this action on the skin is peeling.

Retin A®
Topical vitamin A, also known as tretinoin.

I like to call it *facial dandruff*. We need to help our clients cleanse this peeling with as little irritation and injury to the skin.

Many clients prefer using grains to exfoliate. My experience is that grains have the potential to be damaging to the skin because clients use them too aggressively. I prefer the use of a mask. Papain masks are especially effective. These masks can be used in combination *with* a *fine grain* to help remove the debris. Once the mask is on the face, clients tend to be less likely to push and pull on the skin, causing less harm. Exfoliating should be done *gently* at least three times per week.

ALPHA HYDROXY ACIDS

AHAs are so much more than they were in the 1990s when the application was a simple **gel solution**, the purpose of which was still under investigation. We know more about these acids today, and their use in the skin-care industry is nearly universal in cleansers, moisturizers, and treatment products. For example, AHAs may change the condition of the lipid barrier of the skin allowing a faster penetration of product, which is important. Think about it: a product that will help the absorption of Retin A®, or moisturizers. In fact, some researchers believe that AHAs help relieve dry skin; it helps us understand that a program without AHAs is basically useless or at the very least elementary.

AHAs have gained and sustained popularity in cosmetic products over the last 15 years because of their efficacy, safety, and ease of use. In the beginning, the public had uneasiness about *acids* on the face. More than one client I treated was truly frightened of the idea of acids being applied to the skin, and understandably. Most people think of acids as strong and dangerous. However, let us make a distinction. There are two types of acids: organic (or fruit acids) and mineral acids. Mineral acids are very strong and can be dangerous. These acids include hydrochloric acid or sulfuric acid. The idea of these acids being put on the skin is, in fact, a scary thought. Organic acids, on the other hand, are usually very mild and are commonly found in everyday life. Examples of organic acids are glycolic acid, lactic acid, and even **acetic acid** (vinegar).

Glycolic acids are often selected for use in cosmetics because of the small molecular size and easy penetration into the skin. That AHAs work on both the dermis and the epidermis is now known. In the epidermis, the AHA will "unglue" cells and allow the shedding of keratinocyte at the stratum granulosum.[6] In the dermis, AHAs increase the ground substance and boosts collagen remodeling. Clinically, we observe this phenomenon by an initial dryness followed by a plumpness of the skin.

---

gel solution
Semisolid material that is easily absorbed in the skin without the irritation associated with other cream-based solutions.

acetic acid
A mild organic acid derived from vinegar.

malic acid
An AHA derived from apples.

tartaric acid
An AHA derived from grapes.

citric acid
An AHA derived from citrus fruit (oranges, grapefruit, and so forth).

lactic acid
An AHA derived from milk.

AHAs are fruit acids or organic acids; they are derived from products such as sugar cane (glycolic acid), apples (malic acid), grapes (tartaric acid), citrus fruit (citric acid), and milk (lactic acid).

Aside from the specific AHA (glycolic versus lactic), two other important considerations should be mentioned when selecting an AHA: pH and percentage. If the pH is low and the percentage is high, bioavailability of the acid will be greater. This phenomenon allows the skin to absorb the AHA quickly and efficiently. The pH and the percentage work *hand-in-hand,* and the proper balance is critical to the overall success the product will have on the skin. The pH range should be approximately 3.0 to 4.0, and the percentage should be 12% to 18% for the best result.

Patient Education for Alpha Hydroxy Acids

The FDA evaluated AHA safety in 1997. The information that came from this evaluation gave specific recommendations about the percentages of glycolic acid appropriate for OTC use and salon or spa back bar use. Additionally, the FDA addressed the importance of using sunscreens when using AHAs.

Patient education about AHAs should focus on the application and use of the product. Specifically, the client needs to understand that the *overuse* will cause irritation, **erythema**, and ultimately frustration (Figure 4–2). This educational process is best accomplished by a demonstration on the proper use of the product followed by written instructions.

erythema
A spot on the skin showing diffused redness caused by capillary congestion and dilation.

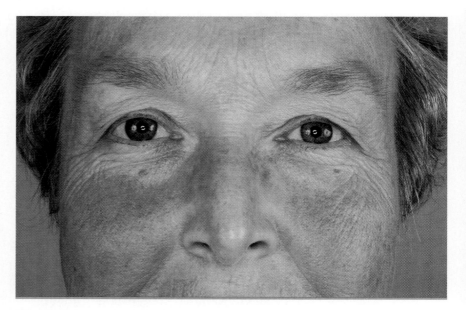

Figure 4–2 Patients can over use AHA, resulting in red, irritated skin.

Table 4–5 Alpha Hydroxy Acids for Specific Skin Types

Skin Type	AHA Formula
Normal	AHAs should be 12%–18%, and pH should be 3.0–3.5.
Oily	AHAs (preferably salicylic) should be 10%–12% and a higher pH, approximately 3.8.
Dry	AHAs (preferably lactic acid) should be eased into program with 8%–10% and a higher pH, approximately 4.0–4.3.
Combination	AHAs should be 12%–18% gels or serums, and pH should be 2.8–3.5.
Sensitive	AHAs (preferably lactic acid) should be eased into program with 8%–10% and a higher pH, approximately 4.0–4.3.

Tell clients that the AHA may tingle or even sting a little. AHA with a pH of 3.0 or under will usually sting or burn, especially on the beginner client. This sting or burn should subside in approximately 60 to 90 seconds. If not, the client should splash it off. Initially, the stinging might happen every day; but if the client uses the product regularly as advised, the stinging will subside over time. If it does not get easier and the client experiences persistent erythema, change the product to a higher pH product. These problems often have less to do with the percentage of the glycolic and more to do with the pH.

Show patients the dose you want them to use. Tell clients to use a "pea-size" amount and then apply this amount onto the back of your hand to demonstrate. Then, lift this amount up and use the fingertips of both hands to apply it to the face. The remaining amount should be massaged into the back of the hands. Let them know, *"This is a medicine, not a moisturizer."* If the skin is feeling dry, apply a little bit more moisturizer or evaluate the moisturizer that is being used. Do not use more glycolic cream (Table 4–5).

free radicals
Molecules lacking an even number of electrons. Free radicals play an important role in tissue ischemia, injury and aging.

■ VITAMIN C

Free radicals cause damage to cells, forcing the aging process into an accelerated pace. Free-radical damage occurs when atoms or groups of atoms have an odd (unpaired) number of *electrons*. Smoking, air pollution, and the sunlight stimulate free-radical damage to the skin. Simply by exposing skin to the sun, the level of vitamin C in the skin drops by 30%,[7] and subsequently, free radicals are formed. *Antioxidants* couple with free radicals to neutralize the unpaired electron. Vitamin C is recognized for its strong antioxidant and *photo-protective* properties,[8] although vitamin C is *never* recommended as a substitute for sunscreen.

Why not just take oral vitamin C to protect the skin? Great idea; but oral vitamin C, whether from food or supplements, is not adequate to perform the necessary antioxidant tasks to improve the skin because the levels of vitamin C required do not make it to the dermis. Recommendations are that all therapeutic programs include a topical vitamin C.

Since topical vitamin C became part of a fundamental skin-care program, controversy has surfaced as to how much and what type is the best. The answer to these questions, as with other subjects within skin care, varies based on the available data and the clinician interpretation of the data. The questions to be asked include, "Should the topical vitamin C be an **ester** or *l*-**ascorbic acid?**" "Should a cream or a gel be used?" "Should a separate application rather than a moisturizer be used?" Answering these questions will initiate the debate.

Topical vitamin C comes in two varieties, *l*-ascorbic (water soluble) and esters (water and fat soluble). The esters and *l*-ascorbic acids are distinctly different. Originally identified at Duke University, *l*-ascorbic acid, penetrates quickly and is used by the skin immediately. However, it deteriorates quickly through oxidation if it is in a light-colored container that is exposed to air each time the patient uses the product. This is why you will often see vitamin C in a dark-brown bottle or an airtight container. Vitamin C esters consist of ascorbyl palmitate and magnesium ascorbyl phosphate. Esters have a longer shelf life and are *time released* on the skin. The time-release phenomenon is the result of the ester waiting for the skin to convert the product into usable vitamin C. Esters have a more even absorption compared with the blast with *l*-ascorbic. Esters are also less irritating. The pH is important with vitamin C: 3.5 pH or lower creates the best environment for the product to absorb.

Patient Education for Vitamin C

Because the use of vitamin C is an extra step in a skin-care program, some clients are reluctant to add the product as a separate component. However, because of its strong antioxidant value, every patient should be on topical vitamin C. A good idea would be to wait until the second or third week to add this step to the program for two reasons. First, vitamin C can be irritating, and when the program starts with AHA and Retin A®, it may be too much for the client to tolerate. Second, let your clients "get into the swing" of a new program and find success with the multisteps before throwing something else into the mix. Add vitamin C to the morning routine after the AHA.

An understanding about percentages is important when dealing with vitamin C because patients will always ask. If the product you are using is *l*-ascorbic, a percentage can be determined. If, on the other hand, you are using an ester, a percentage cannot be determined. Given that the esters are a precursor to the actual vitamin C, in no way can the actual percentage be understood.

---

ester
A fragrant water- and fat-soluble compound formed by the combination of an organic acid and alcohol, removing the water from the compound.

l-ascorbic acid
Topical vitamin C that is both water and fat soluble.

Table 4–6 Vitamin C for Specific Skin Types

Skin Type	Vitamin C Preference	pH
Normal	Both ester and *l*-ascorbic (10% to start)	3.6–3.8
Oily	*l*-ascorbic 12%–15%	3.6–3.8
Dry	Ester in an emollient delivery vehicle	4.0–4.3
Combination	Both ester and *l*-ascorbic (10% to start) in a serum or cream delivery vehicle	3.0–3.5
Sensitive	Ester	4.0–4.3

The *most important* thing for a client to know about vitamin C is its antioxidant powers. Another important fact for the client to know is that the skin, as is the case with the body, can take only as much vitamin C as it can absorb. The remaining amount will sit on the surface of the skin without being absorbed; thus more is not always better (Table 4–6).

▪ MOISTURIZERS

Finding consensus is difficult when defining dry skin. To say that the skin lacks water is far too simple a definition for this complex problem. Some physicians describe dry skin with multifaceted definitions that use the concepts of transepidermal water loss (TEWL) or natural moisturizing factor (NMF). Other physicians define dry skin by the simple appearance of the skin: rough, red, flaky, tender, and so forth.

Skin can be dry for a variety of reasons. Once again, little consensus exists on the *cause* of dry skin. We can, however, agree on several *factors* that *cause* dry skin, among them the lack of humidity in the air, extremes of temperature, diseases of the skin and systemic diseases that *secondarily* cause dry skin, and finally, dry skin that is *created* by the environment through exposure to chemicals that can react on the skin.

We now know (from Dr. Kligman's experiment) that a simple occlusive dressing with water (a wet gauze applied to the skin with an airtight dressing over it) will affect the stratum corneum. Therefore, possibly, moisturizing the skin is easy. This presumption is not necessarily true. Two types of products have been developed that are applied to the skin for the purpose of *moisturizing*. One product is a humectant and one is a lubricant. In this text, a moisturizer will be defined as a humectant, and an emollient will be defined as a lubricant. As discussed, a moisturizer is a product that penetrates the skin and increases the water content (hydration) of the stratum corneum. Lubricants, on the other hand, do not attract water but are more likely to *seal* in the existing water in the stratum corneum. The products most often used in lubricants include petrolatum, beeswax, lanolin, and perhaps some oils. In reality, the best moisturizers are probably a combination of humectants and lubricants.

When we apply a moisturizer to the skin, we notice a change in the appearance and the feeling of the skin. When we are using a moisturizer, as apposed to an emollient, this change is strictly related to the number and blend of humectants in the moisturizer itself and their affect on the skin. Remember that NMF is a blend of *natural* humectants found in the skin. The content of NMF in the skin is directly related to the hydration or water content of the stratum corneum. Lubricants, by comparison, increase the water content of the stratum corneum by simple occlusion; reducing the water loss by use of a sealant.

Creating the perfect moisturizer is not as simple as understanding the composition of NMF and replacing the missing and depleted components to the skin. In fact, water-binding capacities, penetration, and the degree of solvency play a role. In addition to the simple issues of moisturizing the skin, we also want to include other "power punches" to our moisturizers, such as vitamins, antioxidants, and sunscreens. So, how do you choose the perfect moisturizer? Furthermore, is your *favorite* moisturizer the right moisturizer for everyone?

More than Just for Moisturizing

Understandably, consumers can become overwhelmed with the choices that are presented to them in a department store or supermarket. In many cases, people are uninformed about their own skin and which of the many products will best suit them. The power punch in the moisturizer often makes the client buy the product rather than the chemistry of the moisturizer, and why not? Vitamins and antioxidants are far more interesting and simple to understand than the effects of *urea* and *lactate* on the skin.

Composition of Natural Moisturizing[9] (Percentage of NMF)

Amino acids: 40.0

Pyrrolidone carboxylic acid: 12.0

Lactate: 12.0

Urea: 7.0

Sodium, calcium, potassium, magnesium, phosphate, chloride: 18.5

Ammonia, uric acid, glucosamine, creatinine: 1.5

Remainder: unidentified

Several power punches have been developed to moisturizers that should be discussed, and these include vitamin E, selenium, **nicotinamide**, and coenzyme Q_{10} (CoQ_{10}).

Vitamin E is also called *d-alpha tocopherol*. Vitamin E has been shown to have two important benefits for the skin: protecting cellular membranes and inactivating free radicals.[10] Vitamin E has long been considered a good topical for healing scars. However, this presumption is not true, and we should focus our use of vitamin E to its known benefits and use it in a cream form.

Selenium has also been shown to be a powerful antioxidant for the skin. Selenium helps protect the skin from solar-induced skin cancers. However, it functions best when combined with vitamin E.

Nicotinamide, or **vitamin B**, is often found as *niadine* in moisturizers. Nicotinamide has been shown to be successful in the treatment of chronologic aging by decreasing TEWL of the stratum corneum.[11] Studies also point to efficacy in the treatment of acne.

Q_{10}, or **ubiquinone**, can be found both as a separate product serum and as part of the moisturizer. Available documentation of the action of ubiquinone on the skin is limited. However, the few studies that are available are promising. Q_{10} is a cellular antioxidant. It is found in almost all body tissues, including the skin. A recent study demonstrated a 27% reduction of periorbital wrinkles with the application of Q_{10}.

Topical antioxidants are unique and identifiable as free-radical scavengers. A moisturizer that contains all or most of these antioxidants is the power punch we want in a moisturizer (Table 4–7).

nicotinamide
A member of the vitamin B complex that has been shown to decrease TEWL.

d-alpha tocopherol
See vitamin E on page 92.

vitamin B
See nicotinamide on page 102.

ubiquinone
Lipid soluble cellular antioxidant present in virtually all cells.

Table 4–7   Moisturizers for Specific Skin Types

Skin Type	Moisturizers Containing
Normal	Glycerin, hyaluronic acid, and lactic acid
Oily	Water (as main ingredient) and glycerin
Dry	Urea, lactic acid, and hyaluronic acid
Combination	Glycerin, hyaluronic acid, and lactic acid
Sensitive	Hyaluronic acid, no lactic acid

Patient Education for Moisturizers

As we choose moisturizers for our patients, we should assess the status of the client's skin, the impact the AHAs and Retin A® might have, and the end point we are trying to achieve. The client must understand some of the basics about moisturizers and be able to appreciate that the moisturizer you select for them was done so for a specific reason. As we have discussed, two points to ensure that a client understands the moisturizing process are moisturizing versus lubricating and the importance of antioxidants in the moisturizer. Moisturizing is not as simple as spreading a cream on your face, that is, if you want the entire process to be effective.

Moisturizers with Sunscreens

One final stone must be turned when we speak of moisturizers, and that is the concept of moisturizers mixed with sunscreens. In all likelihood, the number of opinions on this subject equals the number of moisturizers and sunscreens. Clients like this blend because it means one less step in the routine. Some clinicians dislike this combination because they believe that these products are not as moisturizing as they would be without the sunscreen component. In reality, produced with plenty of humectants, these products should work just fine and are a great way to simplify a program. Additionally, this combination may be the only way you can get a client to wear sunscreen.

■ SUNSCREENS

Sunscreens are used for the purpose of protecting the skin from **photodamage** resulting from UVA and UVB light. This protection helps reduce photoaging and all of the associated problems such as collagen depletion, dyschromias, and skin cancers. Sunscreens come in two varieties: chemical sunscreens and physical sunscreens. The description of *sun block,* once used to describe these products, has evolved as the FDA has pushed the industry to use the description sun*screen,* recognizing that *block* is a misnomer (Figure 4–3).

Sun protection factor (SPF) is the amount of time you can be in sunlight before you burn. For example, if your skin normally burns in 30 minutes without SPF, applying a 15 SPF theoretically gives you 450 minutes or 7.5 hours of safety.[12] This recommendation assumes that the proper amount of sunscreen has been applied, the individual has not been in the water, and the product is "rub proof." Patients should wear at least a 15 SPF daily. Because SPF is a difficult concept to understand,

photodamage
Damage caused by repeated and unprotected sunlight exposure over time, also called *solar damage.*

sun protection factor (SPF)
The amount of time you can be exposed to sunlight before you burn.

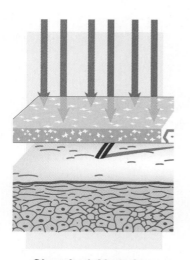

Chemical Absorber

Figure 4–3 Chemical sunscreens absorb the sun's rays as the mechanism for protection.

the FDA is changing the rating for sunscreens to the following levels: *minimum, moderate,* and *high* sunlight protection.

Each of the chemical ingredients found in sunscreen is effective at certain light lengths. Chemical sunscreens absorb UV light. To make sunscreens most effective, manufacturers usually combine a physical block with the chemical block. The chemicals used in sunscreen include **para-aminobenzoic acid (PABA)**, PABA derivatives, **salicylates**, **benzophenone**, **cinnamates**, **dibenzoylmethanes**, **camphors**, **anthranilates**, and other miscellaneous chemicals.[13] **Parsol 1789®** is avobenzone dibenzoylmethane,[14] Parsol 1789® has become a popular and preferred chemical ingredient because of its effectiveness. In the past, Parsol 1789® was believed to destabilize in the bottle, but newer preservatives have solved this problem. If a waterproof sunscreen is the product of choice, be sure it includes a cinnamate. Cinnamates are insoluble in water and are the best ingredient for waterproof sunscreens. Physical blocks such as **zinc oxide** or **titanium dioxide** work by scattering the light rather than absorbing the light. Many of us remember zinc oxide as the white stuff we put on our nose as a child when we were swimming or at the beach. Although physical sunscreens block the sun; they leave a white glob (Figure 4–4).

Patient Education for Sunscreens

Sunscreen is the most important product that you will discuss with your patient. With solar-induced skin cancers increasing at an alarming rate, the clinician must discuss with the patient the importance of sunscreen. Additionally, as you add to the client's program AHAs, Retin A®, and bleaching agents, you put their skin at greater risk of sunburn when exposed to sunlight. Simply stated, we must wear a sunscreen, and our clients must wear a sunscreen. Therefore, whether in a moisturizer or as a separate step, add sunscreens to programs, and be disciplined about their use.

An SPF of at least 15 and preferably 20 should be worn every day. Sunscreen in makeup foundation is not adequate because the protection factor is usually only around 8 SPF. For clients who have not used sunscreen before, this recommendation will be a change. Some clients are annoyed by the way sunscreen "floats" on the skin and is greasy. These patients are better served by a moisturizer with a sunscreen; it is usually less noticeable under these circumstances.

Beyond just adding sunscreen to the skin-care program, clients need to learn to use adequate amounts of sunscreen. Unfortunately,

para-aminobenzoic acid (PABA)
A cousin of the vitamin B complex found in animals other than humans, the most common use of which is that of an effective sunscreen.

salicylates
A salt derivative of salicylic acid, used as a chemical agent in sunscreens.

benzophenone
A chemical absorber that responds to UV light by generating a free radical capable of rapid polymerization.

cinnamates
A derivative of cinnaminic acid, useful for protection against low levels of UVB rays. Also makes sunscreens waterproof.

dibenzoylmethanes
A UVA ray absorber.

camphors
Used topically as an antiitching agent. Derived as a gum from evergreens native to China and Japan.

anthranilates
Weak UVB filters. They absorb mainly in the near UVA portion of the spectrum.

Parsol 1789®
Preferred sunscreen ingredient that protects against photodamage and premature aging of the skin from exposure to UVA light.

zinc oxide
Physical sunscreen that scatters light rather than absorbing or filtering it.

titanium dioxide
Physical sunscreen that scatters light rather than absorbing or filtering it.

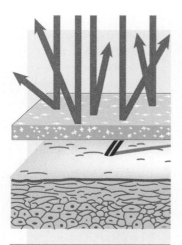

Figure 4–4 Physical blocking agents such as zinc oxide will reflect the sun's rays to protect the skin.

Table 4–8 Sunscreens for Specific Skin Types

Skin Type	Blocking Components	Application
Normal	Combination of chemical and physical—any SPF	After moisturizer, but before makeup
Oily	Chemical with at least SPF 15	Will require behavior modification given that most of these sunscreens will cause breakouts
Dry	Chemical with a lower SPF	Reapply often given that SPF will be lower
Combination	Combination of chemical and physical—any SPF	After moisturizer but before makeup
Sensitive	Physical with at least SPF 15	Reapply often given that physical blockers come off easily

most clients seem to apply sunscreen minimally, with only a small film. The FDA recommends that sunscreen application should be 2 mg/cm^2. This amount is approximately 1 oz for the entire body.[15] In addition, the sunscreen should be applied at least 30 minutes before sunlight exposure to ensure that the chemicals have had the opportunity to bind to the stratum corneum (Table 4–8).

■ HYDROQUINONE

Hydroquinone is a commonly used bleaching agent in the medical spa, available only by a physician's prescription order. Hydroquinone is found naturally in bearberry, cranberry, cowberry, and some varieties of pears. Hydroquinone easily oxidizes (a chemical reaction when combined with oxygen) when exposed to the air and alkaline solutions. Hydroquinone works on melanocytes by inhibiting the production of **tyrosine**, the enzyme that produces melanin at the melanocytes. The overproduction of melanin is associated with melasma and other types of hyperpigmentation. Commercially produced hydroquinone comes in 2% (OTC), 3% (**Melaquin**®), and 4% (**Eldopaque**®).

Kojic acid is a bleaching agent that is often used in combination with hydroquinone. Kojic acid is derived from bacteria on Japanese mushrooms. It is more effective when used with hydroquinone and other therapeutic products. Kojic acid is usually used in 2% solutions.

hydroquinone
A safe, topical bleaching agent that inhibits the production of tyrosine within melanocytes.

tyrosine
An enzyme that produces melanin in melanocytes. Overproduction of melanin is associated with hyperpigmentation.

Melaquin®
A 3% concentration of hydroquinone.

Eldopaque®
A 4% concentration of hydroquinone.

kojic acid
A bleaching agent derived from bacteria on a Japanese mushroom, usually used in conjunction with hydroquinone.

Azelaic acid is an antibacterial usually used for acne treatments, but it has also been shown to decrease discolorations. Used in percentages of 15% to 20%, this product can be as efficacious as is hydroquinone, without the potential for irritation.[16] Similar to hydroquinone, azelaic acid is a prescription medication. When used for significant post-inflammatory hyperpigmentation, azelaic acid should be applied in the morning with AHAs and vitamin C, and use the hydroquinone in the evening with Retin A®. This approach will give the program a real boost and improve the dyschromias faster.

When a bleaching agent is discontinued, a chance exists that the pigment will reappear, especially if the client does not consistently use sunscreen. To solve hyperpigmentation, bleaching agents should be used as *part* of a program.

azelaic acid
An antibacterial agent that is usually used for acne treatment. It also has shown promise in minimizing dyschromias.

All bleaching agents are temporary solutions for the problem of hyperpigmentation.

Patient Education for Hydroquinone

Hydroquinone can be irritating to the skin at higher percentages. In some instances, hydroquinone can actually be the source of irritation rather than the usual suspected culprits, Retin A® or AHA, especially if the percentage you have prescribed is over 6%. I have experienced a delayed redness associated with hydroquinone use that appears the afternoon after the previous evening use. If the client shows this redness, two possibilities for monitoring are *quantity* and *frequency*. First, the client may be using too much. Remember, a pea-size amount is all that is needed. *It is a medicine, not a moisturizer.* Second, using hydroquinone every night may be too much. Evaluating *quantity* and *frequency* is the best way to begin the investigative process to understand the problem.

Hyperpigmentation can occur when using hydroquinone and can happen for two reasons. First, the client fails to wear sunscreen, thinking that the hydroquinone is taking care of the problem, which is simply not true. Patients must be made aware of the importance of using a sunscreen as a condition of treatment. Additionally, patients should be educated on how pigment occurs so they can work *with* you to solve the problem. Second is the phenomenon of postinflammatory hyperpigmentation. For skin types that are very sensitive to postinflammatory hyperpigmentation, the hydroquinone irritation or irritation from any therapeutic product can increase rather than decrease the pigment. The key to avoiding this condition is twofold. Keep the product percentages mild, and keep the application minimal.

Next, include some topical steroid with the application of the hydroquinone. An OTC brand will usually work, but sometimes a prescription is required. This application will make all the difference in the program. The client obviously cannot use the steroid indefinitely, but it

Table 4–9   Hydroquinone for Specific Skin Types

Skin Type	Dosage	Possible Reactions
Normal	6%–8% every evening	Pigment should disappear quickly with minimal reactions
Oily	4% every evening	May result in postinflammatory hyperpigmentation
Dry	3%–5% every other evening	Irritation possible
Combination	6%–8% cream in combination with Retin A®	Pigment should disappear quickly, with minimal reactions
Sensitive	3%–4% every other evening	Irritation possible

is useful to start on the program. Consult with your clinic physician before implementing this step (Table 4–9).

RETINOIDS

Retinoids act by normalizing growth and differentiation in the keratinocytes. Retinoids are vitamin A. Retin A® (tretinoin) is truly *the gold standard* of skin-care products. The efficacy of tretinoin, retinol, or other topical vitamin-A formulations has been shown to have positive effects on the skin.

Retin A® is a *must have* product to help reverse the aging process, specifically photoaging. The groundbreaking work with Retin A® on aging was done by Dr. Albert Kligman in the 1980s when a group of middle-age women being treated for acne noticed an improvement in their fine lines and wrinkles. This observation set in motion the first clinical study, which became the basis for understanding the benefits of Retin A® for aging skin. Tretinoin, interestingly, works not only on the appearance of photoaged skin, but also on the pathologic factors of photoaged skin. Clinical improvement of the skin, such as reduction in fine lines, hyperpigmentation, and lentigines (brown spots), can be seen in as little as 1 month. Stopping the product can cause a reversal of the result. Some clinicians believe that Retin A® can provide a superior result to superficial chemical peels,[17] but combining therapies is the best approach.

Retin A® is a prescription medication. However, vitamin-A derivatives such as retinol and **retinyl palmitate** are available over the counter. The difference between Retin A® and retinol or retinyl palmitate is that

retinyl palmitate
A vitamin-A derivative that must first convert to retinoic acid before it can be useful to the skin. It is also thought to be useful for collagen synthesis.

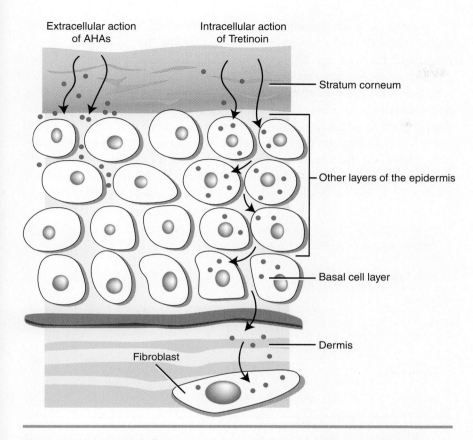

Figure 4–5   Retin A® has intracellular action on the skin versus the extracellular action of an AHA.

the latter two must convert to retinoic acid to become useful on the skin (Figure 4–5).

Patient Education for Retinoids

All retinoids can be potentially irritating. "Overdosing" clients with these products is not in anyone's best interest. The redness, flakiness, and tender skin that present when the product is overused make clients reluctant to carry on a program. Clients' skin need not have the appearance of raw meat to use these products. These products are *medicines, not moisturizers;* instruct your clients accordingly. Use a small pea-size amount on the back of the hand (you can mix in the hydroquinone for a single application). Spread the entire amount over the face and neck. Any extra is massaged into the back of the hand.

Similar to hydroquinone and AHAs, retinoids can cause irritation and erythema. The investigative process remains the same: *quantity* and *frequency*. Patients are likely to be using too much product because getting a pea-size amount around the face and neck is difficult. Mixing retinoids with the hydroquinone helps; but if clients need more volume, add a dab of moisturizer. If this solution does not decrease the symptoms, the problem is frequency. Some practitioners believe that patients should "tough it out" and get through the initial process of flakiness and irritation. However, decreasing the product to every other day is not a problem. In the end, we want the patient to tolerate the treatment and the treatment to be successful. The last option is to change the product

Table 4–10 Retinoids for Specific Skin Types

Skin Type	Dosage
Normal	0.05% Retin A® (0.025% for thinner skin) cream or Renova®
Oily	Differin®
Dry	0.02% Renova® every second or third night
Combination	Retin A® 0.05% cream for aging or 0.025% gel for breakouts
Sensitive	OTC retinol or Renova® 0.02%

Table 4–11 Retin A® Strength and Delivery

Product	Percentage
Retin A® micro	0.1%
Retin A® cream	0.025%
Retin A® cream	0.05%
Retin A® cream	0.1%
Retin A® gel	0.01%
Retin A® gel	0.025%
Retin A® liquid	0.05%
Renova ®	0.02%
Renova®	0.05%

strength or carrier vehicle. Specifically, the carrier vehicle in the case of Retin A® might be a change to **Renova**® or to Micro® to assist with penetration. These products are more moisturizing and have a gentler penetration process (Tables 4–10 and 4–11).

Renova®
A tretinoin that is meant specifically for aging and is recommended for patients with drier-than-normal skin.

Conclusion

Each medical spa should have a protocol on dispensing cosmeceuticals and monitoring patients using cosmeceuticals and topical prescription products. As a clinician, dispensing these products with knowledge and care is your responsibility. Each product should have a separate informational sheet (what the product does), as well as an instructional sheet (how to use the product). The success of the program depends on these simple steps.

▶ ▷ ▷ TOP TEN TIPS TO TAKE TO THE CLINIC

1. The pH of products will make products more intense (lower pH) or less intense (higher pH).
2. A cleanser with a lower pH will keep the skin from becoming too dry. Bath soaps usually have a more alkaline pH.
3. Using a washcloth or facial chamois can cause the skin to be dryer resulting from the laundry detergent residue left in these *implements*.
4. Hydroquinone, Retin A®, or Renova® are necessary to consider the program therapeutic.
5. Vitamin C is manufactured either as an ester (fat and water soluble) or as *l*-ascorbic (water soluble only).
6. Hydroquinone alone will not solve a pigment problem. Sunscreen is necessary to eliminate solar stimulation of the melanin.
7. Products can cause irritation if they are overused; remember the principles of quantity and frequency.
8. Retin A® is vitamin A and is the gold standard for therapeutic programs.
9. A sunscreen of at least 15 SPF and preferably 20 SPF should be worn every day to protect the skin from solar damage.
10. Moisturizers come in two types: humectant (moisturizing) and emollient (lubricating).

CHAPTER REVIEW QUESTIONS

1. What are the key components of a cleanser?
2. What ingredients should be present in a moisturizer?

3. What are cosmeceuticals?
4. Why is the term *cosmeceutical* important?
5. What are the best exfoliating products?
6. What are AHAs?
7. How many AHAs have been developed?
8. From where do AHAs originate?
9. Why is vitamin C used in a skin-care program?
10. Why are sunscreens so important?
11. What is hydroquinone?
12. What are the three important retinoids?

CHAPTER REFERENCES

1. Elsner, P., & Maibach, H. L. (Eds.). (2000). *Cosmeceuticals: Drugs vs. cosmetics.* New York: Marcel Dekker.
2. Elsner, P., & Maibach, H. L. (Eds.). (2000). *Cosmeceuticals: Drugs vs. cosmetics.* New York: Marcel Dekker.
3. Murphy, R. (2003, March). *Cosmeceuticals: Can science support the claims?* [Online]. Available: www.skinandaging.com
4. Draelos, Z. (2002, January 7). *Skin hair and cleansers* [Online]. Available: www.emedicine.com
5. Yosipovitch, G. (2003, March). The importance of skin pH. *Skin & Aging* [Online]. Available: www.skinandaging.com
6. Rubin, M. (1995). *Manual of chemical peels: Superficial and medium depth.* Philadelphia: Lippincott, Williams & Wilkins.
7. American Academy of Dermatology. (2002, February 25). *Vitamins to protect against and reverse aging: The truths vs. the tall tales* [Online]. Available: www.aad.org
8. American Fitness. (1998, November). *C no wrinkles* [Online]. Available: www.findarticles.com
9. Elsner, P. & Maibach, H. L. (Eds.). (2000). *Cosmeceuticals: Drugs vs. cosmetics.* New York: Marcel Dekker.
10. American Academy of Dermatology. (2002, February 25). *Vitamins to protect against and reverse aging: The truths vs. the tall tales* [Online]. Available: www.aad.org
11. Chui, A., & Kimball, A. B. (2003, November 17). Topical vitamins, minerals, and botanical ingredients as modulators, of environmental and chronological skin damage. *British Journal of Dermatology,* 149(4), 681–691.
12. American Academy of Dermatology. (2002, February 25). *Vitamins to protect against and reverse aging: The truths vs. the tall tales* [Online]. Available: www.aad.org

13. Chui, A., & Kimball, A. B. (2003, November 17). Topical vitamins, minerals, and botanical ingredients as modulators, of environmental and chronological skin damage. *British Journal of Dermatology*, 149(4), 681–691.
14. MedicineNet.com. www.medterms.com
15. Bennett, M., & Petrazzuoli, M. (2001, July). What patients should know about sunscreen. *Skin & Aging* [Online]. Available: www.skinandaging.com
16. Bennett, M., & Petrazzuoli, M. (2001, July). What patients should know about sunscreen. *Skin & Aging* [Online]. Available: www.skinandaging.com
17. Bennett, M., & Petrazzuoli, M. (2001, July). What patients should know about sunscreen. *Skin & Aging* [Online]. Available: www.skinandaging.com

BIBLIOGRAPHY

Alster, T. S., & West, T. B. (1998, March). Effects of topical vitamin C on postoperative carbon dioxide laser resurfacing erythema. *Journal of Dermatologic Surgery*, 24(3), 331–334.

American Academy of Dermatology. *(2002, February 25). Vitamins to protect against and reverse aging: The truths vs. the tall tales* [Online]. Available: www.aad.org

American Fitness. (1998, November). *C no wrinkles* [Online]. Available: www.findarticles.com

Baumann, L. (2002). *Cosmetic dermatology practices and principles*. New York: McGraw Hill.

Bennett, M., & Petrazzuoli, M. (2001, July). What patients should know about sunscreen. *Skin & Aging* [Online]. Available: www.skinandaging.com

Breathnach, A. S. (1996, January). Melanin hyperpigmentation of skin: Melasma, topical treatment with azelaic acid, and other therapies. *Cutis*, 57(Suppl 1), 36–45.

Brody, H. J. (1997). *Chemical peeling and resurfacing* (2nd ed.). St. Louis: Mosby.

Chui, A., & Kimball, A. B. (2003, November 17). Topical vitamins, minerals, and botanical ingredients as modulators of environmental and chronological skin damage. *British Journal of Dermatology*, 149(4), 681–691.

Clark, C. P. (2001, October 1). New directions in skin care. *Journal of Clinical Plastic Surgery*, 28(4), 745–750.

D'Angelo, J., Dean, P., Dietz, S., Hinds, C., Lees, M., Miller, E., et al. (2003). *Milady's standard: Comprehensive training for estheticians*. Clifton Park, NY: Thomson Delmar Learning.

Draelos, Z. (2002, January 7) *Skin hair and cleansers* [Online]. Available: www.emedicine.com

Elsner, P., & Maibach, H. L. (Eds.). (2000). *Cosmeceuticals: Drugs vs. cosmetics*. New York: Marcel Dekker.

Fitzpatrick, R. E., & Rostan, E. F. (2002, March). Double-blind, half-face study comparing topical vitamin C and vehicle for rejuvenation of photodamage. *Journal of Dermatologic Surgery, 28*(3), 231.

Gerson, J. (2004). *Milady's standard: Fundamentals for estheticians* (9th ed.). Clifton Park, NY: Thomson Delmar Learning.

Gladstone, H. B., Nguyen, S., Williams, R., Ottomeyer, T., Jeffers, M., & Moy, R. (2000, April). Efficacy of hydroquinone cream (4%) used alone or in combination with salicylic acid peels in improving photodamage on the neck and upper chest. *Journal of Dermatologic Surgery, 26*(4), 333.

Guevera, I. L., & Pandya, A. G. (2003, December). Safety and efficacy of 4% hydroquinone combined with 10% glycolic acid, antioxidants, and sunscreen in treatment of melasma. *International Journal of Dermatology, 42*(12), 966.

Higdon, J. (2003, September 24). *The bioavailability of different forms of vitamin C* [Online]. Available: http://lpi.oregonstate.edu

Humbert, P. (2001, Mar-Apr). Topical vitamin C in the treatment of photoaged skin. *European Journal of Dermatology, 11*(2), 172–173.

Humbert, P., Haftek, M., Creidi, P., Lapiere, C., Nusgens, B., Schmitt, D., et al. (2003, June). Topical ascorbic acid on photoaged skin. *Journal of Experimental Dermatology, 12*(3), 237.

Jan Marini Communications. (1997, Nov-Dec). *News release: Software manages skin care programs, patients* [Online]. Available: www.janmarini.com

Jevelle International. (2004, February 27). *Hydroquinone* [Online]. Available: www.health-and-beauty.us

Krivda, M. (2004, February). *Current therapies for treating photodamaged skin* [Online]. Available: www.skinandaging.com

Kurtzweil, P. (1998, March). Alpha hydroxy acids for skin care. *FDA Consumer Magazine* [Online]. Available: www.fda.gov

Leyden, J. J. (2002, July). Biology behind sensitive skin. *Skin & Aging* [Online].

Lim, J. T. (1999, April). Treatment of melasma using kojic acid in a gel containing hydroquinone and glycolic acid. *Journal of Dermatologic Surgery, 25*(4), 282.

Lowe, N.. & Sellar, P. (1999). *Skin secrets: The medical facts versus the beauty fiction*. New York Collins & Brown.

Mann, J., & Truswell, S. (Eds.). (2002). *The essentials of human nutrition* (2nd ed.). New York: Oxford University Press.

MedicineNet.com. www.medterms.com

Murphy, R. (2003, March). *Cosmeceuticals: Can science support the claims?* [Online]. Available: www.skinandaging.com

Nutrition Research Newsletter. (1998, April). *Vitamins C and E offer slight protection against sunburn* [Online]. Available: www.findarticles.com

Perricone, N. V. (2004, February 17). *Dr. Perricone FAQ: What is vitamin C ester?* [Online]. Available: www.substance.com

Physician's Desk Reference. (2004, February 27). *Retin-A Micro(r) (orthoneutrogena) (tretinoin gel) microsphere 0.1%/0.04%* [Online]. Available: www.pdr.net

Physician's Desk Reference. (2004, March 2). *Drug information: Ascorbyl palmitate* [Online]. Available: www.pdrhealth.com

Physician's Desk Reference. (2004, March 2). *Drug information: Vitamin C* [Online]. Available: www.pdrhealth.com

Pinnell, S. R. (2004, February 26). *Topical vitamin C: How it operates on the skin* [Online]. Available: www.skinceuticals-jp.com

Rolewski, S. L. (2003, December 5). *Clinical review: Topical retinoids* [Online]. Available: www.medscape.com

Rubin, M. (1995). *Manual of chemical peels: Superficial and medium depth.* Philadelphia: Lippincott Williams & Wilkins.

Schardt, D. (2003, Jul-Aug). *The skin game. Nutrition action healthletter* [Online]. Available: http://www.findarticles.com

Sepp, D. T. (2004, February 17). *Skin & the aging process* [Online]. Available: www.skikai.com

Skin Therapy Letter. (1998, May). *Current review of the alpha hydroxy acids* [Online]. Available: www.dermatology.org

Stratus Pharmaceuticals, Inc. (2004, February 17). *Melquin 3 topical solution insert* [Online]. Available: www.stratuspharmaceuticals.com

Spencer, H. (1998, February). *'Age proof' your skin with topical vitamin E. Better Nutrition* [Online]. Available: www.findarticles.com

Spencer, H. (1998, January). *Topical vitamin C for more vibrant skin. better nutrition* [Online]. Available: www.findarticles.com

Tung, R. C., Bergfeld, W. F., Vidimos, A. T., & Remzi, B. K. (2000, Mar-Apr). Alpha hydroxy acid-based cosmetic procedures. Guidelines for patient management. *American Journal of Dermatology, 1*(2), 81–88.

United States Food and Drug Administration. (1997, July 3). *Alpha hydroxy acids in cosmetics. FDA backgrounder* [Online]. Available: www.vm.cfsan.fda.gov

University of Iowa Healthcare. (2004, March 15). *Fluid replacement* [Online]. Available: www.uihealthcare.com

Vermont Soapworks. (2004, March 2). *Sodium laurel sulfate* [Online]. Available: http://www.vermontsoap.com

Wang, C. M., Huang, C. L., & Chan, H. L. (1997, January). The effect of glycolic acid in the treatment of Asian skin. *Journal of Dermatologic Surgery*, 23(1), 23–29.

WebMD. (2004, February 27). *Hydroquinone topical: Usage and dosage* [Online]. Available: www.medscape.com

WebMD. (2004, February 17). *Modulators of environmental and chronological skin damage* [Online]. Available: www.medscape.com

Webster's new world medical dictionary. (2002). New York: Merriam Webster.

Winnington, P. III, (2001, January). *Tips to reduce retinoid sensitivity* [Online]. Available: www.skinandaging.com

Yosipovitch, G. (2003, March). The importance of skin pH. *Skin & Aging* [Online]. Available: www.skinandaging.com

Assessing Patient's Suitability and Predicting Peel Efficacy

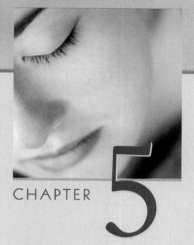

CHAPTER 5

KEY TERMS

actinic keratoses
aging analysis
consultation
deep peels
Fitzpatrick skin typing
Glogau classification of
    aging analysis
health history sheet
Help Us Understand
    You sheet
image business

impression
keratoses
lentigines
moderate peels
patient information
    (PI) sheet
perception
photographs
Rubin classification of
    aging analysis
seborrheic keratoses

skin condition
skin history sheet
skin typing
superficial peels
very superficial
    peels
Wood's lamp

LEARNING OBJECTIVES

After completing this chapter you should be able to:

1. Define and discuss the concepts of skin typing and age analysis.
2. Define and discuss the Fitzpatrick method of skin typing.
3. Define and discuss the Glogau method of aging analysis.
4. Define and discuss the Rubin method of aging analysis.
5. Discuss the consultation process.
6. Describe the process of taking a patient's history.
7. Discuss the indications and contraindications for peel treatments.
8. Discuss how to evaluate and correct patient expectations.

Knowing the *who, when, how,* and *why* before chemical peeling is vital, and skin typing and skin aging analysis will help you answer these questions. The skin typing and skin aging models will address questions such as which skin condition, skin type, and age level will respond to which peel solutions and ultimately help create the plan of action for that patient.

skin condition
A fundamental skin classification in which an individual's skin is grouped according to the degree of moisture retention or its reaction to products and environment, or both.

skin typing
A more detailed skin classification that gives indications as to how a certain skin type will react to various treatment conditions.

aging analysis
An assessment that examines how aging physically presents itself in the skin, particularly, what sorts of damaging conditions to which the skin has been exposed in the past and what the results of that damage are. Aging analysis considers both intrinsic and extrinsic aging modalities.

INTRODUCTION

Responses to most aggressive skin therapies, chemical peels in particular, will vary from patient to patient. Different reasons contribute to such variation, but generally, they are either from clinician technique or from physiologic origins. Biologic variables are accepted and understood in medicine and that includes medical skin care. For example, recommended drug doses are calculated based on the individual patient's weight. Just as a physician or pharmacist would be loathe to dose a full grown man and a little child equally, you would be ill advised to peel everyone who comes through your door the same way. You will need to assess which characteristics and symptoms are best suited for chemical peel treatments. More importantly, you will need to be familiar with the symptoms and afflictions that are inconsistent or exacerbated by performing a peel treatment. By using a combination of categorical systems, taking a complete health history, and making keen observations (and keener documentation), you have all the requisite information needed to ascertain the client's suitability and therefore anticipate the most likely outcome.

This approach might seem complex, understandably. In your very first encounter with a new patient, you have to make a good impression, fish for information, make clinical observations, assess treatment options, and present them with both delicacy and salesmanship, all simultaneously. Although this methodology may seem excessive, your knowledge of the following content will ensure your success and position you as the skin-care authority you will be.

First though, let us start with understanding of the various methods with which skin is categorized. The most general of these categories, **skin condition**, is often deciphered by the patient before he or she even comes into your office (whether he or she is correct or not). Skin condition is classified as normal, oily, dry, sensitive, and combination. To solve the suitability-outcome conundrum, you will have to make a deeper analysis using two important models, **skin typing** and **aging analysis.**

SKIN TYPING

The skin type of a patient does not necessarily convey whether advanced treatments such as microdermabrasion, peels, or laser resurfacing will have a positive outcome. Certainly, the skin type will dictate how a procedure might be done technically; it is seldom the reason your patients will seek your assistance. Problems associated with coloration, texture, and signs of aging are more complex and need to be regarded as such.

Therefore, as a skin-care professional, you will need to understand how individual skin types respond to different treatments, which skin types will allow more aggressive treatments, and which require greater caution. To accomplish this task, you will be using skin typing and aging analysis methods. Clinical research and study has shown that genetics (eye color, hair color, ethnic background, and true skin color) regularly and consistently predict the skin's response to injury.

In 1975, Dr. Thomas Fitzpatrick organized these factors into a classification system, known as **Fitzpatrick skin typing.** This skin typing classification is applied today to predict responses to a variety of therapies from microdermabrasion to carbon dioxide (CO_2) laser resurfacing. Similarly, it also assists the clinician in determining which clients are at a greater risk for complications such as scarring and pigmentary problems.

Fitzpatrick Skin Typing

As discussed previously, in the Fitzpatrick system, each patient is asked a series of questions related to skin color, unaltered eye and hair color, ethnic origins, and response to UV light (without any sunlight protection). Based on a series of questions, we end up with six Fitzpatrick skin types (Fitzpatrick I through VI) that extend from very fair skin to very dark (Table 5–1).

In its simplest form, the Fitzpatrick skin typing says: To get to these classifications, a series of questions are asked of each patient together with your own examination (Tables 5–2 through 5–4). Add up the total scores for each of the three sections for your skin type score. This assessment will give you a better evaluation of the skin type (Tables 5–5 and 5–6).

Now that you have scored yourself, let us delve deeper into the categories and explore the meaning and necessity within the typing matrix.

Skin Color

Skin color is essentially an inherited racial and ethnic characteristic. However, even within the same race and ethnicity, some variability will be found.

When we think of Caucasian, we think white. However, white can come in a variety of shades, and this variation will influence whether the client is a Fitzpatrick I or II or even III. In the Fitzpatrick I type, the ethnic considerations are English, Scottish, Irish, Norwegian, Swedish, and Icelandic. These individuals will present with very fair skin, freckling, green or light blue eyes, and light hair color (Figure 5–1 on page 123).

Dr. Thomas Fitzpatrick was for many years the chairman of the Department of Dermatology at the renowned Massachusetts General Hospital in Boston, Massachusetts. He has been called the father of modern academic dermatology, as well as the most influential dermatologist of the last 100 years. The author of *Fitzpatrick's Dermatology in General Medicine,* he is best known for developing the Fitzpatrick phototype procedure for quantifying skin types and determining an individual's ultraviolet radiation (sunlight) susceptibility. During his career, he was interested in treating many diseases, including psoriasis and vitiligo. His treatment protocol involved the use of ultraviolet A (UVA) light. To quantify the amount of UVA exposure, a system had to be devised to set treatment parameters that would predict the patient's response to UV light, based on his or her type of skin, hence Fitzpatrick skin typing.

Fitzpatrick skin typing
A method of skin typing that considers skin's complexion, hair color, eye color, ethnicity, and the individual's reaction to unprotected sunlight exposure.

Factors regularly and consistently influence the skin's response to injury: genetics, eye color, hair color, ethnic background, and true skin color. The skin's response to these factors defines the Fitzpatrick skin typing system.

Table 5–1 Fitzpatrick Skin Typing Scale

Skin Type	Skin Color	Hair and Eye Color	Reaction to Sunlight	Common Ethnic Considerations
Type I	White	Blond hair and green eyes	Always burns, has freckles	English, Scottish
Type II	White	Blond hair and green or blue eyes	Always burns, has freckles, difficult to tan	Northern European
Type III	White	Blond or brown hair and blue or brown eyes	Tans after several burns, may freckle	German
Type IV	Brown	Brown hair and brown eyes	Tans more than average, rarely burns, rarely freckles	Mediterranean, Southern European, Hispanic
Type V	Dark brown	Brown or black hair and brown eyes	Tans with ease, rarely burns, has no freckles	Asian, Indian, some Africans
Type VI	Black	Black hair and brown or black eyes	Tans, never burns, deeply pigmented, never has freckles	Africans

Table 5–2 Genetic Disposition[1]

	0	1	2	3	4	Score
What color are your eyes?	Light blue, gray, or green	Blue, gray, or green	Blue	Dark brown	Brownish black	
What is the natural color of your hair?	Sandy red	Blond	Chestnut or dark blonde	Dark brown	Black	
What color is your skin (nonexposed areas)?	Reddish	Very pale	Pale with beige tint	Light brown	Dark brown	
Do you have freckles on unexposed areas?	Many	Several	Few	Incidental	None	
Genetic disposition total						

The remaining non-Hispanic Caucasians are usually Mediterranean and Southern European. This group would include Greeks, Middle Easterners, and Italians. These people have darker hair, mainly dark blondes and brown. This category can also present several variations on

Table 5–3   Reaction to Sunlight Exposure[2]

	0	1	2	3	4	Score
What happens when you stay too long in sunlight?	Painful redness, blistering, peeling	Blistering followed by peeling	Burns sometimes followed by peeling	Rare burns	Never had burns	
To what degree do you turn brown?	Hardly or not at all	Light color tan	Reasonable tan	Tan very easily	Turn dark brown quickly	
Do you turn brown with several hours of sunlight exposure?	Never	Seldom	Sometimes	Often	Always	
How does your face react to sunlight?	Very sensitive	Sensitive	Normal	Very resistant	Never had a problem	
Reaction to sunlight exposure total						

Table 5–4   Tanning Habits[3]

	1	2	3	4	5	Score
When did you last expose your body to sunlight (or artificial sunlamp or tanning cream)?	More than 3 months ago	2–3 months ago	1–2 months ago	Less than a month ago	Less than 2 weeks ago	
Did you expose the area to be treated to sunlight?	Never	Hardly ever	Sometimes	Often	Always	
Tanning habits total						

the shades of darker whites and brown skin. They will probably fall into the Fitzpatrick III and IV categories (see Figure 5–1). The eye color is blue, dark blue, and brown.

The Hispanic skin category has darker skin, darker hair, and darker eyes. Their hair is dark brown or black, and their eyes are brown. They will generally fall into the Fitzpatrick IV and perhaps V categories. Their ethnic background is Spanish, Mexican, South American, and Cuban (see Figure 5–1).

Table 5–5 Scores[4]

Summary

Total for genetic disposition
Total for reaction to sunlight exposure
Total for tanning habits
Skin type score

Table 5–6 Your Fitzpatrick Skin Type[5]

Skin Type Score	Fitzpatrick Skin Type
0–7	I
8–16	II
17–25	III
25–30	IV
Over 30	V–VI

The skin types of the African or African-American are darker. However, the skin will vary from light brown (e.g., Hispanics) to a very dark brown or blue or black color. Their hair is always naturally black, but the eyes can be brown to black. In the darkest color, this skin is typically the Fitzpatrick VI, but it might also be Fitzpatrick V as well. Their ethnic background is African (see Figure 5–1). Asian and Pacific Islander skin types are light brown to brown in color; the hair can often be light brown or sometimes a dark red to dark brown. The eyes are brown or dark brown. These skin types have an ethnic background from Japan, China, and the islands of the South Pacific, to mention a few. Native or aboriginal skin types are light brown to brown. The hair color is brown to black. The eye color is brown to dark brown. These people are found in differing parts of the world.

Given that skin coloration has a good deal of variation, an advisable practice is that you avoid making any knee-jerk assumptions that might offend or prove inaccurate. Whether skin coloration appears obvious and the patient has declared it as such, or conversely, the patient is unwilling to disclose or is unknowing, you should still take the following steps to identify the skin color for your purposes in the clinical environment. Begin the analysis of the skin by choosing three areas of the body to evaluate. The best areas for analysis are the face, under the breast or

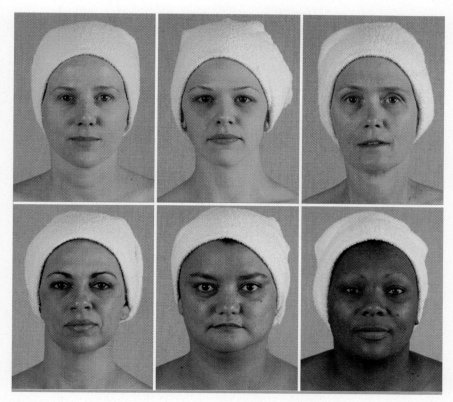

Figure 5–1 Assessing a patient's Fitzpatrick skin color is complicated and challenging.

abdomen, and an arm. The face needs to be clean and free of makeup. Next, look for freckles, telangiectasia, and skin tone. Finally, determine a skin color based on what you see.

Eye Color

As is the case with the skin, eye color is genetically determined. Deciphering eye color is seemingly straightforward at first—but delve further. The three basic eye colors are blue, brown, and green. These colors are further expanded into light blue, blue, blue-green, hazel, light brown, brown, and dark brown or black. Furthermore, a virtual rainbow of colors exists in between. Obviously, the degree of color is determined genetically but also relates to the skin tone. If you are struggling to assess the correct Fitzpatrick skin type, look at the eye color; it will help you make the decision. The eye color is most helpful in analyzing Fitzpatrick I and Fitzpatrick II. These two skin types have varying colors of blue and green eyes that can be confusing to a beginner (Figure 5–2).

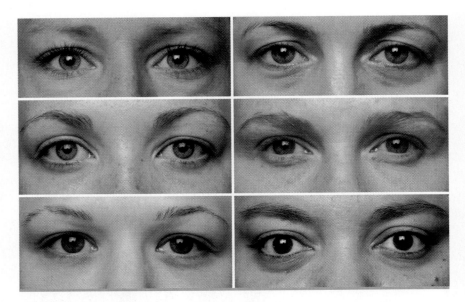

Figure 5–2   Primary eye colors (blue, green, and brown) are quite variable themselves.

Hair Color

Hair color is often a difficult trait to assess. Most women and some men color their hair to some degree, whether it is highlights, full color, or a combination of both (Figure 5–3). Hair color can be determined at the roots, but if the client very recently had his or her hair colored, the roots would tell no secrets. Additionally, the comparison of the colored hair against the natural hair can be deceiving. Given that eyebrows can also be colored, bleached, or otherwise altered, they are not a reliable source for answers either. If you suspect your client's hair color is altered, have him or her describe the natural color as best as possible. Because of the potential for error, you may not want to invest too much time in finding the answer.

Response to UV Light Without SPF Protection

Evaluating the skin's response to UV light is *the* most important indicator of skin type. Given that some people have a hard time owning up to this factor, the manner in which you phrase the questions is critical to the accuracy of the answer. Ultimately, you want to know how the skin responds to sunlight *without* sunscreen. Clients will say, "I never go into the sun" or "I never go in the sun without sunscreen." The better question to ask is, "Did you have a sunburn as a child?" If the answer is yes, then get the details, including whether the sunburn produced blisters. If so, where? If it did not produce blisters, can the client remember how long

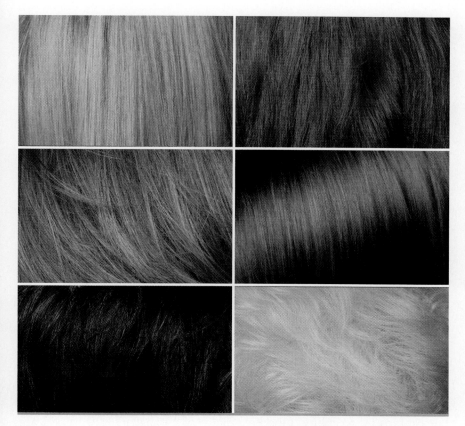

Figure 5–3   Hair color may or may not want to be considered in your assessment because of the prevalence of color processing.

it was sore or red? Time can fade memory, so offer suggestions that might trigger something. For example, "As a child, did you vacation at the beach? How did your skin respond at the beach? As a child, did you swim during the summer? Did you sunbathe in college? Did you use baby oil to sunbathe? What happened to your skin?" The next question involves whether they have ever had a glycolic or trichloroacetic acid (TCA) peel. If the answer is yes, ask for the details. What strength, how long was the peel left on, and what were the results of the peel? Were there any complications from the peel? Remember, Fitzpatrick analysis tells us how the skin responds to advanced skin-care products and treatments.

Evaluating the accuracy of the information the patient has given you about sunlight exposure is done in several ways: physical examination of the skin, patient interview, and analysis of the home products. These three "prongs" will give you a good idea about your patient's sunlight exposure and protection. The patient's willingness to accept sunlight

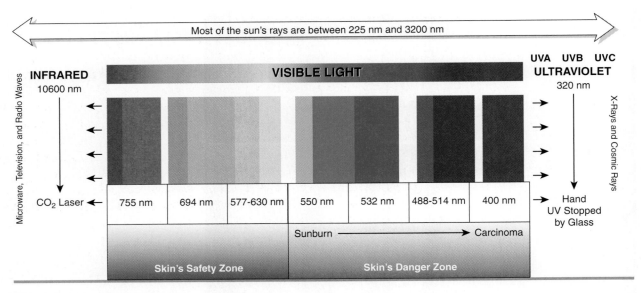

Figure 5—4   UVA, UVB, and UVC light lengths are toxic to the skin.

protection as part of their daily routine will influence the long-term result of the peel and your decision about treatment (Figure 5–4).

Fitzpatrick I is the *very fair*–skinned individual. This person usually has blonde or red hair, light blue or green eyes, and burns within 10 to 15 minutes of being exposed in sunlight without sunscreen. This person tans by freckling. Good examples of Fitzpatrick skin type I are the Irish, English, or Scottish.

Fitzpatrick II is the *fair*-skinned individual. This individual has blonde hair; it will sometimes be *dishwater blonde* with blue or green eyes. The fair-skinned individual may tolerate a slightly longer period in the sunlight before burning, perhaps 30 to 40 minutes. This individual still freckles a lot and has a difficultly tanning. Good examples of Fitzpatrick skin type II are Northern Europeans, those of Swedish, Finish, or Norwegian origin.

Fitzpatrick III individuals are still *white* but tan more easily than do Fitzpatrick I and II persons. These individuals will have fewer freckles than the Fitzpatrick I and II types. Their hair can be blonde but they are more likely to be a light- to moderate-brown color. The eye color is usually dark blue to brown. These individuals can be in sunlight 60 to 70 minutes without sunscreen before they begin to burn. Examples of Fitzpatrick skin type III are German, Northern Italian, and French.

Fitzpatrick IV skin types are *brown;* they tan easily, usually without freckling. These individuals can be in sunlight without sunscreen and will rarely burn. Their hair color is usually brown to dark brown, and the eyes are brown. Examples of Fitzpatrick skin type IV are Greeks, Southern Italians, some Asians, and some Hispanics.

Fitzpatrick V individuals are *dark brown;* they tan easily and generally do not have freckles. They can be in sunlight without sunscreen and will not burn. The hair is usually brown or black, with brown eyes. Examples of Fitzpatrick skin type V include some Asians, some Hispanics, some Africans, and Middle Eastern Indians.

Fitzpatrick VI individuals are *black;* they tan with ease, do not freckle, and are deeply pigmented. Their hair is black, and their eyes are brown or even black. Examples of Fitzpatrick VI are Africans.

Now that you understand in principle what skin types are, we need to delve deeper and understand how these skin types age over time. To do so, you will now layer the skin typing with an evaluation of aging analysis. Doing so will be critical in regard to evaluating the patient for contraindications (discussed later) and treatment efficacy.

■ AGING ANALYSIS

Whereas skin typing will give insights into how the client's skin will likely respond to a particular treatment, aging analysis goes a step further. It examines skin damage that has occurred to date and how that damage presents itself, hence indicating what treatment modality or modalities should be considered to treat the damage with a positive end result. The patient's personal skin-aging patterns, both intrinsic and extrinsic, are considered. You will remember that intrinsic aging refers to the changes that occur to the skin over time, regardless of environmental factors. Extrinsic aging are changes brought on by the effects of the environment, specifically from sunlight exposure, or *photoaging.* Although emphasis is placed on solar damage, aging analysis also considers lines of expression, usually associated with intrinsic aging.

The two aging analysis systems used most commonly are the *Glogau classification* and the *Rubin classification.*

Aging analysis is a method of categorizing clients based on their intrinsic and extrinsic aging factors. The analysis takes into consideration the kinds of lines, solar damage such as keratoses or **lentigines,** and the condition of the stratum corneum. Of the *skin aging systems,* both the Glogau and Rubin systems are widely used and well respected.

The aging analysis is just as important as is skin typing. The aging analysis helps us understand the patient's skin history. Through a group of well-organized questions, we will be able to ascertain the patient's intrinsic aging history and the extrinsic aging history. That is to say, what role the client's genetics are playing and how much sunlight exposure the client has had.

Aging analysis places emphasis on both intrinsic and extrinsic aging processes.

lentigines
Flat brown spots appearing on aged or sunlight-exposed skin. Commonly called liver spots, they are not related to any liver disease.

A facelift may play a deceptive role in the aging analysis because it minimizes the appearance of wrinkling associated with chronologic age; a facelift will not affect overall skin quality.

When the two types of analyses are completed, the clinician will understand how his or her client's skin is going to behave under most circumstances. This understanding will help predict potential stumbling blocks in the program, the possible outcome, and client compliance.

Let us therefore find out how the advanced medical clinicians use skin typing and aging analysis. One method does not give the entire story.

Glogau Classification

Dr. Richard G. Glogau was a clinical professor of dermatology at the University of California, San Francisco, where he is highly regarded in his field. Using an innovative and experienced approach, Glogau garnished national and international recognition for his cutting-edge work in dermatology, specifically in the areas of cosmetic surgery and skin cancer. Dr. Glogau lectures extensively on a wide range of topics in cosmetic dermatology, including soft-tissue augmentation, photoaging, and resurfacing.

The **Glogau classification of aging analysis** measures current damage caused by prior activity. The presenting damage is assigned a numeric *type*. The increasing numeric designations (I through IV) correspond to the increasing degree that age-related damage physically presents.

In the Glogau classification method, skin changes are also designated as being minimal, moderate, advanced, or severe. Classification of each patient is based on the following criteria: the patient's chronologic age, pigment changes, **keratoses,** wrinkles, the use of makeup, and the extent of the acne scarring.

Glogau classification of aging analysis
A system of aging analysis that calculates the degree of aging-related damage and assigning a numeric typing. The Glogau classification considers both intrinsic and extrinsic aging.

keratoses
Horny growths on the skin.

Table 5–7	Glogau Classification	
Damage	**Description**	**Characteristics**
Level one (mild)	"No wrinkles"	Early photoaging
		‣ Mild pigmentary changes
		‣ No keratoses
		‣ Minimal wrinkles
		Patient age: 20s or 30s
		‣ Minimal or no makeup
		‣ Minimal acne scars

Continued

Table 5–7 Glogau Classification—*cont'd*

Damage	Description	Characteristics
Level two (moderate)	"Wrinkles in motion"	Early to moderate photoaging ‣ Early senile lentigines are visible ‣ Keratoses palpable but not visible ‣ Parallel smile lines beginning to appear Patient age: 30s–40s ‣ Some foundation usually worn ‣ Mild acne scarring
Level three (advanced)	"Wrinkles at rest"	Advanced photoaging ‣ Obvious dyschromia, telangiectasia ‣ Visible keratoses ‣ Wrinkles present even when not moving Patient age: 50s or older ‣ Heavier foundation always worn ‣ Acne scarring present that makeup does not always cover
Level four (severe)	"Only wrinkles"	Severe photoaging ‣ Yellow/gray skin color ‣ Prior skin malignancies ‣ Wrinkles throughout; no normal skin Patient age: 60s–70s ‣ Makeup cannot be worn because it cakes and cracks ‣ Severe acne scarring

The Glogau classification is an aging classification used to determine the *past history* of the skin. This classification deals with the appearance of the skin involving both intrinsic aging and extrinsic aging history. Using all of the variables, we end up with four levels of aging. This system can be a little more confusing compared with Fitzpatrick skin typing. Let us therefore talk about the specific categories (Table 5–7).

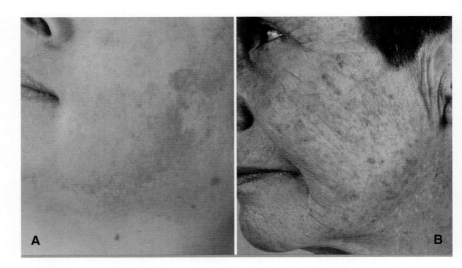

Figure 5–5 *A*, Melasma is a pigment change often thought of as "pregnancy mask." *B*, Solar damage is a pigment change associated with sunlight damage.

Pigment Changes

Pigment changes are those related to sunlight exposure and aging skin (Figure 5–5, *A*). As we know, when the skin is exposed to sunlight, pigment changes are likely. These changes will present as freckles, lentigines, and telangiectasia. Some pigment changes, however, are secondarily related to sunlight and primarily related to medication or pregnancy (Figure 5–5, *B*). The origin of the pigment change is not specifically noted in the classification. If you are using this classification, you will want to note the origin of the dyschromia. In a more subtle way, pigment will also refer to the dull, sallow appearance of the skin that is created over time.

Keratoses

actinic keratoses
Precancerous lesions of the skin, generally from sunlight exposure.

Keratoses are different than pigment changes. Keratoses relate to the skin's response to sunlight by the formation of rough, red, scaling patches. As we know, keratoses can become **actinic keratoses**. Actinic keratoses are sometimes called *precancerous* skin lesions and may develop into skin cancers, specifically basal cell carcinomas and squamous cell carcinomas (Figure 5–6). The number and location of keratoses are important in the aging analysis of the skin. Additionally, we will be interested in the number of previous skin cancers or the suspicion of current skin cancers and their location.

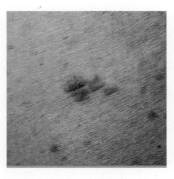

Figure 5–6 Keratoses can be forerunners to basal cell and squamous cell carcinomas.

Wrinkles

In this category, we will be interested to know the number of wrinkles present and in which areas of the face these wrinkles are located. The

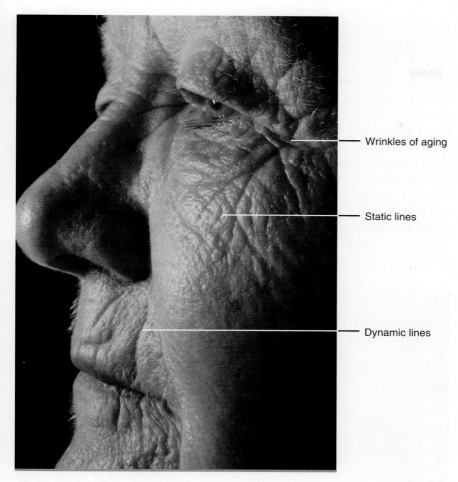

Wrinkles of aging

Static lines

Dynamic lines

Figure 5–7 Wrinkles are most often associated with photo damage. This example of wrinkles includes static and dynamic wrinkles from aging and solar damage.

Glogau classification specifically speaks to the following categories as level one: no wrinkles; level two: wrinkles in motion; level three: wrinkles at rest; and level four: only wrinkles. We will also want to advance our analysis and evaluate whether the wrinkles are fine or coarse (Figure 5–7).

Patient's Chronologic Age

This classification uses the age brackets of 20 to 30 for level one, 30 to 40 for level two, 50 to 60 for level three, and 60 to 70 for level four. The ages represent the patient's actual age, not the age that they appear to be.

Makeup

This category is a tough one within the classification because it is not related to aging, intrinsic or extrinsic. Nevertheless, the Glogau aging classification uses this category. The analysis assumes that more makeup is used as the patient grows chronologically older. As we know, makeup use is a personal choice, whether you are 20 or 70 years of age.

Acne Scarring

The category of acne scars can also be misleading. It assumes everyone has had acne and that the scars get worse as we age. Once again, it is a category within this classification for use (Figure 5–8).

Based on the criteria mentioned, finding fault in its criteria is not difficult. Obviously, too many variables and determining factors exist that may be cultural in nature, having little or nothing to do with photo-damage. For instance, implying that everyone has acne scarring or that

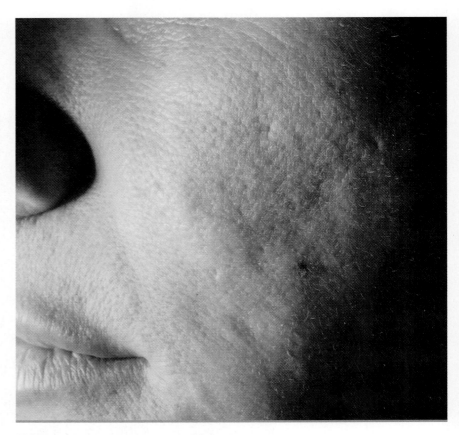

Figure 5–8 Acne scarring in this case will worsen with time as the skin becomes more lax.

makeup gets heavier with age is a generalization. Nonetheless, the majority of the criteria have enough merit to make it worth mentioning. However, it is not the preferred method.

Rubin Classification

The **Rubin classification of aging analysis** is simpler in scope because *actinic keratoses* places emphasis exclusively on aging associated with photodamage (Table 5–8). This feature has great value to you as a clinician. Theorized by Dr. Mark Rubin, the analysis classifies according to "the level of photodamage based on the histologic depth of visible clinical changes."[6] The categories that Rubin uses are pigment changes, texture changes, and wrinkling. This theory of aging analysis helps us understand how *tough* the skin has become based on environmental

Rubin classification of aging analysis
A system of aging analysis that calculates the degree of photodamage and assigns a numerical level. The Rubin classification considers only extrinsic aging.

Table 5–8   Rubin Method of Photodamage Classification

Level	Clinical Signs	Abnormalities	Explanation
Level one (least severe) (Figure 5–9 on page 134)	Alterations in the epidermis only	Pigmentation and texture (freckles, lentigines, a dull rough texture resulting from increased thickness of the stratum corneum)	Freckles, perhaps some lentigines, beginning of a thicker stratum corneum; rarely have wrinkles. We do not define a chronologic age for these patients because this patient can be 20 years of age, or he or she might be 45 years of age, depending on the amount of sunlight exposure.
Level two (more severe) (Figure 5–10 on page 135)	Alterations in the epidermis and papillary dermis	Same as those with level one damage; however, pigmentary and texture charges are more marked. In addition, patients may have actinic keratoses, liver spotting, and definite increase in wrinkling.	In addition to freckles and lentigines, marked change in irregularity of the skin color are present. The stratum corneum is thicker and more irregular. More wrinkles can be found around the eyes and in the naso-labial fold (smile line). Skin will begin to look "crinkled" at this level.
Level three (most severe) (Figure 5–11 on page 136)	Alterations in the epidermis, papillary dermis, and reticular dermis	Same as those with level one and level two damage in addition to a thick leathery appearance and feel, a yellowish tint, and a pebbly texture and open comedones	The skin is wrinkled at rest; many dyschromias are present. The skin is thick and leathery in appearance and to the touch. Yellow, dull, sometimes gray-colored skin. The histologic changes in this category penetrate to the reticular dermis. Solar damage has some open comedones.

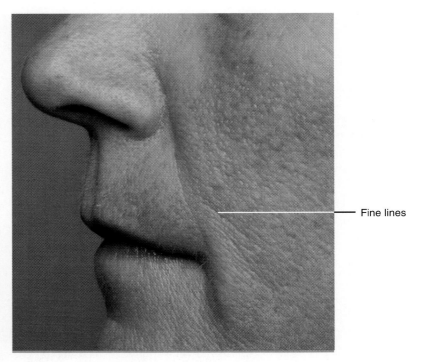

Fine lines

Figure 5-9   Rubin classification for aging level one (see Table 5-8).

Dr. Mark Rubin has been lecturing on cosmetic dermatology and skin rejuvenation at the University of California at San Diego for over 13 years. In addition, he conducts workshops around the country on matters such as cosmetic peeling for physicians. Dr. Rubin has personally trained over 700 physicians from several countries on his techniques for skin rejuvenation. His work has been published in books and medical journals. Currently, he is conducting research at the Lasky Clinic in Beverly Hills on the subjects of chemical peels and laser resurfacing. He is also a diplomat of the American Board of Dermatology and the National Board of Medical Examiners.

First impressions are lasting impressions. Use your knowledge and skills to make your first impression a good one.

damage only. For persons who say their tan is worth the damage, the Rubin classification will prove most useful.

Pigment

Pigment is evaluated in all three categories of the Rubin classification. We know that, as the skin ages, changes in pigment also take place. The Rubin classification analyzes pigment changes that are related to solar damage as opposed to those created by pregnancy, for example. Included in the analysis of the pigment are freckles and lentigines. Sometimes, if the patient is older, the lentigines will be referred to as senile lentigines.

Texture

Texture is a strong marker for the condition of the skin. Evaluation using adjectives such as dull, rough, leathery, and pebbly help us classify the patient into the correct category.

Wrinkling

You now know wrinkling may be static or dynamic, as well as fine, moderate, or coarse. The wrinkling in the Rubin classification is not this detailed.

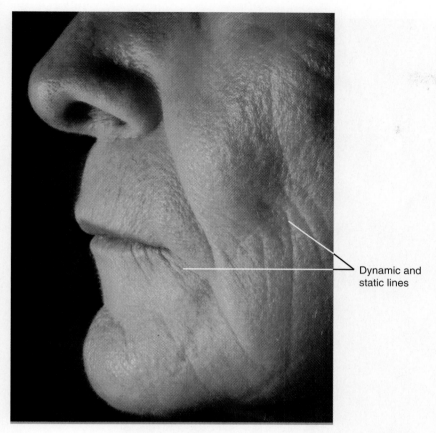

Dynamic and
static lines

Figure 5–10   Rubin classification for aging level two (see Table 5–8).

The classification simply acknowledges that wrinkles exist and gives us the location of the wrinkle. Importantly, you need to take your analysis one step further and define the wrinkles into more detailed categories.

This aging system, when used in concert with Fitzpatrick skin typing, will most effectively evaluate the client's likely response to the appropriate treatment modality, with minimal risks and reliable outcomes.

■ PRACTICAL APPLICATION: CONSULTATION

In most businesses, particularly in the medical and luxury spa businesses, your success will be driven by the **impressions** people have of you and the aesthetic industry. The medical and luxury spa businesses are **image businesses**. The first impression a new patient has of your

impression
A lasting opinion or judgment of something.

image business
The type of business in which the way the public views the company is based largely on how things look—or how they are perceived—more than actual performance.

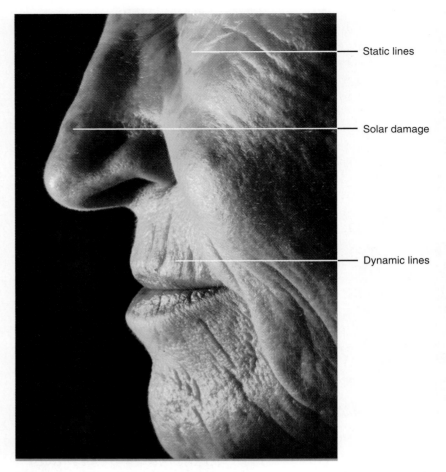

Figure 5–11   Rubin classification for aging level three (see Table 5–8).

office and your expertise is based in part on the cleanliness of the office, the knowledge and friendliness of the staff, and last but certainly not least, your appearance. In the **consultation** or treatment room, patients' ability to listen and hear our information is affected by how comfortable they feel. That *comfort zone* includes how *medicinal* the room appears (this can be intimidating), the seating arrangement, and your professionalism. Professionalism relates to your appearance, knowledge, and command of language. Mastering the skills of friendliness, cleanliness, comfort, professionalism, and communication can influence the patient's first and lasting impressions. Furthermore, the **perception** the patient has of you is one that extends to your physician and his or her partners. The impression the patient has of you and the facility will determine trust, which is the foundation of any relationship.

On the surface, the objective of the consultation is to determine the patient's candidacy for a particular procedure, for example, a glycolic acid peel. Simplifying the objective to a concern only for collecting our information occludes concern for the patient's concerns or fears. Instead, the focus of the consultation should be on building a relationship. For a consultative process to be mutually successful, the patient must be able to communicate his or her fears, concerns, and objectives for the treatment in a safe and trusting environment. Many individuals are nervous when seeking our services. They have concerns of vanity, costs, and scarring. Your success and ultimately that of the patient will be determined by how well you address the concerns and put the patient at ease.

The true mutual objective between patient and clinician is this: improving the patient's appearance. The patient came to you because he or she has a *need* to look better. You are in your position because, through your education and experience, you can *fulfill* that need.

It is important for you to understand your patient, their health history, and their motivations before making any substantive recommendations in consultation.

The **patient information (PI) sheet** is the document that includes all of the social information, e-mail address, and referral sources. This document has a wealth of information: it tells us where the client lives, where the client works (or does not work), if the client is married or has a partner, and what the client's interests are in our business.

The **health history sheet** covers the patient's health. It will address the current chronic or acute diseases, medications that the client may take, and physicians that the client sees. This information will help the clinician determine whether the patient is a candidate for chemical peeling.

The **skin history sheet** compiles a history of the skin conditions, skin treatments, and the products the patient is currently using. It will also have information such as previous product use and skin sensitivities, if any. You will also want this sheet to show information on services the patient has had and the responses to these services.

The **Help Us Understand You sheet** is a communication tool and evaluation tool. The questions on this sheet ask the patient to grade his or her knowledge, communication style, and preferences for skin care. This important tool will help you guide and direct the conversations and educate you in ways to which your patient will be more receptive.

Greeting the Client

The paperwork is finished, and the client is anxious to meet you. This meeting is your opportunity to make a positive, lasting impression

> Think of the consultation process as a *scavenger hunt* for information, and remember, no scavenger hunt is ever the same. Therefore no consultation will ever be the same.

> Aside from the required medical information, the consultation is also a good opportunity to collect other information that will help you better serve the client. To achieve this end, employ several different fact-finding tactics, including a traditional patient information sheet, a health history sheet, a skin history sheet, and the Help Us Understand You sheet.

patient information (PI) sheet
A document used by medical professionals to gather social, personal, and demographic information.

health history sheet
A document used by medical professionals to gather information on past and present health conditions, as well as likelihood for future conditions. This information includes allergies, medical conditions, and prescription information.

skin history sheet
A document used by skin-care professionals to provide information on a client's past and present skin health, including past treatment, sunburns, and conditions that are necessary for treatment.

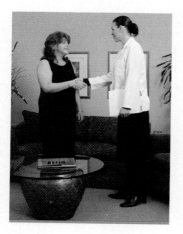

Figure 5–12 The patient greeting is your best opportunity to make a positive lasting impression.

The first time you *meet* a client may be on the telephone. Patients often want to know the answers to questions such as, "How many treatments will it take?" "What products are best for me?" "Will lactic acid work for me?" Obviously, these questions require a face-to-face consultation. Setting an appointment should be the objective of the telephone interview.

(Figure 5–12). Respect for the patient should be your first objective. Always take a quick peek in the mirror before you meet someone new: make sure your hair is neat, your face is clean, and your makeup is evenly applied. When you first make contact with the client, you should introduce yourself and then ask how he or she prefers to be addressed. The conversation should begin with, "Hello, Mrs. Smith. My name is Susan. It is a pleasure to meet you. Do you prefer Mrs. Smith or Lorraine?" The client's preference should be documented in the chart. Remember that the medical office can be a frightening place for many people, even if they are coming in for exciting procedures. Take care to explain the physical layout of the facility: restroom location, which treatment or consultation room you will be using today, and how to exit the facility. A simple tour always helps people feel more at ease and more excited.

Taking a History

Among the assorted documents to be completed by new clients on their first visit will be the *skin history sheet* and the *health history sheet*. Although these two documents sound similar in nature, both will offer you detailed and specific information that is a critical aspect of your responsibilities. These documents are often completed rather quickly and thoughtlessly. As a professional tending to the medical and aesthetic needs of your client, ensuring that the documents are complete and intelligible is ultimately your responsibility.

The skin history sheet is a detailed questionnaire about the patient's skin. You will want to ask questions in the survey that include the past skin health and current skin health. Some of the specific items you will want to know are past and current tanning habits, including sunburns (as a child and as an adult), skin cancer diagnoses, and locations of skin cancers. Additionally, ask the client about moles or lesions that are of concern to the patient, including their location. Information regarding past and current acne concerns, including the medications used (both oral and topical), is vital. You must also be aware of previous skin treatments, x-ray treatments for acne, and UVA (PUVA) treatments for psoriasis, as well as the usual spa treatments such as facials and body treatments and any problems associated with such treatments. You may want to consider using the Fitzpatrick skin typing questionnaires presented earlier to make this information inclusive and complete. Finally, you will want to ask the client about basics such as skin condition (oily, dry, normal, sensitive, combination) and skin type. This document will help you fully understand the patient's overall skin health. It will also give you a clearer history, not just what the patient chooses to tell you verbally.

The *skin history sheet* can also help you understand the segments of your practice. For example, how many patients do you see have had a skin cancer? How many patients do you see with acne? How many patients do you see who tan? Some of this information would be valuable to your marketing department and possible future promotional campaigns.

Make sure that the client completely fills out the health and skin history sheet. This time is a great point to start the conversation. "Mrs. Smith, I am going to take a moment and acquaint myself with your history. Please bare with me a moment while I become familiar with your history." Take a moment and look through the information that the patient has provided, and ask relevant questions to fill in the areas that are incomplete. An incomplete area usually means that the answer to the question is "no"; but sometimes it might mean that the patient did not want to give the information or it was unintentionally skipped. Do not leave any blanks. Ask the patient to finish filling out the document if an area is incomplete. Be sure you review both the health history and the skin history sheets. Add anything relevant as you go through the documents with the client. Make notes on your consultation sheet, not on the documents that the patient filled out. Take this part of the consultation seriously, and make notes that will help you help the patient.

Because people generally like to talk about themselves, and this situation is no different, reviewing this form is a good place to build rapport with a patient. Use this opportunity as an icebreaker to get to know the patient. If your patient is shy or embarrassed, using this technique will help him or her get comfortable with you and the informational exchange. If you review this document in advance of seeing the patient in the treatment room, you lose this momentum.

The *health history sheet* asks about detailed health status. This questionnaire delves into the past and current health of your patient. Included on this document are questions regarding allergies, current and past illness, smoking status, pregnancy status, daily medications, and past surgical events. The objective of the health history is to obtain a detailed "snap shot" of the client's health without spending a lot of time. This form should be set up in a check-box format. Although the client may think that some of the health items are irrelevant, the questions may be important in delivering care, and all boxes should be checked "yes" or "no."

Knowing the medications that the patient is taking is an important step in the long-term result. This information includes regular medications such as birth control pills or antibiotics such as tetracycline. These medications, as well as others, can affect the pigment of the skin. Another important group of medications are those that make the skin sunlight sensitive. You will want to be sure to educate your patient about this group of medications.

A history of herpes simplex is critical for the clinician to know, given that glycolic acid (or any peel for that matter) can stimulate an eruption of a lesion. Medications to control the outbreak of herpes simplex (cold sores) should be a required part of the peel protocol for patients who are susceptible to developing an outbreak.

Health History Updates

Regularly inquire about any changes in patients' health, and update the written documentation yearly. Relevant changes to the client's health include medication changes, new diseases or illnesses, and surgeries and treatments. Updates can be extraordinarily important. Take the example of a client recently diagnosed with breast cancer or diabetes. Health status changes should give the clinician pause in the skin-care setting. Does this new information require an updated consultation, evaluation, and examination? The answer should be "yes." Does the new health status demand a new home program and reevaluation of the treatment plan? Health changes do not mean the client must forego his or her skin care program; in fact, treatments and at-home care may be an important part of the client's emotional healing as he or she copes with the disease. However, for patient safety, the plan needs review.

> Even the slightest or seemingly innocuous changes to the client's health can be extraordinarily important. Updates might include medication or dosage changes, new illness diagnoses, and surgeries and treatments.

Applying Skin Typing and Aging Analysis to Conduct a Skin Analysis

A skin analysis is performed to evaluate the skin condition and determine the skin type and aging analysis. These indicators are important in helping you determine a clinical program that will be best for the client (Figure 5–13). Before beginning, have the client change into a wrap or

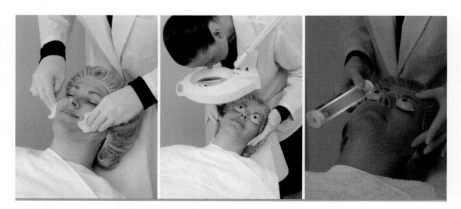

Figure 5–13   Proper analysis of the skin is critical to the success of a peel treatment.

gown, which will allow you a better chance to evaluate the chest and cleanse the face without fear of soiling the client's clothing. With the client changed into a wrap, you will also be able to observe, analyze, and photograph the chest, arms, and hands. This skin analysis is a standardized process, but for review, let us go through the steps.

Step One: Cleanse

Once the client has changed clothes and is made comfortable on the bed, cover the hair with a surgical bonnet or a headband. Using soft gauze or disposable sponge, gently cleanse the face using a mild cleanser and pat dry. Be sure to *gently* cleanse the skin. Our objective is to take off the makeup but not to stimulate the skin. If the skin is overstimulated, observing for skin irregularities such as telangiectasis, for example, will be difficult (Table 5–9).

Step Two: Evaluate Skin Type and Conduct an Aging Analysis

Use a loupe or magnification light to observe the skin. You are looking for hyperpigmentation, telangiectasis, clogged pores, and scars. On a more subjective level, you are evaluating the skin texture and tone, in other words, aging. Take note of the skin's sensitivity; for example, did it turn pink during cleansing? Discuss now any potential areas of concern that were missed in the initial discussion. Hand the patient a mirror, and point out your concerns. Ask the client's opinion.

At first, skin typing and analysis seem straightforward and easy to do. The categories are clear, and the idea of using the definitions to categorize patients seems simple. However, now welcome to reality;

Table 5–9 Skin Analysis	
1. Clean the face	Removal of makeup and debris allows you to see clearly what lies underneath, with minimal obstructions.
2. Analyze and evaluate using Fitzpatrick and Rubin classifications	Use good lighting, magnification, and observation to acquaint yourself with the patient's skin with as much detail as possible.
3. Document	Thorough record keeping will not only include what you see presenting, but also even the smallest details, such as water temperature during cleansing.

nothing is as it appears. How do you put the Fitzpatrick typing scale and one of the aging classifications together and have an understanding of the skin? To understand this process more clearly, let us examine how these classifications will be used in the clinical environment.

A **Wood's lamp** should be used to evaluate the depth of the hyper-pigmentation at this time. Using a Wood's lamp is simple and will take only a couple of extra minutes. Cover the patient's eyes with cotton pads or plastic eye covers. Dim the overhead lights, and turn on the Wood's lamp. Hold the device close to the skin, but avoid touching the skin because it will burn the patient. Then, evaluate the skin conditions you see. Be sure to make a note on the chart.

Using Fitzpatrick skin typing

Now that you have collected all of the information, let us make an analysis of the Fitzpatrick skin type selection by using the following specific definitions. Your determination is based on what you see, the ethnic heritage (geographic origin of forbearers), eye color, and response to UV light. You should also factor in hair color if it is the natural color. The natural tendency is to evaluate primarily skin color when we are typing the skin. Teach yourself to look at all of the characteristics associated with the Fitzpatrick typing chart. The more difficult skins to type will be differentiated by the details of eye color and the skin's response to sunlight (especially as a child).

Using the Glogau classification

Applying the Glogau classification can seem challenging for both the beginner and the advanced clinicians. The first question to ask when using this classification is, "What is my objective?" Within the classification system are multiple objectives, among them evaluation of acne scarring, wrinkling, and solar damage, each one representing a different problem. The numeric type uses two descriptors, one for degree of damage *(mild, moderate, advanced, and severe)* and one specific to wrinkling *(no wrinkling, wrinkles in motion, wrinkles at rest, only wrinkles)*. If you are evaluating the client for a peeling program, your approach might be somewhat different based on the classification you choose. Therefore, if you choose to use this classification, you will need to select the outstanding problem and classify it accordingly. For example, if the client's complaint is aging skin, select only the categories that apply, such as pigment changes, keratoses, wrinkling, and chronologic aging. Your client will be classified by the numeric type that most resembles his or her characteristics, regardless of the other characteristics associated with that typing. In other words, if *moderate* acne scarring is the primary concern, the patient would still be a type II, regardless of smile lines or makeup use.

Wood's lamp
A device that uses UV rays to detect fluorescent material in the skin, which are indicative of certain diseases or conditions.

Interpreting the Wood's lamp information can be challenging. Take these few simple cues to make it easier:
Blue-white spots: normal and healthy skin
White spots: horny layer of the skin (dead skin cells)
Purple fluorescent areas: thin, dehydrated skin
Light-violet areas: dry skin
Bright fluorescent areas: hydrated skin
Orange or coral areas: oily areas of the skin and comedones (seborrhea)
Brown areas: areas of pigmentation—troubles and dark spots

The Fitzpatrick skin typing system has six categories. Your determination is based on what you see and the questions you ask.

Now that you understand the specifics of the categories, let us use some examples. A 40-year-old woman who exhibits yellow, graying skin with actinic keratoses, has not had any skin cancers, and wears little or no makeup would be classified as type III. The overwhelming descriptor that puts her into the type III would be the lack of skin cancers. Let us try a second example: a 35-year-old woman with severe acne scars, visible dyschromias, wears heavy makeup, and has not had any keratoses or skin cancers. This case is a tough one. Does she belong in type II, type III, or type IV? If we let the acne scars be the descriptor, then she belongs in type IV; if we let the solar damage drive the descriptor, we put her into type II. Choose the overriding characteristic, and use it to determine the use of this classification.

Using the Rubin classification

The Rubin classification is easy to apply in practice. With only three specific definitions, and less crossing over between them, patients easily fit into a sensible category. Remember, this classification relates only to extrinsic aging patterns. Depending on the patient and his or her objectives, you might need to create an intrinsic aging analysis for accuracy.

When you are evaluating the patient, use the three categories of texture, pigment, and wrinkling. For example, a woman with mild wrinkling around the eyes and freckles, as well as general dyschromia, will be at level two.

Step Three: Document

Now the time has come for you to document your findings. Documentation is always an important step in any stage of a treatment program. However, it is crucial during the initial consultation. Therefore you would be ill advised to document only the problem areas that have compelled the patient to seek your advice. To this effect, a general rule for documentation is you can never have too much information, especially if a dispute should become litigious. Note the specifics of your findings in the clinical chart. For example, if scars are present, where are they and how large are they? If the patient can elaborate on the history of the scar, document that as well. If an area of hyperpigmentation is seen, note its location and color. Make notes about the skin's texture and tone by describing its appearance. For example, "The skin appears to have solar damage at the lateral jaw line exhibited by *static lines* and roughness." Be sure to note the skin type and condition. If your documentation papers allow for a picture of the face, mark your findings on the picture and make text notes as well. Additionally, record any information that the patient volunteers. Any information that you can put on the form will help you over time with achieving successful treatment results and equally in your own career. Accurate and reliable documentation also has to be noticeable in the next step, photographs.

Taking photographs

Taking **photographs** is perhaps the most overlooked but most important part of patient care. Photographs record how the client appeared on the first visit. Most of the time, we cannot recall with accuracy or clarity exactly how the patient appeared at the beginning of the treatment. After two to four treatments, we often find ourselves raving about the results. The photograph tells the real story. Photographs also may protect us from potential litigation.

A digital photography system with computer storage and color print out is an ideal setup; if not, a sophisticated color Polaroid camera will work just fine.

To ensure the accuracy and consistency in photography, a policy and procedure should be developed. The policy and procedure should include information on *camera specifics, care and maintenance of the camera, flash and lighting techniques, focusing and framing the shot, ensuring accurate photographs, and troubleshooting the camera.*

A Word on Home Care

Home care is an integral component of peeling success. The retinoids and alpha hydroxy acids that are used at home help the skin readily accept the peeling solution in the clinic. Once the peel is complete, the home products penetrate evenly and are more effective. Obviously, sunscreen is part of the daily home-care routine. Makeup should also be considered. Does your patient wear foundation or powder makeup now? Does she want to continue to wear that makeup? How much makeup does she wear? All of these questions should be answered and considered. If the patient is in your chair to improve her skin, the idea of changing or decreasing her makeup should be part of the conversation. If your clinic has a dedicated makeup artist, encourage the patient to have a conversation with this person to evaluate opportunities to update her look and allow her "new skin" to shine through.

■ SELECTING PEEL CANDIDATES

Not every aging or photo-damaged skin problem that is presented to you will be solved with the use of a chemical peeling agent. Similarly, not all acne problems are appropriate for peeling. Therefore what then determines the selection process? Who will be treated and who will not be treated? Aside from the actual indications themselves, a process exists

---

photographs
The reproduction of an image on film. A necessary component of skin-care treatment program that accurately documents the original skin condition so as to prove or disclaim treatment results.

to determine if your patient is a candidate for peeling. The selection process is directly related to the skin condition, skin type, and aging analysis. This process is one that we discussed earlier in this chapter, but we will review and apply specifically to peeling.

Remember that the patient's skin condition (normal, dry, combination, oily and acne prone, or sensitive) should first be determined. If the patient's skin is sensitive, he or she will be immediately eliminated. All other skin conditions move to the next step, which is Fitzpatrick skin typing. Although different peel solutions will work well on different skin types, the preferred skin types are I, II, and III. These skin types have a better response to peeling agents and generally improve more quickly compared with other skin types. Last is the aging analysis determination. Using the Rubin classification of photodamage, we will prefer the candidates to be in level one and two. Those with type III need a more aggressive peel to achieve meaningful results. Regarding acne, superficial peeling is most effective on grades 1 and 2 acne (discussed in Chapter 6). Patients with greater than 25 lesions are candidates for other treatment modalities.

Finally, the issue of realistic expectations must be addressed. Although peels are popular, the caveat must be realistic expectations. Most agents do a good job improving the quality of the skin, but in many cases, lines and wrinkles simply cannot be minimized or eliminated with *repetitive light peels*. Therefore, if the patient is outside the "bull's eye" of the selection process but desires to improve the quality of the skin, color, and texture, glycolic acid will do the job. If, on the other hand, the patient has the desire to *eliminate* lines or wrinkles, another type of treatment will be in order.

Selection Criteria

The selection criterion for chemical peeling is addressed through the patient complaint or indication, the skin typing and aging analysis, the skin condition, and finally the available peeling agents. The best place to start is at the beginning: the indications. For ease of discussion, let us put indications into three basic categories: aging, solar damage, and acne. The next step in the selection process is going to be identified through our skin analysis: skin condition, Fitzpatrick skin typing, and Rubin aging analysis. Finally, based on the other information that has been collected, a peel solution can now be selected. The peel depths that respond to the specific solutions that we will be discussing fall into four categories. The categories are **very superficial peels** (glycolic acid and designer peels), **superficial peels** (glycolic and salicylic acids and Jessner's solution) **moderate peels** (TCA), and **deep peels** (phenol and pyruvic acid).

Listen to patients and their desires. If they are looking to improve fine lines, even the color, and improve the skin tone, chemical peels are a beneficial treatment.

very superficial peels
A peel depth that does not achieve erythema or flaking and thus is ineffective.

superficial peels
A peel depth that extends into the stratum granulosum.

moderate peels
A peel depth extending into the papillary dermis.

deep peels
A peel depth extending into the papillary dermis or upper reticular dermis. Most notable of deep peels are phenol.

Table 5–10   Indications and Peeling Agents
Lines and Wrinkles
Irregular texture
Dyschromias
Mild acne

Many peeling agents will be in your armamentarium, including glycolic acid, salicylic acid, Jessner's solution, TCA, and designer peeling options. The use of each of these agents (except deep-peeling agents) will be covered in detail later in the text; for a moment, then, let us consider the indications and contraindications for using peel agents.

seborrheic keratoses
A benign skin tumor common in older adults, thought to develop from prolific epidermal cells.

Indications for Peel Treatments

Indications are the conditions for which peels will be effective, assuming the selection process has been accurate. The indications for peeling are lines and wrinkles, irregular texture, dyschromias, and mild acne. Lines associated with Rubin level one and two aging are most appropriate for peeling. Irregular texture is usually epidermal in nature when found in Rubin level one and two but may extend into the papillary dermis. The uneven texture is associated with solar damage and can include mild actinic keratoses, **seborrheic keratoses,** and lentigines. Dyschromia or pigment changes associated with solar damage are evident in level one and two. Because these pigment problems are mainly in the epidermis (especially with Rubin level one), they will respond nicely to superficial peeling. Superficial peeling also works well on mild acne. The process helps exfoliate the surface, removing debris that might otherwise find its way into the sebum and pores. The slightly deeper lines and solar damage associated with Rubin level two will need attention with a moderate peeling agent such as TCA (Table 5–10).

Contraindications for Peel Treatments

Contraindications are conditions that eliminate peeling from the list of possible treatments. On the standardized list of peel contraindications are sunburn, active facial rashes, active herpes simplex (cold sore), open lesions of the face, immediate post-facelift or facial surgery, and current use of Accutane. Additional consideration should be given to pregnant and lactating women, patients suspected of body dysmorphic disorder, and grade 3 acne (Table 5–11).

Table 5–11   Contraindications for Peel Treatments
Sunburn
Active facial rashes
Active herpes simplex (cold sore)
Open lesions of the face
Immediate post-facelift or facial surgery
Current use of Accutane

Evaluation and Correction of Client Expectations

Obviously, setting expectations is part of the consultation process. However, exactly what are realistic expectations for glycolic peeling? Several points need to be discussed with the patient before beginning a peel program. The discussion points should include the improvement possibilities, the repetitive nature of the treatment, the possible downtime, and the importance of home care.

The improvement possibilities should be discussed in concert with the patient's desires. Letting patients know that you might not be able to achieve the result they are seeking is acceptable. This approach is much better than overpromising and underachieving.

Some patients become discouraged with the bi-weekly or monthly visits to the clinic. The patient must be educated about the skin: the monthly turnover of cells and the need for regular stimulation to keep the skin looking good. Monthly visits to the clinic have to become part of the patient's routine, just as is getting hair coloring or waxing. Use the example of exercise. Regular exercise will get the body in great shape, but failure to continue will lead the body to deteriorate the improvement. The skin is much the same.

Times will occur when the results of a peel are more than you anticipated. The dryness of a patient's skin or overuse of home-care products can cause a peel to take up faster than you anticipated. Whatever the reason, the peel will cause the patient a little downtime. Sometimes, this condition will appear as "rug-burns"; other times, it is just excessive "facial dandruff." The patient needs to be educated about this possibility in advance, so when it happens (and it will happen), you can remind him or her of the conversation and help the patient get through this short period of inconvenience.

Using home-care products is just as important as is the peeling process. The products that are used at home help the peeling agent to penetrate and the skin to improve. Persons who do not use a therapeutic home-care program including Retin A® and hydroquinone are not getting the full benefit of the glycolic peel.

Examples

Let us take the time to explore our knowledge. The following examples give you a photograph and the details of the individual's sun history and skin-care regimen. Read through the examples and try to determine the skin type. Additionally, do an aging analysis. Finally, decide which peel treatment might work best for this candidate and explain why.

Example #1

Jill is a 50-year-old mother who spent her early years in the sun (Figure 5–14). She comes to the office today seeking a consultation for her skin and options for improvement. She is concerned about her crow's feet and the deep lines around her mouth. While you note the crow's feet and naso-labial lines (smile lines) around the mouth, you also notice other areas of aging. On examination, you note that she has extensive telangiectasia across her cheeks and around the nose. At the forehead, she has a scar from an excision of basal cell carcinoma. Her eyes are blue-green, and her hair is reddish brown. She states that she will burn almost immediately if she is in the sun without sunscreen, but since the basal cell carcinoma, she wears sunscreen everyday. Although she has crow's feet, you also notice that she has fine lines on the cheeks and lines of expression on the forehead. Her solar damage presents in fine lines, loose skin, and a very irregular texture. What Fitzpatrick skin type is she? What is her Rubin and Glogau classification? What home-care products will have the greatest impact on her appearance?

Example #2

Janet is a 45-year-old mother of three (Figure 5–15). She had a facelift and eyelid lift 2 weeks ago. The purpose of her visit today is postsurgical skin care. Her eyes are still swollen from the surgery, and the sides of her face are swollen as well, most notably on her earlobes. Her current healing phase should influence the decision of the type of care she will receive in the beginning. She has brown eyes and brown hair and rarely burns in the sun. She usually tans deeply, without much attention to her skin. She had lots of little fine lines around the sides of her face, before the lift. These lines are not apparent now. She also had crow's feet before the surgery, opting many times for Botox® treatments. She spends time outside playing tennis in the summer. She also hikes in the mountains when she gets the chance. She wants to sustain the facelift result, but she does not want to give a lot of time and effort to the

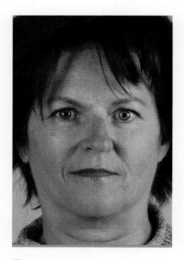

Figure 5–14
Example #1—Jill.

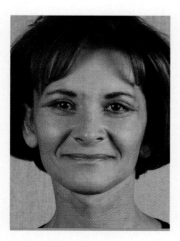

Figure 5–15
Example #2—Janet.

process. What Fitzpatrick skin type is she? What Rubin or Glogau classification is she? What is the best home-care program for her today? What is the best long-term program for her?

Example #3

Joe is a 25-year-old student with brown hair and brown eyes but has a tendency to burn quickly in the sun (Figure 5–16). He has grade 1 acne and is a picker. He has grown a beard to cover some of the breakouts that occur in that area. When he is studying at school or is stressed with finals, he breaks out more frequently and with larger pustules. He does absolutely nothing for his skin right now, but his girlfriend has encouraged him to seek your help. What is his Fitzpatrick type? What is his Rubin or Glogau aging analysis?

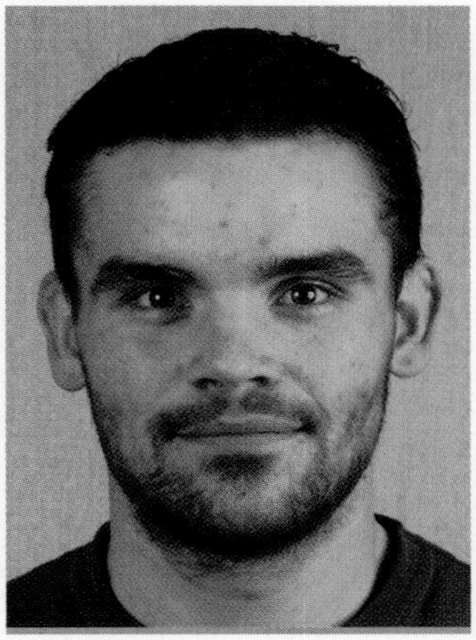

Figure 5–16
Example #3—Joe.

Conclusion

Now we understand the method by which all medical professionals collect information about the skin's color, aging, and condition. Our own analysis will help us choose our peel patients wisely. The skin color analysis tells us who will tolerate and benefit not only from superficial treatments, but also from moderate treatments. We also must determine which patient tans and how much time they normally spend in the sun, an important part of the compliance component of medical skin care treatments.

Patients in the deeper aging categories (level two+) have problems that are going to be successful based primarily on the strength of the particular peel solution selected. These patients should be advised that the outcome is going to be based on the strength of the type of peel solution and the related downtime. Some patients may want the option of minimizing their results because of limited available time.

When we meld the two classifications together—skin color analysis and aging analysis—we can select our peel candidates with ease, knowing that we have an understanding of the predictable outcome. These analyses also help us determine the solution choice and as such create a plan of action that can be shared with the patient. This approach provides a mutually agreed on arrangement that minimizes misunderstandings and improves patient results.

> Patients in the *deeper aging categories* (level two+) have problems that are, for the most part, not going to be *solved* by microdermabrasion. Our choice to treat these patients will come with the caveat of realistic expectations.

> > > **TOP TEN TIPS TO TAKE TO THE CLINIC**

1. The Fitzpatrick skin typing process is a commonly accepted method of measuring the skin's response to UV light.

2. The Fitzpatrick skin typing process can predict the skin's response to chemical peeling, laser treatments, and microdermabrasion.

3. The Fitzpatrick skin typing method should be used on every patient to ensure that the proper treatment plan has been selected.

4. The clinician must inquire about the client's ethnic history and sunlight exposure history to find the right Fitzpatrick assignment.

5. Eye color and natural hair color are indicators for Fitzpatrick assignment.

6. A Glogau classification or a Rubin classification is necessary to complete the client analysis.

7. Melding an aging analysis and a skin typing assessment will determine who is best suited for peel treatments. Usually skin types I, II, and III have the best results with peels.

8. The Rubin classification is easier to use compared with the Glogau classification.

9. Generally, most skin types are "mixed" and require study to ascertain the correct typing.

10. Asking questions about the skins response to sunlight as a child will help determine the accurate skin type.

CHAPTER REVIEW QUESTIONS

1. What is Fitzpatrick skin typing?
2. What is the Glogau aging analysis?
3. What is the Rubin aging analysis?
4. Why do we skin type before chemical peeling?
5. Why do we do an aging analysis before chemical peeling?
6. Does an aging analysis identify chemical peel candidates?
7. What are the most important components of the Rubin aging analysis?
8. What can be the consequences of failing to do skin typing and aging analysis?
9. How do you identify the skin type of someone who is tanned?
10. How do you identify the skin type of someone with colored hair?

CHAPTER REFERENCES

1. Fitzpatrick Skin Typing Chart (part 1: Genetic Disposition). Used with permission of the Medical Procedure Center, P.C., and adapted from multiple sources.

2. Fitzpatrick Skin Typing Chart (part 2: Reaction to Sun Exposure). Used with permission of the Medical Procedure Center, P.C., and adapted from multiple sources.
3. Fitzpatrick Skin Typing Chart (part 3: Tanning Habits). Used with permission of the Medical Procedure Center, P.C., and adapted from multiple sources.
4. Fitzpatrick Skin Typing Chart (part 4: Scoring). Used with permission of the Medical Procedure Center, P.C., and adapted from multiple sources.
5. Fitzpatrick Skin Typing Chart (part 5: Your Fitzpatrick Skin Type). Used with permission of the Medical Procedure Center, P.C., and adapted from multiple sources.
6. Rubin, M. (1995). *Manual of chemical peels*. Lippincott Williams & Wilkins Philadelphia: Lippincott Williams & Wilkins.

BIBLIOGRAPHY

American Society of Plastic Surgeons. (2003, December). *2002 quick facts on cosmetic and reconstructive surgery trends* [Online]. Available: http://www.plasticsurgery.org

APA Optics, Inc. (2004, March 18). *Personal UV monitor* [Online]. Available: www.apaoptics.com

Berryhill, D. (2002, May). *Capturing patients' enthusiasm* [Online]. Available: www.skinandaging.com

Brody, H. J. (1997). *Chemical peeling and resurfacing* (2nd ed.). St. Louis: Mosby.

Coleman, W. P., & Lawrence, N. (Eds.). (1998). *Skin resurfacing*. Baltimore: Williams and Wilkins.

D'Angelo, J., Dean, P., Dietz, S., Hinds, C., Lees, M., Miller, E., et al. (2003). *Milady's standard: Comprehensive training for estheticians*. Clifton Park, NY: Thomson Delmar Learning.

Gail, S. (2003, May 1). *Managing your patients' expectations: A fresh approach* [Online]. Available: www.cosmeticsurgerytimes.com

Gail, S. (2004). *Milady's the clinical esthetician*. Clifton Park, NY: Thomson Delmar Learning.

Genetree. (2004, February 28). *Genetree eye color inheritance chart* [Online]. Available: www.genetree.com

Institute for Medicine, Physics, and Biophysics. (2004, February 27). *Definitions* (Working Group UVR) [Online]. Available: i115srv. uvwein.ac.at

The Lasky Clinic. (2004, March 1). *Mark Rubin, M.D.* [Online]. Available: www.laskyclinic.com

MGH Hotline. (2003, August 22). *In memoriam: Thomas B. Fitzpatrick, M.D., Ph.D.* [Online]. Available: www.mgh.harvard.edu

Parks, J., & Pierce, M. (2002, May). *Effectively treating ethnic skin* [Online]. Available: www.skinandaging.com

Random House Dictionary. (1992). New York: Random House.

Rubin, M. (1995). *Manual of chemical peels: Superficial and medium depth.* Lippincott, Philadelphia: Williams & Wilkins.

San Francisco Dermatology. (2004, March 1). *Richard Glogau, M.D.* [Online]. Available: www.sfderm.com

Science Education Partnership. (2004, February 28). *The genetics of human eye color* [Online]. Available: www.seps.org

Thomas, C. L. (Ed.). (1997). *Taber's cyclopedic medical dictionary* (Vol. 18). Philadelphia: F. A. Davis.

Understanding Chemical Peeling

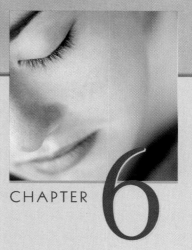

CHAPTER 6

KEY TERMS

atopic dermatitis	flash injuries	rhytids
Baker-Gordon solution	folliculitis	ringworm
blanch	frost	salicylate toxicity
body surface	fungal infection	secondary intention
area (BSA)	glabella	Septisol®
burns	hormone replacement	static rhytids
cautery	therapy	tinea corporis
cellulitis	impetigo	tinnitus
croton oil	malignant	vesiculation
dynamic rhytids	predisposed	yeast infections
etiology	pseudofolliculitis barbae	

LEARNING OBJECTIVES

After completing this chapter you should be able to:

1. Discuss the principles of chemical peeling.
2. Discuss chemical wounding.
3. List the peel solutions.
4. List the contraindications for peels.

INTRODUCTION

Chemical peeling has been used for centuries with only a minimal understanding of the *best* processes, the probable outcomes, and the potential complications. Only recently, as of 1960, has chemical peeling become prominent in plastic surgery literature.[1] In the last 35 years, physicians, both plastic surgeons and dermatologists, began to study and accumulate data that has helped us *really* understand what the chemicals *do* when they are applied to the skin. The studies and the subsequent documentation give us an understanding of the possible effects and potential outcomes of chemical peeling on the skin. The *principles of chemical peeling* are specific concepts associated with controlled skin wounding, the idea that peeling is, in fact, a *controlled burn* of the skin. Chemical peeling principles also include the concepts of peel depth and how the depth of the injury affects the skin and creates the final result. That is to say, a single light peel with light wounding will have a minimal effect compared with a deeper peel creating deeper wounds. Each peeling agent has its advantages and disadvantages; many times, the choice of agent is based simply on the practitioner's preference rather than factual data. Discussions about chemical peeling should include which indications are best suited for particular types of chemical peeling and which conditions are considered contraindications. Among these indications that are especially responsive to chemical rejuvenation are **rhytids** (wrinkles), solar damage, and dyschromias. Conditions that are considered contraindications include excessively sagging skin, postsurgical facelifts, and excessive telangiectasia. A balanced discussion and complete understanding of all the indications and contraindications is required before beginning a career in chemical peeling.

rhytids
The clinical name for wrinkles.

■ PRINCIPLES OF CHEMICAL PEELING

The principles that are to be taken into consideration before peeling the skin are *the skin condition, the skin type, the aging factor,* and *the patient's general health.* These important variables assist the clinician in selecting the proper candidates for peel treatment, as well as the appropriate solution to meet everyone's goal. The *skin condition* includes not only the five definitive categorizations with which we are familiar—normal, dry, oily or acne prone, sensitive, and combination—but also skin problems. Additional descriptors of skin problems are necessary, that is, dyschromias, wrinkles, aging, and acne. This additional descriptor will assist us in determining possible indications and contraindications for the peel.

Remember, indications or contraindications are *conditions* that *are* or *are not* appropriate for chemical peeling. As you consider a patient for treatment, an important step is to determine if the skin conditions you wish to treat will be affected by the peel treatment you choose or, for that matter, by peeling at all. Just as important is the *skin type*. A Fitzpatrick skin typing analysis must be done to determine if the patient is likely to have a positive treatment outcome. Similarly, an aging analysis must be done. The skin typing and age analysis exercise should answer the following questions: will the skin have a propensity for hyperpigmentation, will the skin peel evenly, what chemical will be necessary to achieve the result, and finally, will the skin actually improve? Lastly, and not to be disregarded, is the patient's health status. Unlike a simple microdermabrasion treatment, chemical peels are more likely to be affected by the patient's health status. Because the chemical peel is a *controlled burn*, the clinician must understand the impact of a burn on the body. From your first-aid classes, you might recall the three types of burns: first degree, second degree, and third degree (Table 6–1). Additionally, percentages are assigned to areas of the body to determine the amount of the body that has been burned. For our purposes, we need to review and be aware of both categories (Table 6–2).

The face constitutes approximately 5% of the body surface; therefore a significant insult is applied on the body when a chemical peel is

Table 6–1 Types of Burns

Type of Burn	Appearance	Structures Affected	Usual Cause
First-degree burn	The skin is pink or red and very sensitive.	Epidermis involvement only	Sunburn, chemical peels
Second-degree burn	Skin is red with oozing blisters. The area might **blanch** when touched.	Epidermis and partial dermis involved	**Flash injuries** Chemical peels
Third-degree burn	Skin is leathery, white, black, or red.	Epidermis, dermis, and hypodermis	Burning clothing, house fire

blanch
A rapid loss of coloration.

flash injuries
A tissue injury caused by a sudden and rapid exposure to electricity, heat, cold, or chemicals.

body surface area (BSA)
A term used to represent an amount when calculating the percentage of the body burn.

Body Area	Percentage Based on Body Surface Area (BSA)[2]
Head and neck	9%
Anterior trunk	18%
Posterior trunk	18%
Upper limbs	9% each
Lower limbs	18% each
Genitalia/perineum	1%

Table 6–2   Body Surface Area Percentages for Burns

done, especially if the injury is into the upper papillary dermis. This situation means that the patient needs to be healthy and fully capable of healing the wound. Even patients with a cold or influenza, for example, should not be treated with chemical peeling agents. When peeling the face is combined with peeling the arms and hands, for example, the patient needs to be healthy, and the clinician must have respect for the insult he or she is foisting on the patient.

Patients who should be carefully considered before chemical peeling include patients with diabetes, patients with cancer who are undergoing chemotherapy or radiation, and patients who are taking oral or inhaled steroids. Take a careful health history, and consult your clinic physician if you are concerned about the patient's ability to heal from a chemical peel.

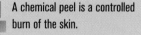

A chemical peel is a controlled burn of the skin.

Controlled Skin Wounding

As previously stated, the process of chemical peeling is a *controlled wounding process;* other controlled wounding processes include carbon dioxide (CO_2) laser or erbium laser. The wounding itself is defined by two components: the type of agent and the depth of the wound. The type of agent defines, in part, the potential of the wound. Chemical wounds are created by different types of chemical peels, such as glycolic acid, Jessner's solution, salicylic acid, trichloroacetic acid (TCA), and designer peels. Each of these products creates a wound depth that is either epidermal or papillary dermal. Wounding is also further delineated by the definitions of superficial, medium, or deep chemical peeling (Table 6–3).

The ability to control the wound is also determined by other factors such as the pretreatment routine, the length of the pretreatment routine,

Table 6–3   Definitions of Peeling Depth

Type of Peel	Depth of Peel	Usual Agents
Superficial peels	Epidermal	Glycolic, salicylic acid, resorcinol, Jessner's solution, 10%-20% TCA
Medium-depth peels	Epidermal into papillary dermis	70% glycolic with 35% TCA, 35% + TCA, Jessner's solution + TCA, erbium lasers
Deep peels	Papillary dermis into the upper reticular dermis	Phenol, CO_2 lasers

and the in-clinic skin preparation. As we move forward in the text, all of these components will be discussed, and we will refer to them as *controlling the depth of the wound*.

Depths of Chemical Wounding

A skilled clinician must able to predetermine the depth of a peel before applying the peeling solution. Depending on the type of peel, this determination can be difficult. In fact, the skill to determine the depth of the peel and the projected outcome of the peel speaks to the experience and ability of the clinician. Clinicians who put chemicals on the patient, knowing little and hoping for the best, are in grave danger of creating a serious complication. The ability to ascertain the potential depth a chemical peel will have on the skin is dependent on a list of variables and the knowledge to understand these variables. Among these variables are the wounding agent (peel solution) itself, the percentage and pH of the peel solution, the number of coats of the solution, the length of time the agent has been left on the skin, the preparation of the skin at home, the preparation of the skin in the clinic, and finally, the aftercare. In many cases, the ability to evaluate and determine the endpoint for the superficial peel can be more challenging than it is for medium-depth peels, largely because lighter peels often do not have a defined clinical sign signifying the endpoint. Rather, the lighter peel uses erythema and **vesiculation** as the endpoint, while medium-depth peels use a **frost** to determine the endpoint. The erythema and vesiculation are often patchy and can go deeper in certain areas, depending on the clinical preparation of the skin. Frosting is the phenomenon of protein coagulation in the skin. This action occurs with Jessner's solution, TCA, and phenol

vesiculation
The process of forming blisters.

frost
Coagulation of protein in the skin that turns the skin a white color.

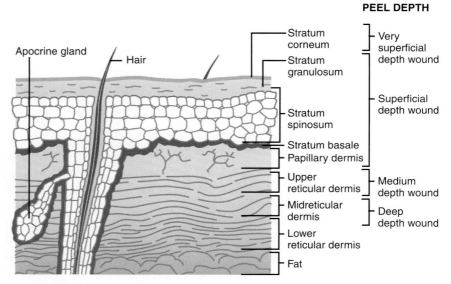

Figure 6–1   Peel depths vary from very superficial to deep depth wounds as depicted in this illustration.

peeling agents. The depth of the peel also has the caveat of skin condition; for example, an open pustule that is covered with 50% glycolic acid will become a dermal injury.

Different wounding agents, as predicted, have different wounding depths. As previously noted, these depths are defined as superficial, moderate, and deep (Figure 6–1). The percentage of the peeling agent and the pH are especially important in alpha hydroxy acid peeling agents, such as glycolic acid. Percentage also plays a part in TCA peeling solutions. Each solution is prepared differently and has important factors that can affect its depth. The clinician should be aware of this information before its use. Let us start at the beginning: the home preparation of the skin.

The preparation of the skin at home is going to affect the depth of the peel significantly. For example, a dry-skinned patient who has been using glycolic acid and Retin A® every day is going to take up the peel more quickly than would an oily skinned patient who has not been using any home-care products. Furthermore, if the oily skinned patient were using Retin A®, the thin dry-skinned patient would still have a potential to take up more quickly. Next, the preparation in the clinic before peeling should never change. Your routine should always be the same, regardless of the home preparation, skin type, or skin condition, which will allow greater predictability. If you are always changing the preparation process, you will not know what to expect from the peel. Lastly, the aftercare can be a variable in the depth of the peel. Poor care, picking, allergies, or cold sores are all reasons the peel might have deeper results than predicted.

Epidermal Wounding

Epidermal wounding is an injury that moves only into the epidermis (Figure 6–2). It would, in reality, be defined as a first-degree burn. The wound will be tender to the touch, red or pink, and it may swell slightly. Agents that are generally considered epidermal wounding agents include 20% to 50% glycolic acid, Jessner's peels, salicylic peels, and some light TCA applications, 10%, for example. However, you should be reminded once more that the selection of the peeling solution alone does not determine the depth of the peel.

Wounding that is superficial is limited to the stratum granulosum through the basal layer and will heal quickly through cutaneous appendages. You will remember that the appendages—the hair follicles and sweat glands—house epidermal cells that are recruited during the healing process. These types of light peels will create little, if any, downtime and can be a great peel for individuals who are seeking little downtime and have patience in achieving results. Worth noting, however, peels that *do not* achieve *erythema* or *flaking* of any kind will not achieve any clinical change.[3] Therefore achieving a level of erythema is important to promote flaking and the obvious subsequent result.

> Epidermal wounding is a peeling injury that is limited to the layers of the epidermis: stratum corneum, stratum granulosum, stratum spinosum, and basal layers. The injuries are very superficial to superficial and heal within days.

Dermal Wounding

Dermal wounding is the injury that passes through the epidermis and into the papillary and upper reticular dermis. Although these peels will not exhibit blisters as a traditional burn would, the skin will swell and ooze. The depth of this peel would be defined as a second-degree burn. The agents that create dermal wounding include 70% glycolic acid, TCA in 20% or higher concentrations, and phenol. For the clinician reading this text, any wounding through the papillary dermis will be a significant peel that will require the assistance of your clinic physician or at least policy and procedure to guide your patient. This practice will ensure that the patient recovers without scarring or complications. Remember, the healing of dermal wounds happens through the process of **secondary intention**[4] at this depth. These peels will take longer to heal but provide a more substantial result compared with the lighter epidermal peels previously discussed. The dermal wounding peel will improve collagen remodeling, improve blood flow to the dermis, and increase the ground substance. All of these changes improve the appearance of the skin.

secondary intention
The process of healing that includes coagulation and inflammation, reepithelialization, granulation tissue formation, angiogenesis, and collagen remodeling.

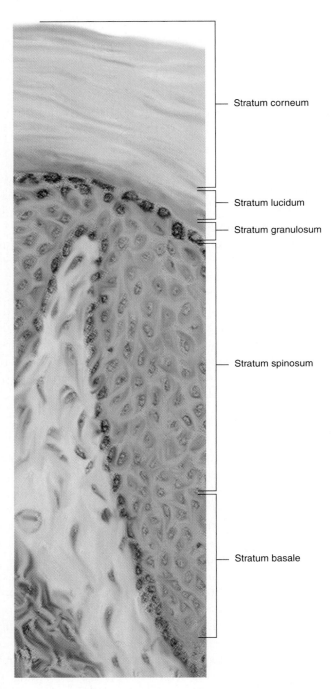

Stratum corneum

Stratum lucidum

Stratum granulosum

Stratum spinosum

Stratum basale

Figure 6–2   The epidermis has five sublayers: the stratum corneum, the stratum lucidum, the stratum granulosum, the stratum spinosum, and the stratum basale.

■ TYPES OF PEELING AGENTS

Many different types of peeling agents have been produced. Among the familiar agents are glycolic acid, Jessner's solution, salicylic acid, TCA, and phenol. Each agent has its own advantages and disadvantages as a peeling agent. Additionally, each one is technique sensitive, meaning that the end result is dependent on the knowledge and skill of the clinician. As in any clinical procedure, the more often you perform the procedure, the better you get at the process of the treatment and as such the end result for the patient. Each peeling agent has a specific action on the skin and therefore may be best indicated in certain conditions. Knowing the available peel solutions, their actions, and your patient's skin will decrease the variability of peeling. When you analyze your patient, the skin condition or problem, skin type, and aging analysis, you will be able to determine which peeling solution will best suit the situation (Table 6–4).

Glycolic Acid

Glycolic acid is a *fruit acid* derived from sugar cane. Once prepared naturally, glycolic acid is now usually prepared synthetically for clinical use. It is used in the home-care program and as a peeling agent. When it is used as a peeling agent, glycolic acid comes in three basic strengths (although the percentages can be varied to meet the clinician's needs): 30%, 50%, and 70%. Just as important as the percentage of the acid is the pH of the product. Usually, the solution for peeling should be at a pH of 2 or less. Glycolic acid is indicated for photodamage, exhibited as dyschromias, fine lines, or rough textures. Glycolic acid is also used for acne treatments, usually grade I and grade II. Glycolic acids are available through product vendors, but many offices have the product made by a compounding pharmacy. Glycolic peels are a common choice in the

Table 6–4   Peeling Agents

Treatment	What It Does	What It Does Not Do
TCA peels	Flattens scarring	Reduces pore size
	Reduces rhytids	Eradicates all rhytids
	Corrects photodamage	Removes telangiectasia
	Improves hyperpigmentation	Removes deep scarring
Jessner's solution and glycolic acid peels	Reduces rhytids	Reduces pore size
	Corrects photodamage	Eradicates all rhytids
	Eradicates all rhytids	Removes telangiectasia
		Removes deep scarring

medical spa. They are usually light, safe, nontoxic, and generally have few complications. Since the rise in popularity of microdermabrasion, glycolic peels have become less popular. This trend is unfortunate because glycolic peels have a specific and useful place in treating skin superficially. Glycolic acid and microdermabrasion have also been combined, providing an excellent result for the patient.

Jessner's Peel

Jessner's peel solution is a combination of three different acids: 14% salicylic acid, 14% resorcinol, and 14% lactic acid in an ethanol base. Attempts to increase the percentages of the salicylic in this solution are often made to increase its efficacy in treating acne. However, any increase in the salicylic acid will lead to clumping and debris in the solution. Therefore the best course of action is to stick with what is known as 14%-14%-14% to keep the peel solution from separating. Jessner's solution will provide a superficial peel, focusing on exfoliating and digestion of the debris. Because of this action, Jessner's solution is a great choice for the patient with acne. Jessner's solution is also frequently used in combination with other acids to potentate the result, usually with TCA. Jessner's solution is also combined with glycolic acid to provide a deeper peel, but this approach is far more risky because of the need to neutralize the glycolic acid to stop the action of the peel. If the clinician chooses to prepare the skin with glycolic acid before using the Jessner's peel, it should be done with a lower percentage and always neutralized before applying the Jessner's solution.

Salicylic Acid (Beta) Peel

Salicylic acid is a hydroxybenzoic acid found in willow bark, though it is manufactured synthetically from sodium phenolate. The salicylic acid or "beta peel" usually comes in two peeling strengths, 20% and 30%, although other strengths are certainly available from a compounding pharmacy. This peel is most effective for the treatment of acne and should be directed accordingly. Salicylic acid is also found in some medical offices as a 50% paste and is used for treating solar damage on the extremities. This peeling process is highly specialized and the decision should be left to the physician for two reasons: the use of an unfamiliar peeling paste and the potential for **salicylate toxicity**. Although the clinician will not likely be faced with a salicylate toxicity, he or she should understand the symptoms, which include headache, dizziness, vomiting, and **tinnitus** (ringing in the ears). Should your patient develop these symptoms during or within 24 hours after a peel, your clinic physician should be contacted.

salicylate toxicity
Absorption of too much salicylic acid, resulting in ear ringing, dehydration, and possible convulsions.

tinnitus
Ringing in the ears.

Trichloroacetic Acid

TCA is a common peeling agent in the medical spa. It comes in a variety of strengths, usually increasing incrementally 5%, 10%, 15%, 20%, 25%, and so on. TCA has many benefits: it is nontoxic, stable, easy to use, and has the ability to create a variety of results. The most commonly recognized TCA peel is the Obagi Blue Peel™, which usually uses 30% TCA. The TCA is then diluted with blue dye, which causes it to be reduced to 15% or 20%. TCA penetrates to the papillary dermis or the upper reticular dermis when a full frost is achieved. The frost is the result of the chemical (TCA) coagulating the protein in the skin. When the chemical is applied to the skin, it acts as a **cautery** in coagulating the protein.[5] TCA is easy to use and provides a predictable medium-depth peel.

Designer Peels

The definition for designer peels may fluctuate from one spa to the next. In reality, the term designer peel has a specific definition and indication. Designer peels are a combination of multiple solutions, usually herbal and homeopathic substances. Common ingredients are azelaic acid, lactic acid, mulberry root, bearberry, Echinacea, gotu kola, azela, lavender, licorice, or kojic acid. These peels are often used in conjunction with microdermabrasion treatments or facials.

Other Solutions

Other peeling solutions we have not explored but are important to note include phenol, pyruvic acid, and lactic acid. The most commonly used deep-peeling agent is phenol, or the **Baker-Gordon solution**. The Baker-Gordon solution is a combination of phenol, **Septisol®**, and **croton oil**. This combination results in a 45% to 55% concentration of phenol.[6] This peel will penetrate to the reticular dermis and, as with TCA, coagulate with the proteins in the skin, giving a frost. The Baker-Gordon phenol peel is used for deeper lines and aged skin. It will always (except in a rare case) leave the skin permanently hypopigmented.

Pyruvic Acid

Pyruvic acid is a keto-acid and is rarely used. The safety and efficacy have not been established for this solution, and only rare documentation can be found evaluating its importance as a peeling agent in the medical spa. Because of the unknown factors, recommendations are that other more familiar agents be used in the medical spa setting.

cautery
Tissue destruction, usually done using electricity.

Baker-Gordon solution
A phenol deep-peel solution.

Septisol®
An antibacterial cleansing agent.

croton oil
A fixed oil extracted from the croton plant (castor oil).

To avoid disappointment, a full consultation with the patient is necessary. This consultation should include a discussion of desired results, downtime, health status, and the patient's current skin-care program. The clinician should also evaluate the indications for peeling at this time.

Lactic Acid

Lactic acid, as we know, is a component of the natural moisturizing factor (NMF). Additionally, lactic acid increases the glycosaminoglycans (GAGs) and, as such, the ground substance of the skin. In the past, lactic acid has not been used as a peeling agent; but recently, it is finding its way into the clinic as a component of designer peels.

BEST RESPONSES TO CHEMICAL PEELING

Chemical peeling has many benefits that cannot be duplicated by other spa or clinical treatments, among them are increasing the GAGs in the ground substance of the skin, thickening the epidermis, and increasing collagen remodeling in the dermis. These improvements result in a healthier skin that appears more vibrant and youthful. The best responses to chemical peeling are achieved when the patient's objectives, the peel solution, the skin indications, and the clinician's ability all coincide. The patient's objectives should be ascertained at the initial consultation or during a peel consultation. Included in this discussion should be the patient's desired end result, the amount of downtime available, and the health status. The clinician should also evaluate whether the patient will be able to follow the postcare instructions. Chemical peels can be ugly during the healing process, and some patients cannot emotionally tolerate their appearance. Ascertaining whether the patient is a good "emotional" candidate is important. Other information that is collected includes the indications and contraindications. This information will drive some of the decision about the peel solution selection. Remember, the depth of the peel is directly related to the end result. Therefore, if you are trying to remedy deeper rhytids, a deeper peel is in order. On the other hand, if you are trying to resolve fine lines, lighter repetitive peeling will work fine.

An important point to understand, before treatment, is what a peel can do and what a peel cannot do. This level of clarity will alleviate misunderstandings with the patient and frustration on the part of the clinician. Among the indications for light chemical peeling are dyschromias, rough textures, fine lines, and acne grades I and II. Indications for medium peeling are rhytids, dyschromias, and rough textures. Patients with loose skin and deeper lines (who do not choose facial surgery) will benefit from a deep phenol peel. Knowing that the indication and the patient expectation drive the peel solution, let us look at the possible indications and the recommended peeling solutions.

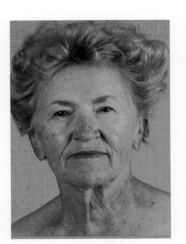

Figure 6–3 Wrinkling is the result of prolonged exposure to gravity and the sun's harmful rays.

Rhytids

As we age, wrinkles are the most obvious change we see in our skin (Figure 6–3). These lines, known as rhytids, will respond to both superficial and moderate chemical peeling, depending on the depth of the wrinkle. Rhytids can be divided into three classes: fine, medium, and coarse. The rhytids are further classified as static rhytids (those that occur without reference to facial movements) and dynamic rhytids (those related to facial movements). Rhytids are the number one complaint of clients and the first sign of aging. Proper evaluation of the rhytids includes an understanding of how they occur and which chemical peel will resolve or minimize their appearance (Table 6–5).

Static Rhytids

Intrinsic and extrinsic aging create **static rhytids**. Static rhytids are those found in the morning after sleep, from sunlight exposure (usually on the sides of the face), and from the effects of gravity (Figure 6–4). Static rhytids are present in the passive face and are not a result of facial movement. Deeper rhytids in this category are a result of skin laxity. In this case, a deeper peel may be required to achieve a smooth face. In some instances, the combination of a medium-depth peel and dermal filler is a good choice for these clients. Patients with deeper rhytids who choose moderate-depth peels (for whatever reason) are less likely to be satisfied with the end results; therefore adjusting their expectations is important before treatment.

static rhytids
Wrinkles that show without movement.

Table 6–5 Peel Solutions and the Effect on Lines

Solutions	Dynamic Fine Lines	Dynamic Medium Lines	Dynamic Deep Lines	Static Fine Lines	Static Medium Lines	Static Deep Lines
Glycolic acid	X	X		X	X	
Salicylic acid	X			X		
Jessner's solution	X			X		
Designer peels						
TCA	X	X	X	X	X	X
Phenol solutions	X	X	X	X	X	X

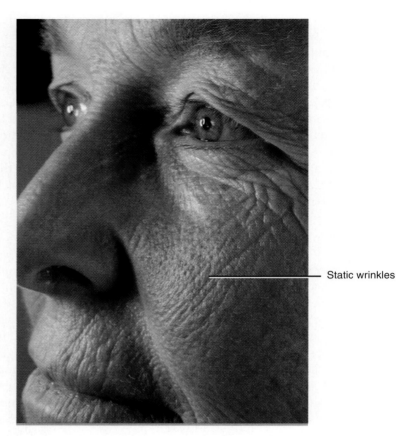

Static wrinkles

Figure 6–4 Static rhytids are caused by both intrinsic and extrinsic aging factors.

Dynamic Rhytids

dynamic rhytids
Wrinkling that occurs as a result of facial movement.

glabella
The area between the eyebrows.

Dynamic rhytids are lines that are created by muscle movement over time. Patients with expressive faces and animated features have far more lines than do those with stoic faces. These rhytids usually appear in the forehead (especially the **glabella**, or frown line), the sides of the face from robust smiles, and on the upper and lower lip from pursing (Figure 6–5, *A* and 6–5, *B*).

These lines are deeper and correspond to the muscle groups underlying the skin, dimpling the area. Continued muscle movement makes effectively treating these lines with peeling difficult. A phenol peel will sometimes dramatically improve the appearance, but even then, the deep dynamic line will not completely resolve. More importantly, the minute the expression begins after the peel has healed, the line will begin to reform. These situations will often respond best if treated with

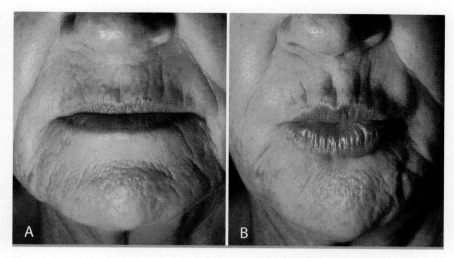

Figure 6–5 **A**, Dynamic rhytids are lines that are created by muscle movement over a time period. Evaluate this woman in the resting position. **B**, Now compare the lines in movement.

Botox® before the peel. In some cases, such as at the side of the face, the use of Botox® is not indicated, and dermal fillers are used. Additionally, the use of Retin A® long term is highly recommended. The good news is that peels will still improve dynamic lines, even without the use of Botox® or dermal fillers, but proper expectations are required.

Fine Rhytids

Fine rhytids are the first lines to appear in the aging face. These lines are usually found at the eye area and are referred to as crow's feet. Crow's feet can be seen on individuals as young as 18 or 19 years of age, especially if they have had moderate sunlight exposure (Figure 6–6). Fine rhytids can also be seen along the sides of the face and are either static or dynamic in nature, either from solar damage or smiles. Fine lines, either static or dynamic, are perfect for peeling treatment. Using Botox® and dermal fillers as an adjunct to this treatment will improve the result.

Solar Damage

Solar damage is a current and expanding problem for the general population. Many of us sat for hours in sunlight with baby oil using aluminum foil reflectors to enhance our tans. Now it is time to pay the price. Solar damage can be as simple as fine lines associated with the deterioration of dermal health, or it can be more severe, resulting in hyperpigmentation, actinic keratoses, and superficial and invasive skin cancers (including melanoma).

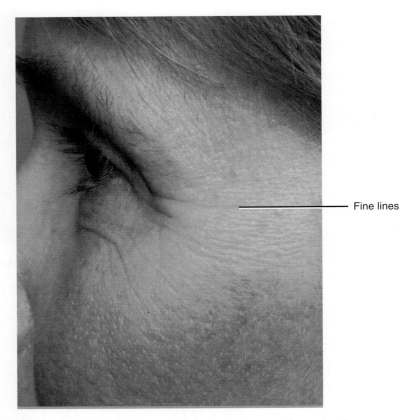

— Fine lines

Figure 6–6 Fine rhytids are the first to appear in the aging face, sometimes as early as the late teen years. Fine rhytids are most commonly seen in the crow's feet.

Sunlight exposure and the subsequent damage that occurs before the age of 18 is the leading cause of skin cancer and accelerates the aging process (Figure 6–7). As a result, many young men and women will appear significantly older than their chronologic age. The skin types at greatest risk are the Fitzpatrick types I, II, and III.

Peel therapy is an excellent choice for these patients. However, a full program would not be complete without an educational program to implement behavior modification. This part of the program will be the most difficult if your client is a "sun worshipper." The patient should be encouraged to use sunscreens, hats, and umbrellas. Even sun protection factor (SPF) clothing is worth considering. Without behavior modification, the associated peel treatments and home care will not have the desired long-term results. When your clients are truly committed to making a change in their skin, it can be done, but it requires effort, expense, and hard work, both inside and beyond the clinic.

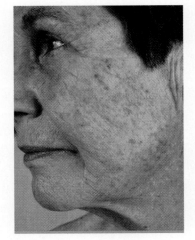

Figure 6–7 Sun exposure and the subsequent damage that occurs before the age of 18 is the leading cause of skin cancer and accelerates the aging process.

Hyperpigmentation

Hyperpigmentation occurs when the enzyme tyrosine triggers the over-production of melanin (Figure 6–8). Hyperpigmentation has a variety of causes, specifically, prolonged unprotected sunlight exposure, birth control pills, hormone replacement therapy, pregnancy, some antibiotics, and even skin irritation in certain individuals. Hyperpigmentation is often difficult to treat because the source of the problem may remain a constant, such as birth control pills. Monthly peels can be an effective tool in the treatment of hyperpigmentation. For a compliant client, a peel program with the proper adjunct therapy can usually solve the problem, depending on the depth of the pigment.

Melasma

Melasma is the hyperpigmentation that is located on the cheeks, chin, and forehead. It is usually hormone related and may be triggered by a change in the hormone status, such as during pregnancy or when using birth control pills. When the melasma is caused from pregnancy, it is called chloasma, or the "mask of pregnancy." **Hormone replacement therapy** for menopause has not been shown to create melasma. Melasma is made worse by sunlight exposure. In some instances, even protected sunlight exposure or strong fluorescent light bulbs can stimulate melanin.

Rough Texture

Rough texture is usually the result of unprotected sunlight exposure but may also be inherited. This phenomenon can be described as the "orange peel look" or a "pebbly" appearance.[7] Rough texture is many times accompanied by congested pores and is usually found on older individuals. The condition can be described as "golfer skin." Rough texture responds very well to peels. The peels can be medium-depth TCA peels, or, if the client has patience, biweekly glycolic peels will also improve the situation. The most important thing a patient will need to do is to wear sunscreen because rough textures arise from unprotected sunlight exposure.

Keratoses

Keratoses are described as horny growths: an abnormal overgrowth of cells. Many different types of keratoses have been identified, but for our purposes, we will focus on seborrheic keratoses and actinic keratoses. Seborrheic keratoses are related to aging, and actinic keratoses are related to sunlight exposure.

The most common type of keratoses are seborrheic keratoses, and these lesions do not become **malignant**.[8] A seborrheic keratosis is

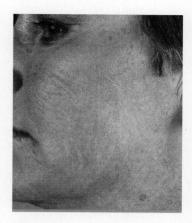

Figure 6–8 Hyperpigmentation occurs as a result of the overproduction of melanin.

hormone replacement therapy
A therapeutic replacement of natural and synthetic hormones as a means to counter the side effects of their absence, usually given to postmenopausal patients.

malignant
Cancerous or harmful to one's health.

thought to develop from prolific epidermal cells.[9] They vary in color and are more common on sunlight-exposed areas of the body.[10] These lesions seem to increase with age and can be problematic to the patient. In fact, seborrheic keratoses are so unsightly, patients and clinicians can become preoccupied with the lesion and overlook a more serious actinic keratosis or melanoma. A clinical program of monthly peels can reduce or eliminate seborrheic keratoses, especially when combined with a home-care program of Retin A® and alpha hydroxy acids.

Actinic keratosis (AK) is a lesion that has become premalignant. These lesions develop from the solar damage and are sometimes referred to as solar keratoses. AKs may come and go on the face, ears, neck, shoulders, and arms, but most commonly on the hands. They are pink in color and sometimes peel. AKs evolve into squamous cell carcinomas (SCCs) or basal cell carcinomas (BCCs). If you suspect that your patient has AKs, have your clinic physician evaluate this patient before peeling.

A program of 5FU® (Efudex) or surgery may be an appropriate treatment for actinic keratoses. Following treatment, these patients are candidates for peeling because of their significant solar damage and need for treatment and regular evaluation.

Grades 1, 2, and 3 Active Acne

Acne is described in grades 1, 2, and 3. Half grades also exist (i.e., 1.5, 2.5). Grade 1 is described as a few lesions, usually fewer than 10, over the entire face (Figure 6–9). Grade 2 acne is moderate and will have at least 20 lesions on the face (Figure 6–10). Grade 3 is 40 lesions or more over the entire face. When the patient is in consultation, the grade should be documented. Furthermore, as the treatments progress, the grade should continue to be documented (Table 6–6).

CONTRAINDICATIONS FOR CHEMICAL PEELING

Contraindications are conditions that are not appropriate for peeling. These conditions are usually quite obvious but bear discussion. Among the contraindications for peeling are excessive telangiectasia, infections, rashes, open lesions, and sunburns. Additionally, a patient who has just had a facelift or eyelid lift should not be a candidate for skin peeling. Finally, the patient who has been on Accutane® in the last year is not a candidate for facial peeling. Each of these contraindications is uniquely individual discounting the patient as a candidate for treatment based on the specific reason. Read on to find out more.

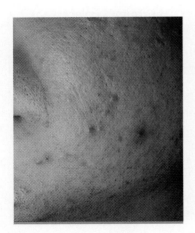

Figure 6–9   Grade I acne is described as mild lesions under 10 lesions at any one time.

Contraindications for peels include sunburns, open lesions (such as a cold sore), a rash (of any kind), or an infection on the face.

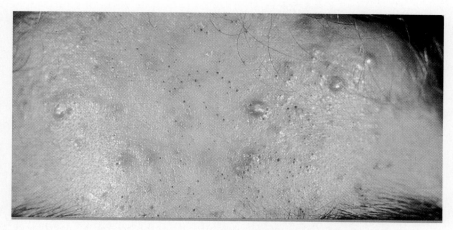

Figure 6–10   Grade 2 scattered lesions of 20 at any one time.

Table 6–6   Global Severity Score[11]

Grade	Description of Severity
3	Severe: large number of lesions in any one area or many areas of the face; a total of greater than 40 inflammatory acne lesions on the patient's face
2	Moderate: scattered acne lesions in several areas of the face; a total of approximately 20 inflammatory acne lesions on the patient's face
1	Mild: few acne lesions; fewer than 10 inflammatory acne lesions on the subject's face
0	Clear: no acne present; no acne lesions present on the subject's face; possible presence of residual pigmentation or scant macular erythema (or both)

Excessive Telangiectasia

Skin with large patches of telangiectasias should not be treated with peeling because the treatments may make them worse or more visible (Figure 6–11). Patients who fall into this category are usually Fitzpatrick types I or II. They are the classic ivory skinned with red hair color. Telangiectasias are treatable and should be treated with laser or other therapies before peeling therapy. Once the condition is treated, the peel program can be implemented. However, use care because these

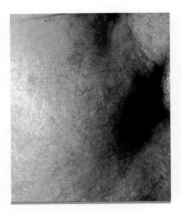

Figure 6–11
Telangiectases are tiny
blood vessels on the face
that can become more
apparent after
microdermabrasion or

predisposed
Possessing attributes that increase the
likelihood of an event taking place.

cellulitis
A potentially serious infection of the
skin.

impetigo
A skin infection from staphylococcal or
streptococcal bacteria.

folliculitis
An infection of the hair follicle, such as
"in-grown hairs."

**pseudofolliculitis
barbae**
In-grown hairs.

fungal infection
Any infection caused by the kingdom of
organisms, which includes yeasts and
molds.

patients are **predisposed** to these vessels and can have a reoccurrence.
The patient should be made aware of this fact.

Bacterial Skin Infections

Bacterial skin infections occur when a break in the skin occurs and bacteria
from the skin's surface or from the environment enter the opening. Most
skin infections are warm to the touch, red, inflamed, and tender. These
infections may also ooze. The presence of bacterial skin infections constitute
a contraindication for peel therapy. Examples of skin infections that the
clinician might see include **cellulitis**, **impetigo**, and **folliculitis**. All infections require medical attention and antibiotics. If the clinician should suspect any skin infection, refer the patient to the clinic physician.

Impetigo is an infection commonly thought to be a childhood
affliction, but it can also be seen in adults and occasionally after spa
treatments, especially microdermabrasion and peels. Impetigo is group
A Streptococcus or Staphylococcus infection. The most commonly
affected area for impetigo is around the nose and mouth. Impetigo presents as blisters of varied appearance, depending on the bacteria.
Impetigo itches and is contagious. If the clinician suspects impetigo, the
treatment should not be provided, and the patient should be referred to
a physician for antibiotics and care.

Cellulitis is a potentially serious infection of the skin. Cellulitis initially appears as a small red area surrounding a skin injury, for example a cut
or bite. The skin is red and warm to the touch, and red streaks may
appear. The infection can quickly involve the underlying tissues, creating
an emergency situation called necrotizing fasciitis or "flesh-eating strep."
Clients at risk include older adults and persons with a compromised
immune system (patients with immunodeficiency virus [HIV] or those on
chemotherapy), diabetes, chickenpox, and herpes. Peel therapy must not
be done, and the client should be referred to a physician for care.

Folliculitis is an infection of the hair follicle. The hair follicle is irritated and erythremic, with pus found in the center. Each infected follicle
will have a pimple at the base. Several types of folliculitis have been
identified; the most common to the clinician is **pseudofolliculitis
barbae**, which is found after shaving or waxing in certain individuals.
Refer the patient to the clinic physician for treatment with either topical
or oral antibiotics before any treatment.

Fungal Infections

Fungal infections of the skin are usually found in the moist, dark
areas of the body, for example, the space between the toes. Less

frequently, fungal infections can also be found on more exposed areas of the body such as the face. Examples of fungal infections include ringworm and yeast infections. Patients with fungal skin infections should not be treated with chemical peeling until their fungal infections are cleared.

Several different types of **ringworm** have been identified. The type of ringworm most concerning to the clinician in the medical spa environment is **tinea corporis**, or body ringworm. The fungus presents itself as a rash and can appear on the body or the face. Ringworm is circular and has raised edges. The center becomes less red as the lesion grows. The clinician should be alert for ringworm in geographic areas of high humidity and high temperatures. Exposure to ringworm is increased when a family has pets that may carry the disease. Ringworm must be treated by a physician before chemical peeling can begin.

When **yeast infections** are considered, one generally does not think of the face, yet small yeast infections can occur at the corners of the mouth. Yeast is normally not a detrimental component of the skin; however, a yeast infection can appear in patients with a depressed immune system. The clinician should be alert to cracks or tiny cuts in the corners of the mouth. To diagnosis this problem, a scraping of the skin must be taken and examined under the microscope. The physician may recommend medicated ointments to cure this problem. If a yeast infection is suspected, the patient should be referred to a physician before chemical peel treatments begin.

ringworm
A popular term for dermatomycosis caused by a species of fungi from the Microsporum family.

tinea corporis
Body ringworm.

yeast infections
A viral infection caused by several unicellular organisms that reproduce by budding. Oral yeast infections are common in persons with compromised immune systems.

Viral Infections

Viruses are parasitic organisms that invade and attach to living cells to survive and reproduce. Viruses cannot be treated with antibiotics. Rather, antiviral medications are the only successful treatments. The most common viral infections of the skin are herpes simplex, shingles, and flat facial warts.

Active Herpes Simplex

Active herpes simplex virus 1 (HSV-1) is the virus that causes cold sores. These viral infections appear as small clear blisters on the face, most commonly around the mouth. After the lesion has healed, the virus will be dormant in the body, periodically reactivating. Herpes is contagious, and persons with open sores should avoid contact by kissing or other means of person-to-person contact (Figure 6–12). Chemical peels should not be done when a patient has active herpes simplex (cold sores).

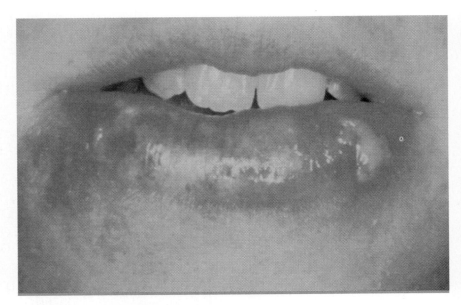

Figure 6–12   Herpes simplex.

Open Lesions and Rashes

Open lesions, rashes, and **burns** are obviously not appropriate for chemical peels. Open lesions include areas of surgical treatment such as a keratoses treated with liquid nitrogen. Rashes are generalized skin eruptions that are erythremic and raised, for example, poison ivy, allergic reactions, or sun rashes. Burns include sunburns, as well as other types of burns. Skin that is compromised in any way should be healed through appropriate pathways before peeling is considered. Once the skin is healed, having clear guidance from the physician is important before beginning treatments.

Sunburns

No matter how minor, sunburn is still a skin injury and should not be treated with a chemical peel. Patients will often be resistant to your refusal to treat them, but this decision is in their best interest. Healing a simple sunburn is just a matter of time and care. Instruct the client to avoid therapeutic products for the next 2 to 3 days, and moisturize aggressively. Sunburns can be second-degree burns if blisters appear. If the sunburn is serious, the patient should see a physician for further care.

Atopic Dermatitis

Atopic dermatitis is a rash of unknown **etiology** and can be a frustrating problem. In many instances, these problems will appear as acne,

burns
Thermal or electrical injuries that wound the skin.

atopic dermatitis
A skin irritation or rash of unknown origin.

etiology
The cause of a disease.

with small pustules but without comodones. Dermatitis usually comes from contact with soaps, cleanser, fabrics, or other products such as toothpaste. If your client has a facial rash, investigative work is important. Ask the patient, "When did the rash start?" "Does it itch?" "Does it hurt?" "Did you change any home product such as laundry detergent?" Prompting the client with different scenarios will help both of you understand the potential cause. Has the client been using topical steroids, new facial products, or a new sunscreen? Did the client change toothpaste? Does the client let the toothpaste ooze out of the mouth onto the skin when teeth are being brushed? These are all important investigative questions. If this problem is significant and does not respond to discontinuation of products, then refer the client to a physician who can implement further treatment. Do not perform chemical peels on a client with atopic dermatitis.

Accutane®

Accutane® is prescribed for severe unresponsive acne. Accutane® is isotretinoin and is related chemically to retinoids and retinol, forms of vitamin A. It decreases the sebaceous activity in the skin by shrinking the oil glands. The decrease in the sebaceous activity is related to the dose of Accutane® and the duration of treatment. As the activity in the sebaceous glands is decreased, the skin's healing action is slowed. Accutane® can have minor side effects such as dry and chapped lips, dry skin and hair, but can also have significant side effects, including birth defects, depression, intracranial hypertension, and acute pancreatitis. Therefore Accutane® treatment should be reserved for the most recalcitrant cases of nodular acne. Patients taking Accutane® should always be under the care of a physician. The standard of care for patients who have taken Accutane® is a waiting period of 1 year before being treated with chemical peels.[12]

Immediate Post Operative Facelift, Blepharoplasty, or Neck Lift

Patients who have had facial surgery are always excited to get back to their skin-care program. Persons who have not been involved in a program are often energized to begin one after surgery. However, the clinician and patient must take care to avoid potential complications by starting the program too early. Bruising will be present for up to 10 days, and hematomas can develop even 2 weeks after surgery. Numbness can last up to a year in certain areas; consequently the clinician must be careful because the client will not feel the chemical peels. The time for beginning a skin-care program for the patient after plastic surgery is at the sole discretion of the plastic surgeon.

Deep Dynamic Rhytids

Deep dynamic rhytids, though not a contraindication, should be treated with the caveat of realistic patient expectations. Deep dynamic wrinkles usually come with jowls and sagging skin; and although peels can improve the texture and quality of the skin, this patient may be a surgical candidate, and the discussion of the appropriate treatment needs to be open and frank to avoid patient disappointment.

▶ ▷ ▷ TOP TEN TIPS TO TAKE TO THE CLINIC

1. Skin peeling is a controlled burn of the skin.
2. The three conditions especially susceptible to chemical peeling are rhytids, solar damage, and dyschromias.
3. Keep in mind the skin type, skin condition, and aging analysis when choosing a peel solution.
4. When you choose a peel solution, know its benefits and limitations for the problem you are trying to treat.
5. The deeper the wound is, the more significant the outcome will be.
6. The peel solution alone does not determine the depth of the peel.
7. Know the contraindications for chemical peeling.
8. Cutaneous appendages assist in epidermal wound healing.
9. Treatment of dynamic lines with Botox® before peeling will improve the results of the peels.
10. A cold sore may develop after chemical peeling in patients who carry the virus.

CHAPTER REVIEW QUESTIONS

1. What are the principles of skin peeling?
2. How deep do peel solutions go into the skin?
3. Is peeling the right treatment for all rhytids?
4. What is the right treatment for someone with telangiectasia?
5. Is peeling the right choice for solar damage?
6. What are the contraindications for peeling?
7. What are the peel treatments for acne?
8. What are the different types of designer peels?
9. What is the most common peel solution in the medical spa?

CHAPTER REFERENCES

1. Caputy, G. (2002, April 3). *Skin surfacing and chemical peels* [Online]. Available: www.emedicine.com

2. O'Connor, R. (2004, April 21). Medicine in Traveller: Regulating body temperature, *Freelance Traveller* [Online]. Available: www.freelancetraveller.com

3. Coleman, W. P., & Lawrence, N. (1998). *Skin resurfacing.* Baltimore: Williams & Wilkins.

4. Coleman, W. P., & Lawrence, N. (1998). *Skin resurfacing.* Baltimore: Williams & Wilkins.

5. Rubin, M. (1995). *Manual of chemical peels: Superficial and medium depth.* Philadelphia: Lippincott, Williams & Wilkins.

6. Coleman, W. P., & Lawrence, N. (1998). *Skin resurfacing.* Baltimore: Williams & Wilkins.

7. Rubin, M. (1995). *Manual of chemical peels: Superficial and medium depth.* Philadelphia: Lippincott, Williams & Wilkins.

8. Blitzner, A., Binder, W. J., Boyd, J. B., & Carruthers, A. (Eds.). (2000). *Management of facial lines and wrinkles.* Philadelphia: Lippincott, Williams & Wilkins.

9. Balin, A. K. (2002, February 27). *Seborrheic keratosis* [Online]. Available: www.emedicine.com

10. Balin, A. K. (2002, February 27). *Seborrheic keratosis* [Online]. Available: www.emedicine.com

11. Goldman, M. P., & Boyce, S. M. (2003). A single-center study of aminolevulinic acid and 417nm photodynamic therapy in the treatment of moderate to severe acne vulgaris. *Journal of Drugs in Dermatology, 2*(4), 393–396.

12. Bernard, R. W., Beran, S. J., & Rusin, L. (2000). Micro-dermabrasion in clinical practice. *Clinics in Plastic Surgery, 27*(4), 571–577.

BIBLIOGRAPHY

Azer, M. (2002, March 1). *Salicylate toxicity* [Online]. Available: www.emedicine.com

Balin, A. K. (2002, February 27). *Seborrheic keratosis* [Online]. Available: www.emedicine.com

Bernard, R. W., Beran, S. J., & Rusin, L. (2000). Microdermabrasion in clinical practice. *Clinics in Plastic Surgery, 27*(4), 571–577.

Blitzner, A., Binder, W. J., Boyd, J. B., & Carruthers, A. (Eds.). (2000). *Management of facial lines and wrinkles.* Philadelphia: Lippincott, Williams & Wilkins.

Breathnach, A. S. (1996, January). Melanin hyperpigmentation of skin: Melasma, topical treatment with azelaic acid, and other therapies. *Cutis,* 57 (Suppl 1), 36–45.

Brody, H. J. (1997). *Chemical peeling and resurfacing* (2nd ed.). St. Louis: Mosby.

Caputy, G. (2002, April 3). *Skin surfacing and chemical peels* [Online]. Available: www.emedicine.com

Coleman, W. P, Lawrence, N. (1998). *Skin resurfacing.* Baltimore: Williams & Wilkins.

Deitz, S. (2004). *Milady's the clinical esthetician.* Clifton Park, NY: Thomson Delmar Learning.

Del Rosso, J. Q. (2003, October). Shining new light on rosacea. *Skin & Aging,* Oct(Suppl 1), 3–6.

Goldman, M. P., & Boyce, S. M. (2003). A single-center study of aminolevulinic acid and 417nm photodynamic therapy in the treatment of moderate to severe acne vulgaris. *Journal of Drugs in Dermatology,* 2(4), 393–396.

HealthandAge.com (2004). *Aging skin: Blemishes and nonmelanoma skin cancers* [Online]. Available: www.healthandage.com

Healthsquare.com. (January 15, 2004). *Accutane* [Online]. Available: www.healthsquare.com

Kang, W. H., Chun, S. C., & Lee, S. (1998, September). Intermittent therapy for melasma in Asian patients with combined topical agents. *International Journal of Dermatology,* 25(9), 587–596.

Leffell, D. (2002, February). *New advances in treating actinic keratoses* [Online]. Available: www.skinandaging.com

Lim, J. T. (1999, April). Treatment of melasma using kojic acid in a gel containing hydroquinone and glycolic acid. *Journal of Dermatologic Surgery,* 25(4), 282.

MayoClinic.com. (2004, February 25). *Cellulitis* [Online]. Available: http://www.mayoclinic.com

MedicineNet.com. (2003, December 5). *Medical dictionary: Melanocyte* [Online]. Available: www.medterms.com

Merck Pharmaceutical Company. (2004, February 25). *The Merck Manual: Second Home Edition* [Online]. Available: http://www.merck.com

Merck Pharmaceutical Company. (2004, February 25). Folliculitis, skin abscesses, and carbuncles. *The Merck Manual: Second Home Edition* [Online]. Available: http://www.merck.com

Merck Pharmaceutical Company. (2004, February 25). Shingles. *The Merck Manual: Second Home Edition* [Online]. Available: http://www.merck.com

Merck Pharmaceutical Company. (2004, February 25). Viral infections. *The Merck Manual Second Home Edition* [Online]. Available: http://www.merck.com

Merck Pharmaceutical Company. (2004, February 25). Warts. *The Merck Manual: Second Home Edition* [Online]. Available: http://www.merck.com

O'Connor, R. (2004, April 21). Medicine in Traveller: Regulating body temperature. *Freelance Traveller* [Online]. Available: www.freelancetraveller.com

Perez-Bernal, A., Munoz-Perez, M. A., & Camacho, F. (2000, September–October). Management of facial hyperpigmentation. *American Journal of Clinical Dermatology* 1(5), 261–268.

Roche.com. (2004, January 15). *Accutane product information* [Online]. Available: www.rocheusa.com

Rubin, M. (1995). *Manual of chemical peels: Superficial and medium depth*. Philadelphia: Lippincott, Williams & Wilkins.

Skin Cancer Foundation. (2004). *Actinic keratosis: What you should know about this common precancer* [Online]. Available: www.skincancer.org

Thomas, C. L. (Ed.). (1997). *Taber's cyclopedic medical dictionary* (Vol. 18). Philadelphia: F. A. Davis.

Tuleya, S. (2003, October). Melasma update. *Skin & Aging*, 11(10), 89–91.

University of Maryland Medicine. (2003, May 14). *Dermatology health guide: Candidiasis (yeast infection)* [Online]. Available: http://www.umm.edu

University of Maryland Medicine. (2003, May 14). *Dermatology health guide: Cellulitis* [Online]. Available: http://www.umm.edu

University of Maryland Medicine. (2003, May 14). *Dermatology health guide: Folliculitis, boils, and carbuncles* [Online]. Available: http://www.umm.edu

University of Maryland Medicine. (2003, May 14). *Dermatology health guide: Fungal infections of the skin* [Online]. Available: http://www.umm.edu

University of Maryland Medicine. (2004, February 25). *Dermatology health guide: Skin infections* [Online]. Available: http://www.umm.edu

Glycolic Peels

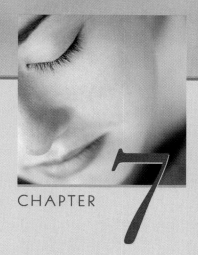

CHAPTER 7

KEY TERMS

acetylcholine
bicarbonate solution
Clostridium botulinum
Collagen®
consent form
defatted

epidermolysis
Hylaform®
naso-labial folds
neutralization
occlusion
peel percentage

Radiesse®
Restylane®
solid carbon dioxide
Valtrex®

LEARNING OBJECTIVES

After completing this chapter you should be able to:

1. Discuss the indications and contraindications for glycolic peels.
2. Discuss the pretreatment necessary for glycolic peels.
3. Discuss the anticipated results for glycolic peels.
4. Name the reasons to contact your clinic physician when doing glycolic peels.

INTRODUCTION

Chemical peels, especially glycolic or alpha hydroxy acid peels, have become a popular form of skin rejuvenation. In the early 1990s, glycolic acid competed for consumer market share with trichloroacetic acid (TCA) and phenol, the more traditional peeling agents. Given that so few studies had been conducted and little history of its use, the belief was that glycolic peels, or "lunchtime" peels, were of little value and did not provide improvement to the epidermis or dermis. Since that time, however, glycolic acid has become a well-studied and frequently used peeling agent. We now know that, even with their repetitive *light* nature, glycolic acid peels have the ability to improve both the epidermis and the dermis. This ability is the result, in part, of the short carbon chain common to lactic and glycolic acid.[1] The short chain is also responsible for the penetration rate common to glycolic and lactic acid. **Epidermolysis** (the separation of epidermal cells) occurs with glycolic acid, especially higher percentages of glycolic acid, within minutes, depending on the skin's preparation in the clinic and at home.

Glycolic acid is often thought of as a benign, natural agent that comes from sugar cane. In reality, glycolic acid *as a peeling agent* is neither benign nor natural. Manufactured synthetically, glycolic acid can be among the trickiest acids in the peeling armamentarium. It must be neutralized to *end the peeling action*; therefore it can peel quite deeply when left on the skin too long. Glycolic acid also has a tendency to peel the skin irregularly, deeper in areas of aggressive skin preparation. This preparation can be related to the home care, for example, overuse of Retin A® on the upper lip. Clinical preparation before peeling can also cause deeper peeling, for instance, in areas where the skin is **defatted** more aggressively, such as the forehead.

epidermolysis
Separating of the epidermal cells.

defatted
The use of isopropyl alcohol or acetone to remove all oils from the skin, which will allow peel solutions to work evenly.

■ GLYCOLIC PEELS

Knowing that glycolic peels are not a simple, risk-free peel, we can also assume they are not the easiest peel for clinicians to perform. Many variables factor into creating a superior result using glycolic acid. Among these variables are the pretreatment program, the clinical preparation, determining which solution to use and why, anticipating the skin's response to the peel, and being prepared for potential complications, to name a few.

The pretreatment program requires at least 2 weeks of use with the prescribed home-care products to prepare the skin properly. Any time less than 2 weeks will not allow an even penetration of the peel solution. Some clinicians will do a peel at the consultation, to get the patient "started." Nothing can be a bigger waste of time. The peel cannot penetrate evenly or effectively when the stratum corneum is built up from years of abuse. If the patient comes to your office and is currently using Retin A® but has not been on your program, the stratum corneum can be uneven and irregular, causing a potential "rug burn" or, worse yet, a deeper injury.

The clinical preparation is an important step in creating a smooth, even peel. The clinician must understand the importance of cleansing and preparing the skin before the peel treatment. Furthermore, understanding how glycolic acid behaves on the skin, and knowing which solutions to choose, will ultimately be the difference between success and failure for the patient and the clinician.

Finally, understanding and being able to treat complications is part of the knowledge bank of the experienced clinician. This information can make the difference between a good result and a problem that should be referred to the physician.

Pretreatment Preparation

The pretreatment preparation refers to the home-care program that the patient will be doing 2 weeks before the peel treatments begin. This program is usually a combination of at-home alpha hydroxy acids (glycolic or lactic), vitamin C, Retin A® (or retinol), hydroquinone, sunscreen, and "power" moisturizers. As you know, the organization of the home-care program is critical to the success of the peel product penetration. The treatment program should be done daily unless an irritation problem exists that precludes the patient from performing the treatment. Home care programs should also include an exfoliating program. The exfoliating program should be done every third day. However, the patient should never use grains or an exfoliating product of any kind on the morning of the peel treatment. What about using other therapeutic products such as alpha hydroxy acids or Retin A® the day before the treatment? Yes, by all means, patients should stay on their program. Only the exfoliating product (especially grains) can make a difference in the stratum corneum landscape, which will affect an uneven pick up of the peel solution.

The minimum pretreatment is standardized in the medical community as 2 weeks. If the patient cannot get in for the first treatment until the 3-week mark, that is fine, but not before 2 weeks. Seeing the patient at 1 week is a good idea for several reasons. First, the clinician has an opportunity to evaluate the product use. Is it working for the skin? Is it too harsh or just right? Does the patient have any questions about the product use? Second, it is a great time for a facial. The facial will help exfoliate any skin that is "stuck" and will help keep the patient motivated.

Clinical Preparation

Not enough can be said about keeping your treatment room clean and organized. If you use more than one glycolic peel strength, the bottles should be marked when they are received by highlighting the percentages with colored markers—yellow highlight for 30% and pink highlight for 50%. If pH levels are different, these need to be identified as well. This process will help eliminate any possible unintentional use of the wrong peel solution. The bottles should be organized on the counter so they are easily seen. Any necessary peel supplies should also be set out on the counter, close at hand. These supplies include application supplies (gauze, brushes, cotton-tipped applicators, small medicine cups), a bowl of water, eye wash, cleansers, moisturizers, neutralizing solutions, and sunscreens. At least two of each product category are usually on the back bar to provide selection to the clinician. Additionally, you will need a small motorized fan to help the patient's skin cool during the treatment. Lastly, a bonnet or head band to protect the patient's hair is included. Standardizing the treatment room helps cut down on potential mistakes when the clinician is peeling.

Obtaining a Consent

All peels have a risk of complication; therefore the patient must be informed about the procedure and sign a **consent form**. The consent form is part of our legal protection in the event that the patient ever decides to sue or if a conflict exists. The consent has several important sections: the introduction, the disclosure of allergies, chronic medical conditions, the facts of the procedure, the potential results, and the risks and complications. Consents that are used in your facility should be reviewed by your clinic legal counsel before use.

Solution Percentage

Choosing the **peel percentage** is as much an art as it is a science. Among the facts to be considered when choosing a solution percentage are the dryness of the skin, the adherence to the home therapy, the level of irritation, the patient's social or business schedule, and the result of the last peel.

The dryness of the skin is important because the peel will quickly absorb into dry skin. Think of a dry kitchen sponge that is dropped into

---

Keep the treatment room clean and orderly. This practice portrays an organized and professional image and helps keep the clinician from making mistakes.

consent form
Required clinical documentation in which associated risks, complications, and presumable outcomes are outlined in association with a given procedure. This document gives permission by the patient to the clinician to provide the procedure.

peel percentage
The amount of bioavailability of the active ingredient, not to be confused with pH.

Consent forms are the tool that is used to inform the patient about the risks and complications of a procedure. This document also makes the clinician aware of the patient allergies, expectations (through discussions), and chronic medical problems. The clinician should make sure that a consent form accompanies each procedure that is performed.

water. The skin will behave similarly when you put the peel solution on; so bear in mind the percentage you will use. When the skin is oily, the solution may not absorb quickly or may float on the surface of the skin. This phenomenon will be especially true if the patient has not been using the home-care program.

The adherence to the home-care therapy also will be a consideration. If the patient has not been faithful to the program or uses the program intermittently, the skin will not be as responsive to the peel solution. The surface of the skin will be irregular. The T-zone will take up the peel solution more quickly, and the lateral aspects of the face will be slow to respond, which makes achieving a uniform, effective peel difficult.

Conversely, if the patient has been overusing the products, the skin may be irritated; this situation will cause the peel solution to take up more quickly, and the peel may become deeper than was anticipated, perhaps into papillary dermis (Figure 7–1).

Also important to take into consideration is the patient's schedule. Patients are sometimes very busy and cannot afford the possibility of downtime. The choice of solution will also be affected in this circumstance. Finally, recall the results of the last peel: was it a lot or little? Are we achieving the desired end result? These questions need to be answered before selecting the peel percentage.

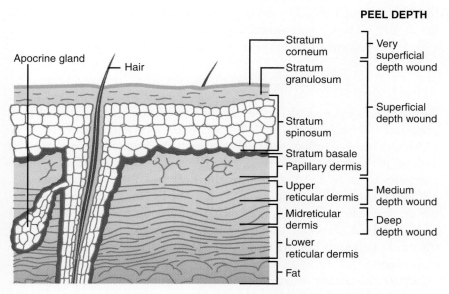

Figure 7–1   The glycolic peel solution can penetrate into the upper papillary dermis as shown by this diagram.

20% to 30%

The 20% and 30% glycolic peel solutions are very mild. They should have a low pH to help the solution penetrate. A pH of approximately 0.5 is sufficient. These percentages should be chosen if the clinician is concerned about dryness, if the patient has some product irritation, or if the patient does not want to risk having excessive flaky skin over the next few days. Although the results will be minimal, these percentages will still be effective; therefore administering the peel is never a waste of time.

40% to 60%

Glycolic peel solutions in the 40%-to-60% category are the mainstay of the glycolic peeling inventory. These solutions provide the most noticeable results over a period of months. Because these solutions are higher percentages, and presumably lower in pH, the clinician should carefully evaluate the skin before choosing one of these solutions. Additionally, the clinical preparation will be critical to controlling the peel. Therefore, if the skin is dry or otherwise likely to take the peel solution quickly, lower the percentage to avoid a potential problem.

70% and Above

Clinicians who use 70% and above should be expert peelers. The beginner peeler should not consider using 70% glycolic acid. Observing for the end point of a glycolic acid peel takes a trained and qualified eye. Do not move into this higher percentage until you have extensive experience with lesser percentages; 70% glycolic acid can and will scar.

Peel Application

The key to a successful peel is the peel application. How the skin is prepared, the choice of the application device, and the method of **neutralization** all affect the peel outcome. Additionally, repeating the process the same way each time, regardless of skin type, will also make a difference as to the outcome of the peel and ultimately the result. Different application devices can be used: a brush, gauze, or a cotton-tipped applicator. Folded gauze seems to provide the best control and is a preferred method. Folded gauze also works well to neutralize the peel, although cotton balls and sponges have also been used to neutralize.

After the patient is made comfortable on the bed, the hair is protected, and the chest is draped with a towel, you are ready to begin cleansing the skin. However, first, look around. Is your room completely

neutralization
A process by which active agents lose their potency, either with the addition of another agent or the loss of time.

stocked? Is the fan on the counter? Do you have the peel solution you want? Do you have your neutralizer? Now that you have done a quick supply-inventory check, you are ready to begin. Using a mild cleanser on *soft gauze*, cleanse the face until all of the makeup and debris has been removed. This process may take two applications of cleanser. Next, de-fat the skin with acetone. This process will take away all of the oils on the skin, allowing the peel solution to penetrate. When the process of de-fatting the skin is not done well, the peel solution will get hung up on oily patches of the skin (usually on the T-zone), which can cause an uneven peel. Once the face is clean and dry, you are ready to begin peeling.

Loading peel solution on to the folded gauze can be done in two ways. The preferred method is by using a medicine cup. You can find the appropriate type of cup at a medical supply company. These cups are usually made of glass. The Obagi Blue Kit™ also comes with a small cup that can be washed and reused. The other option is to pour the solution on the gauze from the bottle. The benefit of using a medicine cup is control. The folded gauze can be dipped into the solution, and any extra can be squeezed out against the side of the medicine cup. When the solution is poured out of the bottle onto the gauze, it can become too saturated. The excess solution can be dangerous because drops may go into the patient's eyes. Once the gauze is loaded with peel solution, you are ready to begin the application process.

To apply the solution, begin on the forehead and make vertical strokes, beginning at the eyebrows and moving to the hairline. Then, repeat the process horizontally. This application will help ensure that all the skin is covered. Once the forehead has been treated, both horizontally and vertically, move to the upper lip. Again, use horizontal and vertical application. Resoak your gauze as necessary to make sure that you are applying an even coat of peel solution. Next, move to the lower eyelid, which is always an area of concern for patients, so be sure you apply a reasonable coat of solution. The next step is to cover the lateral face and finally the nose. Remember, all areas get two coats, one that is vertical and one that is horizontal. Pay attention to the thinner-skinned areas, most notably the eyelids, which will be an area that you will probably want to neutralize first, given that it is likely to be "cooked" first. Patients often complain that the upper lip stays hot. Pay attention to this area. Although the skin is thick and the likelihood of a deep peel is rare, patients seem to have a lot of discomfort in this area. If a patient complains that the area is stinging and hot, the peel solution is still working. Keep neutralizing until the patient is more comfortable (Figure 7–2).

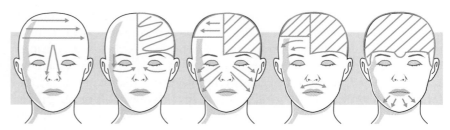

Figure 7–2 The application of the glycolic peel solution should begin on the forehead where the skin is thicker and continue around the face as indicated.

Response to Peel Solutions

The skin will initially turn pink when the solution is applied. Many times, the pinkness is spotty and uneven, which is normal. If you are pressing hard, some of the pinkness is caused by the pressure of your hand. In some instances, you may want to press hard or maybe even "scrub in" the solution to achieve a deeper and more even peel; but just be aware that part of the erythema is associated with the application technique. The patient's skin may tingle or itch while the solution is active. This is normal.

The longer the peel solution stays on the skin, the pinker the skin will get. The skin will eventually turn red. If the solution is allowed to stay on the skin longer, the skin will begin to turn white in some areas as it combines with the protein in the papillary dermis.

Always watch the skin. Some clinicians or instructors advocate the use of time as a determining factor for neutralizing glycolic peels. The reality is that glycolic peels can progress quickly. Therefore your eye should be on the skin, not on the clock. You are looking for pinkness or redness, depending on the intended depth of the peel. Spots of frost usually occur around the eyes and chin; therefore watch these areas carefully. Be aware that glycolic acid can work quickly and that it will continue to work until it is *completely neutralized*. Therefore beginning the neutralization process slightly *before* the intended result is wise. If you wait until you see exactly what you want, it may be too late, and by the time the peel is neutralized, a deeper peel than intended will have occurred.

As the peel begins to "cook," some areas will need to be neutralized before other areas. This situation is normal. Keep your neutralizer lotion and gauze close at hand. Begin to spot neutralize as you see the skin "come up," but be prepared to neutralize the full face, if necessary. A variety of solutions can be used for neutralization. Some clinicians like to use a simple homemade **bicarbonate solution**. The preferred choice

bicarbonate solution
Any salt containing bicarbonate anion; pH above 7.

is a professional solution that is intended for glycolic neutralization. If the neutralization solution has a pH that is too high, the neutralization process will sting and ultimately cause the skin to be redder and dryer than is necessary.

Once the neutralization process is complete and the skin is cool, examine the treated area. If you notice an area of frost that you did not plan, do not despair; help is available. Be sure to have on hand a product called Vigalon®. When applied to a glycolic peel wound, this gel sheeting will help "draw out" the heat of the peel and abbreviate the injury. The sheet comes with *both sides* covered in a paper-thin plastic. Be sure to remove both sides of the protective plastic before applying to the area of concern. The gel will be sticky, which is normal. Once you apply the gel on the skin, it will stick to the warm skin and cool the area. Patients can be sent home with this product on their face with instructions to remove it in a couple of hours. Some patients report that it will fall off in about an hour, which is just fine. Once the Vigalon® is removed, the patient needs to apply an anti-inflammatory gel. Do not use Aquafor® or Vaseline® because they will occlude the wound and may cause the heat to continue to injure the skin.

Before the patient is discharged, chart your notes regarding the procedure. Areas that absorbed a greater amount of peel solution and therefore will most likely peel more deeply or aggressively should be noted. Also note how the patient responded to the treatment or any other specific considerations. Finally, make sure that the patient has the proper postcare instructions and an appointment for followup.

Use of Occlusion

Occlusion can be used if the peel was neutralized too soon and you would like to drive the peel a little deeper. The heat that was created during the peeling process will continue to injure the skin if the peeled area is covered with Vaseline® or Aquafor® immediately following. The occlusion is a gentle way of creating a slightly deeper peel.

Solid Carbon Dioxide

Some clinicians like to use **solid carbon dioxide** ice after peeling. This practice can be dangerous and should be attempted only by persons with experience. The injury to the skin has already occurred with the peel solution, and further injury with a substance such as solid carbon dioxide can create a dermal wound and possible scarring. The practice is embraced by some clinicians and used with some frequency. Be extremely careful when applying the dry ice. Move quickly and do not let the ice touch any skin surface for too long. The ice can also hurt (burn the skin) if you are lingering too long in any one spot.

occlusion
The state of being closed.

solid carbon dioxide
The clinical name for dry ice.

Posttreatment

The posttreatment for a glycolic acid peel is simple. Available agents on the market that are antiinflammatory in nature will cool and moisturize the skin. An agent such as this should be used in the first 12 hours. After the first 12 hours, the skin should be kept soft with a moisturizer that is specifically designed for postpeeling. If any "hot spots" or "rug burns" develop at this time, these areas need to be kept soft with Aquafor®. By the third day, the skin should be exfoliated. An enzyme mask exfoliant is preferred over one with grains, the former of which is gentler and does not subject the skin to potential scratches.

On the day of the peel and the day after the peel, the patient should avoid therapeutic home-care products such as alpha hydroxy acids and Retin A®. These products may be too irritating and may cause the skin to become erythemic and sensitive. The best approach is to place the patient on a "peel kit," which includes a gentle cleanser, an emollient moisturizer, a sunscreen, and an exfoliant, in other words, the products you prefer for patients to use in the postpeeling phase. The usual protocol is to begin the usual home-care program on the second to third day after the peel (Table 7–1).

Anticipated Results

The results of the glycolic peel can be dramatic or minimal, depending on the strength and intensity of the peel. Seeing an improvement in dyschromia and texture with just one peel is not usual. Over the course of a peeling series, say five to eight peels, a noticeable difference will be seen in fine lines, wrinkles, and the effects of solar damage. The patient (and the clinician) must realize that glycolic peeling is a progressive treatment and that a mutually agreeable result will not be achieved with one or even three peels. With this circumstance in mind, the patient will begin to "feel" immediate results. The skin will be softer, and it will begin to

Table 7–1   Posttreatment for Glycolic Acid Peel

Antiinflammatory gel	First 12 hours
Postpeel moisturizer	After the first 12 hours
Aquafor®	Treatment of "hot spots" or "rug burns"
Enzyme mask exfoliant	On the third day
Usual home-care program	Second to third day after the peel

"glow" after even the first peel. These results are often so subtle that only the patient will know the skin has changed. Eventually, however, both of you will see the difference, and the patient will soon be getting compliments from friends and family (Figures 7–3 and 7–4).

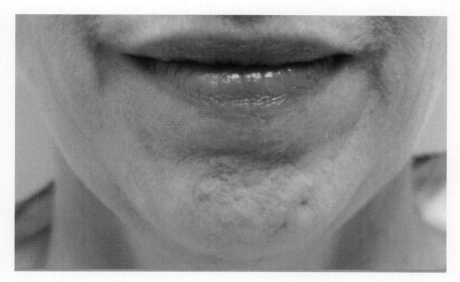

Figure 7–3 Before a glycolic peel.

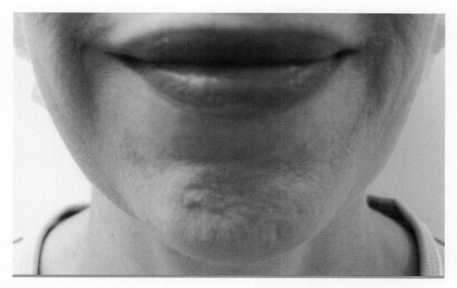

Figure 7–4 After the glycolic peel. Note the improvement in the quality of the skin: tone, texture, and color. Also note the improvement in the lines at the sides of the face.

Complications

The complications of glycolic peeling are directly related to the length of time the solution is left on and the strength of the solution. Remember that the termination of a glycolic is complete even *after neutralization*. If the peel is not completely neutralized, it will continue to work, and this could cause a papillary dermis injury. Generally, 30% and 50% solutions do not risk scarring. However, with 70% glycolic peel, scarring is possible. Other complications that are possible with glycolic acid include the overuse of triple antibiotic ointment, irritation, dry skin, allergy, cold sore breakout, and infections (Table 7–2).

You will remember that bacteria live on the skin and protect us from the environment. If the bacteria count is disrupted, a rash or irritation will occur. This phenomenon can occur when triple-antibiotic ointment is used on closed skin. The clinician must not occlude closed skin. In other words, if the epidermis is still intact, an ointment is not indicated. A moisturizer will work just fine to hydrate the skin. Specific moisturizers have been developed that are intended for postpeel use to ensure that the skin will be lubricated and hydrated; using one of these moisturizers is the best choice (Figures 7–5 and 7–6).

Irritation from the peel is also possible, which usually occurs when the patient returns to his or her therapeutic program too quickly. If the patient's skin is red and dry, additional peeling will usually follow. A topical 2% hydrocortisone application will help with this problem.

Dry skin is common after peeling, especially around the mouth. Extra moisturizer will help. Giving the patient a facial is also helpful. This hydrating process will alleviate the dry skin and exfoliate the loose skin.

Allergies, though rare, do occur with glycolic acid. The patient will usually become very irritated, erythemic, and sometimes exhibit a rash. Obviously, an allergic response dictates removal of the culprit from the

Table 7–2   Possible Complications for Glycolic Peels
Scarring
Overuse of triple antibiotic ointment or Aquafor®
Allergy
Irritation
Herpes simplex breakout
Bacterial or viral infections

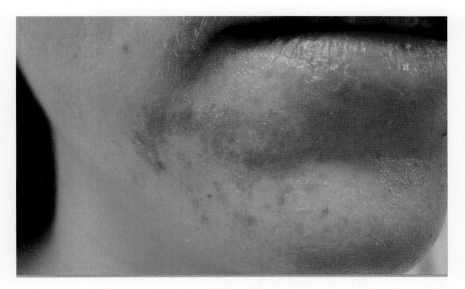

Figure 7–5   Glycolic rash or irritation.

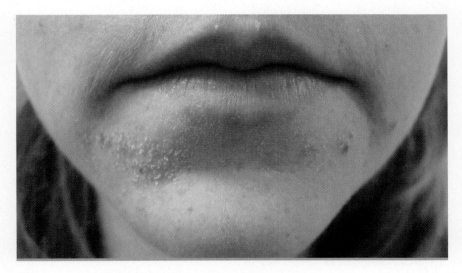

Figure 7–6   Glycolic irritation 4 days later.

skin-care and peeling routine. In some instances, the culprit is the actual peeling solution: glycolic acid.

Infections can occur with glycolic acid peels, especially when the peels are slightly more aggressive. If an infection occurs, it is usually in an area where the skin is compromised. Sometimes, even impetigo can occur after a peel, which is discussed in the previous chapters. If the clinician suspects impetigo, chemical peeling should not be done, and the patient should be referred to a physician for antibiotics and care. If impetigo *occurs* or you suspect an infection, you will need to have the patient see your clinic physician for evaluation and antibiotics.

A glycolic peel can precipitate herpes simplex (cold sores). Patients who are predisposed to herpes simplex should always have an antiviral such as **Valtrex**® on hand. For patients who are very sensitive, a wise course of action would be to have them begin Valtrex® 2 days before the peel and continue 3 days after the peel. Active herpes simplex is explained in previous chapters. Most patients who get cold sores know it, and they hate them. These patients are usually quite cooperative with you about taking medications or postponing a peel.

Acne breakouts can occur after a peel, usually isolated to individuals with oily or acne-prone skin. A topical antibiotic is helpful to control the breakouts, and, if necessary, an oral antibiotic can be used. Also useful for this patient is to be scheduled for a facial 1 week after the glycolic peel to avert an increase in breakouts.

Hyperpigmentation and hypopigmentation can be consequences of glycolic peeling. Choosing candidates carefully and applying a conservative treatment will create a buffer of protection against postinflammatory hyperpigmentation. Additionally, making sure that the home-care program includes hydroquinone and insisting that the patient wear a sunscreen are important defensive actions against postinflammatory hyperpigmentation. If hyperpigmentation occurs after the peel, aggressively treat the problem with a home-care regiment for at least 2 to 3 weeks before considering another peel treatment. Hypopigmentation is a serious consequence of peeling, which usually means that the patient was picking at the skin, that a deeper than expected peeling took place, or that cold sores or infections progressed the skin injury. Little can be done for hypopigmentation. In the areas of hypopigmentation, the melanocytes are no longer functioning and have been irrevocably damaged.

Combining Glycolic Peels with Other Treatments

Glycolic peels are only one isolated treatment in an antiaging protocol. Most patients have many other antiaging treatments to augment the results of the glycolic peel. The treatments are sometimes simultaneous and other times independent of the peel. Glycolic peels are commonly partnered with dermal fillers and Botox®, for example. Glycolic acid is also simultaneously used with microdermabrasion to achieve an advanced result. Facials and glycolic acid peels are also a winning combination. Knowing all of the options available for your patient gives

Valtrex®
An antiviral treatment for herpes simplex.

you the opportunity to make recommendations that will enhance the result of the glycolic peel.

Injectables

Injectables are familiar in any medical spa and a terrific way to improve a patient's appearance without surgery. The most popularly used injectable right now is Botox®. Botox® allows for the treatment of fine lines and wrinkles through the paralysis of specific muscle groups. Among the other injectable treatments that can be combined with peels are a cascade of dermal fillers, including **Restylane®**, **Hylaform®**, **Radiesse®**, and SCULPTRA®. Careful scheduling of these treatments is required to ensure that the treatments occur in the proper sequence and will suit the aftercare required of each treatment. For example, having the patient lie down after Botox® therapy is generally unadvisable. Therefore the peel treatment should be done before the Botox® treatment, if it is to be done on the same day. Restylane® or Radiesse® treatments should also be done at separate appointments. The skin is somewhat sensitive and perhaps slightly swollen after the peel. This swelling may cause the misplacement of the dermal filler. Waiting a day or two is best to provide the best result for the client. The preferred course is to administer the peel treatment first and follow with the injection therapy a few days later, after the peeling is complete. As aesthetic skin-care programs have advanced, they have become multipronged, using many options to achieve the desired end result, which is certainly true for glycolic peeling and dermal fillers.

Botox®

Botox® (Allergan, Irvine, California), *Clostridium botulinum* toxin type A,[2] is used to paralyze muscles groups by inhibiting the release of **acetylcholine** at the neuromuscular junction. Once the active muscles are treated and begin to relax, the glycolic peel therapy will be much more effective in areas of active movement. The areas treated will result in smoother skin and a reduction of lines, specifically, in the glabella, crow's-feet, and forehead, the areas most commonly treated with Botox®. These areas of animation are difficult to treat with glycolic peeling alone; therefore the combination of the two treatments provides an excellent outcome. Botox® is safe, and no nervous system effects[3] have been reported with this product. Botox® is a *temporary* solution, and patients should be aware that the treatment needs to be repeated every 3 to 6 months (Figures 7–7 and 7–8).

Restylane®

Restylane® is the newest dermal filler and is injected to wrinkles and fine lines, as well as augment the lips for a fuller lip line. Manufactured as a biodegradable non-animal stabilized hyaluronic acid (NASHA) gel,

Restylane®
Trade name for the first FDA approved hyaluronic acid for dermal filling.

Hylaform®
An injectable hyaluronic acid manufactured from rooster combs.

Radiesse®
A calcium hydroxylapatite (a dermal filler).

Clostridium botulinum
The bacteria derived for Botox®.

acetylcholine
An enzyme found in various tissues and organs, associated with muscle movement.

Collagen®
A dermal filler and the trade name for injectable bovine collagen.

Botox® and glycolic peeling are good partner procedures. Botox® will minimize the muscle movement and improve the appearance of dynamic lines, and the peel will smooth the skin and encourage collagen remodeling in the dermis.

Restylane® is the newest dermal filler, gaining popularity over Collagen®. It was approved by the U.S. Food and Drug Administration (FDA) in November of 2003.

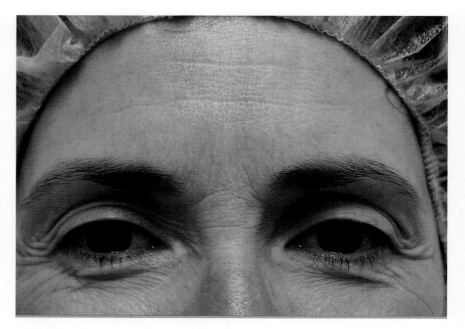

Figure 7–7 Glycolic peel result without the benefit of Botox® therapy.

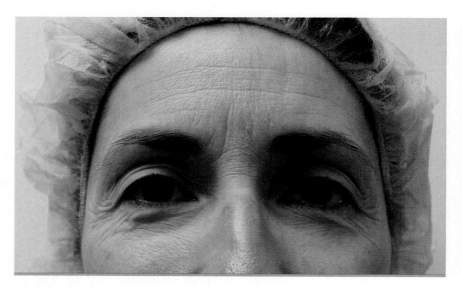

Figure 7–8 Glycolic peel result with the benefit of Botox® therapy.

Restylane® is hyaluronic acid. This newest dermal filler does not require a skin test and is very durable. Restylane® is versatile and provides many options to the nurse or physician (Figures 7–9 and 7–10).

Using a small fine-gauge needle, the product is injected into the areas of defect. The process takes approximately 30 minutes to 1 hour. The patient may exhibit some bruising and swelling that evening and into the next day, generally resolving within a week. On a rare occasion, lumps and bumps can form, but these usually resolve within a week. The treatment will need to be repeated every 8 to 10 months. Restylane® can be combined with Botox, as well as chemical peeling, for an outstanding result.

Radiesse®

Radiesse® is calcium hydroxylapatite suspended in a gel[4] for injection. This product has had many uses over the years and has been found to be reliable and durable. The FDA has not approved Radiesse® (as of this writing) for cosmetic uses. However, recently, plastic surgeons have begun to use this product for cosmetic uses because of its long-term stability of approximately 18 months to 2 years. This use, of course, is not illegal because of FDA amendment 6: "Nothing in (FD & C) shall be construed to limit or interfere with the authority of the healthcare practitioner to prescribe or administer any legally marketed device to a patient or any conditions or disease within a legitimate healthcare practitioner-patient relationship."[5] Radiesse® is effective for use in the lips and deeper **naso-labial folds** (smile lines). Once this product is approved, it will no doubt become far more popular with physicians and patients alike.

Facials

Facials and peels go together; it is just that simple. After a peel has been done and the patient begins to shed, nothing can feel as good as a facial. A facial is the perfect treatment to help the skin through the exfoliation process and to help hydrate the skin. Facials also help the patient relax and enjoy their new skin.

Microdermabrasion

Microdermabrasions and glycolic peels are often used concurrently to gather the benefits of both treatments. Although some clinicians use the peel after the treatment, the best results come when the glycolic peel solution, in low strengths, is used as a keratolic agent before the microdermabrasion treatment. Glycolic peels that are used after microdermabrasion increase the risk for uneven uptake and possible unintentional deep peeling in the areas where the microdermabrasion abraded the skin aggressively.

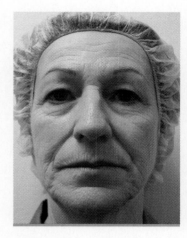

Figure 7–9 Glycolic peel result without the benefit of Restylane® therapy. Although the skin is smooth and even in color as a benefit of the glycolic treatment, lines are still present around the mouth and at the sides of the face.

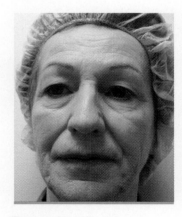

Figure 7–10 Glycolic peel result with the benefit of Restylane® therapy. Note the improvement around the mouth.

naso-labial folds
The area of skin connected to the nose and lip.

Radiesse® is not FDA approved for cosmetic uses, but some physicians still use it for cosmetic purposes.

Regiment of Clinical Treatments

Glycolic peels are meant to be a progressive treatment program. You know now that one or two glycolic peels will not provide a meaningful result. Therefore creating a program of visits that keeps the patient focused on a regular regiment will provide the best results. This effort requires a two-pronged approach: peel packages and regular scheduling. Developing a package of peels and facials, for example, makes sense; it allows the patient to be financially committed to the peel program, and because of the treatment variety of facials and peels, the patient is more likely to schedule appointments. Patient retention is the key to treatment success. The more often the patient is in the clinic, the more likely the result will be one with which the client will be happy and of which you will be proud.

Number of Treatments

No correct number of treatments has been established to achieve a desired result with glycolic peels. Patients are usually seen every other week for three to four treatments and then on a monthly basis thereafter. When the peels are performed lightly, as would be indicated with this frequency, they are sometimes referred to as "lunchtime" peels. If, on the other hand, the peels are more aggressive, then scheduling them on a 6-week rotation is appropriate. This process is individualized and should be engineered to meet the patient's needs. The time between peels should be set up to allow for the skin to heal and new cellular growth to occur. Eventually, the peel should be done on a 4- to 6-week rotation in rhythm with the skin's natural process.

Alternation with Other Treatments

Glycolic acid is a good peeling agent that provides improvement to both the dermis and the epidermis. The most meaningful results are achieved when the defects are mainly in the epidermis; this is especially true of the hyperpigmentation. However, greater benefits can be derived from glycolic acid peels when they are combined with other treatments. Among the treatments that can help improve the glycolic acid result are intense pulsed light therapy and facials.

Alternating intense pulsed light (IPL) or Photo Facial® with glycolic acid peeling can be of great benefit. IPL can improve telangiectasia uncovered by peeling or assist with the treatment of hyperpigmentation.

Not enough can be said about the benefits of facials. These procedures, whether done with steam or via a heat mask, can provide vitamins, antioxidants, and hydration to the skin. Alternating the glycolic peel with a facial will ultimately provide a better result than would just the glycolic acid peel alone.

■ WHEN TO CONSULT YOUR CLINIC PHYSICIAN

An important and delicate part of a physician-clinician relationship is to know when to consult about the patient's progress. This is, in large part, a function of the detailed policy and procedure manual. However, the rapport is also the relationship that the clinician and physician create. In the medical spa setting, physicians consider you a professional and expert; and although physicians are generally performing procedures and caring for patients at the level they were trained, they should always be available to you. A clinician should never feel uncomfortable or embarrassed to ask the assistance of the clinic physician.

Glycolic peeling itself is such a safe treatment, we rarely think about the idea of *precautions*. However, all procedures, including glycolic peels, have precautions. When treating patients with glycolic peels, the clinician should have a heighten awareness when the following issues are encountered: body dysmorphic disorder, sensitive skin, chronic sunlight exposure, hepatitis, immune deficiencies such as acquired immune deficiency syndrome (AIDS) and human immunodeficiency virus (HIV), pregnant or lactating patients, or patients with suspicious lesions or lupus (Table 7–3).

Table 7–3   Appropriate Times to Talk with the Physician

Concern	Discuss with Physician
Truthfulness of a client	X
Concerns about the ability to achieve desired results	X
Indications for a possible surgical procedure Concerns about body dysmorphic disorder	X
Efficacy of the care plan	X
Patient has need for prescription medications	X
Clarification of medical conditions	X
Indications for chemical peel treatment	X
Possibility of an ongoing disease process	X
Need for advance acne treatment	X
Suspicious lesions	X

▶ >> TOP TEN TIPS TO TAKE TO THE CLINIC

1. Glycolic peels are not as easy as they seem and should be respected.
2. Epidermolysis can occur quickly with glycolic acid; be aware of this possibility.
3. Glycolic acid peels can appear spotty, depending on the preparation in the clinic and at home.
4. Keep the treatment room neat and organized.
5. To achieve the best results, the patient should be on a home-care program 2 weeks in advance of the clinic peel program.
6. The peel application technique can affect the outcome of the treatment.
7. Do not peel patients with cold sores.
8. Know the complications of glycolic peels, and do not disregard a patient telephone call.
9. Botox® and injectable fillers improve the results of glycolic acid peels.
10. Patients should be seen on a monthly basis to achieve and sustain the best results.

CHAPTER REVIEW QUESTIONS

1. What is glycolic acid?
2. How does glycolic acid work to peel the skin?
3. What are the best indications for glycolic acid?
4. How does glycolic peeling interface with other treatments?
5. How do you choose the strength of the peel solution?
6. What are the important components of a consent for treatment?
7. What is the pretreatment protocol for glycolic peels?
8. What are the skin's normal response to glycolic peels?
9. What are the objectives of glycolic peels?
10. What are the potential complications of glycolic peels?

CHAPTER REFERENCES

1. Brody, H. J. (1997). *Chemical peeling and resurfacing* (2nd ed.). St. Louis: Mosby.
2. Fagien, S., & Brandt, F. S. (2001). Primary and adjunctive use of botulinum toxin type A (Botox) in facial aesthetic surgery: Beyond the glabella. *Clinics in Plastic Surgery*, 28(1), 127–161.
3. Fagien, S., & Brandt, F. S. (2001). Primary and adjunctive use of botulinum toxin type A (Botox) in facial aesthetic surgery: Beyond the glabella. *Clinics in Plastic Surgery*, 28(1), 127–161.

4. Bioform Medical. (2004, April 11). *Product characteristics: Radiesse* [Online]. Available: www.bioforminc.com

5. Nassif, P. S. (2004, April). Radiesse: An injectable calcium hydroxylapatite. *plasticsurgery.com* [Online]. Available: www.plasticsurgery.com

BIBLIOGRAPHY

A Board Certified Plastic Surgeon Resource. (2004, April 7). *Chemical peel: Find a chemical peel surgeon near you!* [On line]. Available: http://www.aboardcertifiedplasticsurgeon.com

Alam, M., Omura, N., Dover, J., Amdt, K. (2002, June). Glycolic acid peels compared to microdermabrasion: A right-left controlled trial of efficacy and patient satisfaction. *Dermatologic Surgery, 28,* 475.

Alam, M., Omura, N., Dover, J., Amdt, K. (2002, June). *Glycolic acid peels compared to microdermabrasion: A right-left controlled trial of efficacy and patient satisfaction.* [Online]. Available: http://www.ncbi.nlm.nih.gov

American Society for Dermatologic Surgery. (2004, May 13). *Chemical peel: Patient fact sheet* [Online]. Available: http://asds-net.org

American Society of Plastic Surgeons. (2004, May 12). *Procedures, chemical peel* [On line]. Available: http://www.plasticsurgery.org

Ancira, M. A. (1998). Chemical peels: An overview. *Plastic Surgical Nursing, 19,* 179.

Bioform Medical. (2004, April 11). *Product characteristics: Radiance* [Online]. Available: www.bioforminc.com

Brody, H. J. (1997). *Chemical peeling and resurfacing* (2nd ed.). St. Louis: Mosby.

Brody, H. J., Geronemus, R. G., & Faris, P. K. (2003, April). Beauty versus medicine: The non-physician practice of dermatologic surgery. *Journal of Dermatologic Surgery, 29*(4), 319–324.

Caputy, G. (2002, April 3). *Skin surfacing and chemical peels* [Online]. Available: www.emedicine.com

ClevelandClinic.org. (2004, April 21). *Facial rejuvenation: Lotions, potions, lasers, and peels* [Online]. Available: www.clevelandclinic.org

Daresbury Imaging Group. (2005, May). Collagen [On line]. Available at: http://detserv1.dl.ac.uk

Fagien, S., & Brandt, F. S. (2001). Primary and adjunctive use of botulinum toxin type A (Botox) in facial aesthetic surgery: Beyond the glabella. *Clinics in Plastic Surgery, 28*(1), 127–161.

Goldberg, G. (2004, January 15). *Chemical peels* [Online]. Available: www.pimaderm.com

Guttman, C. (2002, August). Histologic studies: Chemical peels, not just superficial. *Cosmetic Surgery Times* [Online]. Available: http://www.cosmeticsurgerytimes

Koch, R. J., & Hanasono, N. M. (2001, August). Chemical peels. *North American Journal of Facial and Plastic Surgery,* 9(3), 377–382. Also available: http://www.aesthetic.lumenis.com

Merck Pharmaceuticals Company. (2004, April 21). *The Merck manual: Second home edition, section 24: Accidents and injuries: Burns* [Online]. Available: http://www.merck.com

Nassif, P. S. (2004, April). Radiance: An injectable calcium hydroxylapatite. *PlasticSurgery.com* [Online]. Available: www.plasticsurgery.com

Obagi, Z. (2000). *Skin health restoration and rejuvenation.* New York: Springer-Verlag New York.

PlasticSurgery.com. (2004, May 13). *Chemical peel: How is a chemical peel performed?* [Online]. Available: www.plastoicsurgery.com

Rubin, M. (1995). *Manual of chemical peels: Superficial and medium depth.* Philadelphia: Lippincott, Williams & Wilkins.

Sengelmann, R. T., & Tull, S. (2004, May 14). Dermal fillers (excerpt). *eMedicine Specialties: Dermatology* [On line]. Available: http://www.emedicine.com

Sepp, D. T. (1998, December). *Alpha hydroxy acids* [Online]. Available: www.shikai.com

Skin Therapy Letter. (1998, May). *Current review of the alpha hydroxy acids* [Online]. Available: www.dermatology.org

U.S. Food and Drug Administration. (1997, July 3). *Alpha hydroxy acids in cosmetics. FDA Backgrounder* [Online]. Available: www.vm.cfsan.fda.gov

Wang, C. M., Huang, C. L., & Chan, H. L. (1997, January). The effect of glycolic acid in the treatment of Asian skin. *Journal of Dermatologic Surgery,* 23(1), 23–29.

Whitaker, E. (2003, December 2). *Chemical peels* [Online]. Available: www.emedicine.com.

Jessner's Peels

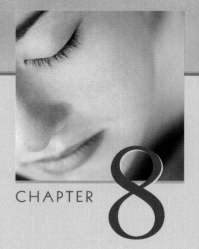

CHAPTER 8

KEY TERMS

5FU® pulse peeling
body dysmorphic
  disorder (BDD)

resorcinol
universal precautions

LEARNING OBJECTIVES

After completing this chapter you should be able to:

1. Discuss the "recipe" for Jessner's peel solution.
2. Discuss the neutralization process for Jessner's peels.
3. Discuss the indications and contraindications for Jessner's peels.
4. Discuss the anticipated results for Jessner's peels.

INTRODUCTION

J essner's solution was pioneered by Dr. Max Jessner, a German-American dermatologist. To create superficial peeling without the toxicity, Dr. Jessner combined **resorcinol** and lactic and salicylic acids in percentages of 14% suspended in an ethanol base. The Jessner's peel solution is a preferred peeling agent for oily, acne-prone skin and hyperpigmented skin because of its safety (nontoxic), superficial (does not need to be neutralized) nature. "Overpeeling" with Jessner's solution is difficult because of the mild percentages associated with the acid combinations. It is safe in almost any clinician's hands but still requires a knowledge base that allows the clinician to anticipate the potential problems and to treat them accordingly.

Anecdotal evidence tells us that repetitive Jessner's peeling improves the quality, tone, and texture of the skin. The solution is frequently used in concert with other solutions such as trichloroacetic acid (TCA) and glycolic acid. It is versatile, safe and a commonly used product for peeling the skin.

■ JESSNER'S PEELING

Jessner's peeling creates a controlled injury to the skin at the epidermal level. The skin regeneration that follows the peel improves both oily and acne-prone skin, as well as hyperpigmentation. Several important points need to be considered when using Jessner's solution, among them are the pretreatment, the clinical preparation, the peel application, and the skin's response to the peel. All of these considerations are keys to the final outcome, and none should be taken for granted.

The pretreatment preparation speaks to the home-care program the patient is using. An important point to remember is that home-care programs should be designed in a fashion that allows superior penetration of each step of the program. In setting up such a program, the clinician can be assured that the skin will be prepared to accept the peel solution.

The peel application is the process by which the peeling solution is applied and, obviously, has everything to do with the final outcome of the treatment. Understanding the importance of de-fatting the skin, choosing the solution (a variety of Jessner's solutions are available, aside from the traditional mixture), and the proper application of the solution to the skin make the difference in a quality result. Finally, the ability to understand what one is seeing on the skin as the peel begins to work

resorcinol
Equal parts of hydroquinone and catechol, a peeling agent with similarities to phenol.

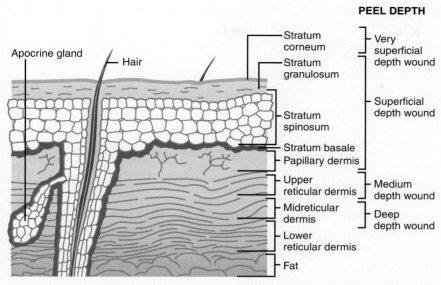

PEEL DEPTH

Stratum corneum
Stratum granulosum
Stratum spinosum
Stratum basale
Papillary dermis
Upper reticular dermis
Midreticular dermis
Lower reticular dermis
Fat

Apocrine gland
Hair

Very superficial depth wound
Superficial depth wound
Medium depth wound
Deep depth wound

Figure 8–1 Jessner's peels can penetrate into the upper papillary dermis as shown.

requires a skilled clinician. Knowing what to *expect* based on the previously discussed variables and how to *predict* the peel solution's behavior on the skin is what you will learn in this text.

Jessner's peels are considered superficial but, compared with other superficial peels, have the tendency to slough more skin (Figure 8–1). For these reasons alone, a Jessner's peel will be selected, hardly the variables that one should use when rendering patient care. Nevertheless, it happens. This chapter will discuss the Jessner's peel process in depth and address indications, predictable outcomes, and possible complications.

Pretreatment Preparation

As with any superficial peeling agents, the work done at home is just as important as the peel that takes place in the clinic. This process means that the patient should be on at least 2 weeks of a suitable alpha hydroxy acid (AHA, glycolic 8%+ or lactic acid), Retin A® or retinol, and hydroquinone. Additionally, remember that, although the aforementioned products are familiar to a therapeutic program, they are not the *only* products necessary for a great result. Do not forget to add the sunscreen and moisturizers. Make sure that patients have the proper organization of the products in the home routine so they will get the best result. Also be sure that patients understand that the use of facial grains on the day of the peel is *not* indicated. Finally, remember to instruct patients to continue using the home-care products every day before the peel.

Moderately devised home-care programs can cause the skin to become red and irritated, even peel, especially if the patient is a first-time Retin A® user. This patient should be brought to the clinic for a facial before the peel series begins. This step can keep the patient from becoming discouraged because he or she is peeling, irritated, and may look worse than when the program began.

Clinical Preparation

As with any peel, make sure the room is properly set up and the supplies are within reach. If you keep any variations of the Jessner's peel solution, such as a different percentage of resorcinol or salicylic acid, these bottles need to be clearly marked. The peel solution that you are going to use needs to be set out and available for you. Additional supplies are also needed, including application tools (gauze, brushes, cotton-tipped applicators, and a small medicine cup), a bowl of water, eyewash, cleansers, moisturizers, and sunscreens. Additionally, a small motorized fan is necessary to help the patient's skin cool during the treatment. Lastly, a bonnet or headband should be used to protect the patient's hair. Once the room is prepared, bring the patient into the treatment room and begin the procedure.

Obtaining the Consent

As we have previously discussed, all peels have a potential for problems; therefore, regardless of the type of peel, a consent form is always necessary. Such is the case whether you are in a medical office, medical spa, or for that matter, a luxury spa setting. Remember, the consent will be a part of your protection in a dispute. You can get a consent form from a book, and it may appear sufficient for your situation. However, remember, every facility is different, and the consent form you choose to use should be reviewed by your clinic attorney. This precaution ensures you are well protected for your individual situation.

Choosing the Solution Percentage

When using a standard Jessner's solution, consideration should be given to the clinical preparation of the skin, the adherence to the home-care therapy, any irritated spots on the skin, and the social consequences of skin shedding for the next 7 days.

Consents are the tools that are used to inform the patient about the risks and complications of a Jessner's peel procedure. This document also makes the clinician aware of the patient allergies, expectations (through discussions), and chronic medical problems. The clinician should make sure that a consent form accompanies each procedure performed.

When considering the clinical preparation of the skin for Jessner's peeling, be aware that cleansing the skin and applying the solution will *not* provide the best result. When using Jessner's solution, de-fatting or stripping the skin is important. The minimum preparation that is recommended is 70% isopropyl alcohol. Some clinicians prefer 90% isopropyl alcohol; others use acetone. Remember, these agents are flammable; therefore follow the necessary precautions associated with such product use. The use of rough gauze is effective in scrubbing the skin and will help de-fat the skin. This process will affect the stratum corneum, especially around the eyes and corners of the mouth. If you are trying to provide improvement on the upper lip, be sure to prepare this area well.

The adherence to the home-care therapy is also a consideration. If the patient has not been faithful to the program, the skin will not be as responsive to the peel solution. When the home-care regimen has not been followed exactly, the surface of the skin may be irregular, and the peel solution will not penetrate evenly. If, on the other hand, the patient has been overusing the products, the skin may be irritated, which will cause the peel solution to take up more quickly and possibly penetrate deeper than was anticipated.

One consideration in choosing the peel and the peel percentage is the amount of shedding or peeling the patient can tolerate in the coming week. This concern may seem silly, but understand that every appointment the client makes has a period of downtime, which can be discouraging to the patient to the point of giving up. Remember that continuity in a treatment plan is important for successful results. Therefore take seriously the patient's schedule and his or her social and business considerations.

Lastly, always check the results of the previous peel and the progress of the home-care program. What is the patient reporting to you? Did the patient peel a little or a lot? Are the areas of concern improving? Is the patient tolerating the program? Finally, what are you seeing? Taking before and after pictures may be useful to ensure that what you think you see is actually what you see.

Jessner's solution and other additives

As with any great treatment, variations on the theme can be found. Traditional Jessner's solution is commonly called 14%-14%-14%, denoting the ratio of the three acids that comprise the solution (resorcinol, lactic acid, and salicylic acid). Green tea, Paraguay tea, and kola nut are known antioxidants and have sometimes been added to the Jessner's solution to create a "power punch" to the standard Jessner's peel. This addition can help the skin rejuvenate and control free radicals in the process.

Choosing the peel solution is as much an art as it is a science. Knowing the skin and predicting how it will react to the peel solution comes with experience and knowledge. Creating the result you want for a patient with a peel solution is a real art.

Peel

As with any clinical process, the technique of the clinician is an important factor in the results of a peel. Such is the case with Jessner's peeling. The choice of preparation processes, the gauze or sponge that is used to clean the skin, the application device, and the cooling process all make a difference to the end result.

Several different application devices can be used: a brush, gauze, or a cotton-tipped applicator. The best results come from using folded gauze. This approach allows the greatest control and the least amount of splashing or dripping of the peel solution.

Make sure your patient is comfortable on the bed; having the patient change into a spa wrap or patient gown is sometimes helpful, especially if you plan to treat the neck and chest. If the patient does not change into a gown or wrap, be sure to put a towel over the patient's chest to protect the clothing from becoming soiled. Be sure that the hair is placed in a surgical bonnet or held back by a spa headband. The blue bonnet is really the easiest way to keep the hair neat and yet protected from the solution, water, or the breeze from the fan.

Now you are ready to begin. However, first, take an inventory. Is your room completely stocked? Is the fan on the counter? Do you have the correct peel solution? Is the eyewash solution close at hand? Do you have a bowl of water to cool the skin? Now that you have done a quick check of supplies, you are ready to begin. Using a mild cleanser with *soft gauze*, cleanse the face until all of the makeup and debris have been removed. This process may take two applications of cleanser. Follow cleansing by de-fatting the skin as previously discussed. Next, pour the selected Jessner's solution into a small medicine cup or similar container. Dip the folded gauze into the peel solution. Squeeze out any extra solution against the side of your medicine cup; *your gauze should not be dripping with peel solution.* To apply the solution, begin on the forehead and make vertical strokes, beginning at the eyebrows and moving to the hairline. Then, apply the solution to the upper lip. If the gauze becomes dry, use new gauze and continue the peel. Next, turn your attention to the lower eyelid and crow's-feet; follow this with application to the sides of the face. Always apply two coats, one vertically and one horizontally. This application method helps ensure that the solution has been evenly distributed on the skin surface (Figure 8–2).

Skin's Response to the Peel

The skin will initially turn pink when the solution is applied, then the skin will begin to turn red, and, finally, it may frost. The potential of a frost is based on several variable factors: how well the skin was defatted,

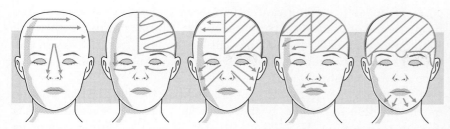

Figure 8–2   The application of the peel solution should be methodical as indicated by this diagram.

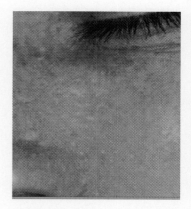

Figure 8–3   A common appearance of frost with a Jessner's peel. This color can also be a salicylate precipitate that can be wiped away. Be sure you have a frost by gently wiping the area to ensure it is not a salicylate precipitate.

the home-care preparation, and the number of coats applied to the affected area. The frost of a peel solution on the skin is a phenomenon seen with Jessner's peels, glycolic peels, and with TCA peels. Frost occurs when the peel solution reacts with the "major protein of the epidermis, keratin, precipitating the protein and forming a frost."[1]

The frost can be challenging to identify. Watch for the pinkness to turn red, which should then be followed by an appearance of a white haze. A salicylate or crystallization of the peeling products may sometimes appear on the skin (Figure 8–3). Do not be fooled: this is not a frost. If the whiteness on the skin moves or can be wiped off, it is not frost. You may need to wait up to 5 minutes for a frost to occur with Jessner's solution. Frosting will usually occur in the thinnest skin first: around the eyes, for example, or in the driest areas such as on the upper lip (Figure 8–4). If a frost is not desired, apply only one rather than two

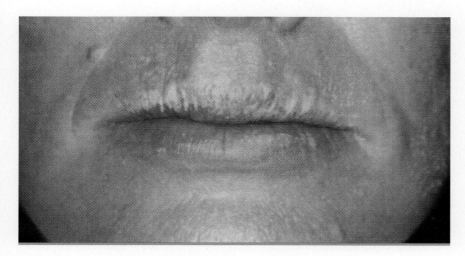

Figure 8–4   A frost on the upper lip.

Figure 8–5 Commonly, Jessner's solution will cause a speckling on the skin rather than a complete frost.

coats. If the skin is significantly damaged by sunlight exposure or the proper home or clinical preparations to the skin are not made, then the solution may actually repel and bead up on the skin (Figure 8–5). In this case, the solution can be massaged with gloved hands or rough gauze to encourage penetration.

Talk to the patient as you are applying the solution and ask what he or she is feeling and where. In the areas that are hotter, you should see a quicker response on the skin. Remember, Jessner's solution cannot be neutralized; it can only be diluted. Be sure that the number of coats you apply is appropriate for the wounding you intend.

When you are ready to cool the skin, you will be diluting the solution. Physicians, in general, do not dilute or cool Jessner's peels but simply send patients home. However, cooling the skin and making patients more comfortable before sending them home is appropriate. Once the skin has reached the appearance you desire, begin the cooling process. Dip soft gauze into cool water or saline and apply the sponges to the face. Be careful to avoid dripping the water down the patient's neck and back. You want to be professional and not messy. Keep washing down the face until the patient has some relief. All of the burning will not go away. The skin will remain hot for a couple of hours, which is perfectly normal. Once the cooling process has occurred, use an antiinflammatory gel, and follow with a sunscreen.

Use of occlusion

Occlusion can be used with the Jessner's peel, just as with glycolic peeling. If the peel did not come to a frost, to achieve a deeper peel, apply an occlusive dressing. This dressing would be either Vaseline® or Aquafor®. Keeping the heat in the tissues will continue to cause a minor injury, thus increasing the peel depth. The increase in the peel depth will be very slight, so do not be misled that it will significantly increase the skin's injury.

Posttreatment

The posttreatment for a Jessner's peel is easy and similar to a glycolic peel. Begin with the application of an antiinflammatory product that will cool and moisturize the skin. Many such agents are on the market. Inflammatory gel should be used in the first 6 hours to cool and soothe the skin. After the first 6 hours, the skin should be kept soft with Aquafor® to avoid any potential cracking and subsequent early peeling. On the second day, especially if a frost occurred, the skin will turn a brown color, similar to a tan. The skin should continue to be lubricated with Aquafor® to prevent early peeling. The home-care program should be avoided until the sloughing is complete, which will take approximately 5 days.

At the third day, the skin will begin to peel. The patient should be instructed to avoid picking because this behavior can result in scarring and infections. For some patients, picking is *so* tempting and difficult to avoid. Education about picking is an important part of the clinician's job. Once the skin begins to peel, on the evening of the fourth day, the patient should exfoliate the skin (Figure 8–6). A very fine grain is the best choice. In the shower, let the face get very warm and soft; then use the grain to exfoliate (Table 8–1).

Anticipated Results

Jessner's peels can be quite dramatic, especially for patients with acne-prone or hyperpigmented skin. Jessner's peel, similar to glycolic acid peel, is a progressive treatment that will not provide a final result with one peel. The usual course is bi-weekly for patients with acne-prone skin and once a month for patients with hyperpigmented skin. Obviously, the frequency has to do with the depth of the peel and the length of the peeling process. Patients will not tolerate a sloughing face all the time (Figures 8–7 and 8–8).

Complications

For the most part, Jessner's peels are safe and self-limiting. Surprisingly, Jessner's peels rarely progress past the expected depth, considering the erythema associated with the process. For aestheticians who are becoming familiar with peeling solutions and processes, this peel feels

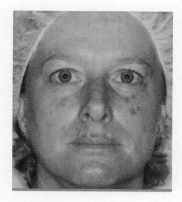

Figure 8–6 The patient before a Jessner's peel.

Table 8–1	Posttreatment for Patients with Jessner's Peels	
Day one	Antiinflammatory gel Aquafor® (for open skin), moisturizer (for closed skin)	First 6 hours following Jessner's peel Hours 6-24
Day two	Aquafor® (for open skin), moisturizer (for closed skin)	Damaged skin tissue begins to appear brownish in color.
Day three	Aquafor® (for open skin), moisturizer (for closed skin)	Noticeable peeling starts. Advise against picking.
Day four	Fine-grain exfoliant	Necrosed skin should be gently removed.
Day five	Return to normal home-care treatment	

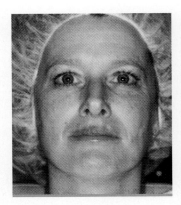

Figure 8–7 Patient
4 days after a Jessner's peel.

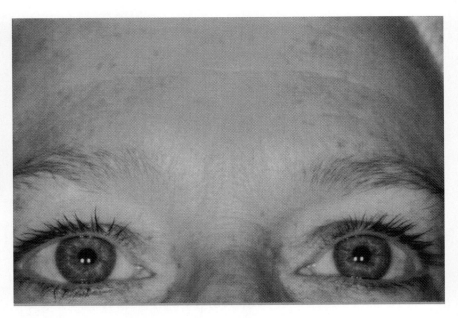

Figure 8–8 The patient after a Jessner's peel.

comfortable because it goes on uniformly. This characteristic contrasts with glycolic peels in which the peel solution will take up on different areas of the face, causing a blotchy peel. Another reason that clinicians prefer Jessner's solution is that it provides peeling, rather than flaking associated with glycolic peels. Nevertheless, complications can arise from the use of Jessner's solutions. Among these complications, of which the clinician should be aware, are infections, herpes simplex outbreaks, dry skin, product sensitivity and allergies, and acne outbreaks.

Bacteria live on the skin and protect us from the environment. If the bacteria count is disrupted, a rash, irritation, or even an infection will occur. The clinician must not occlude the patient's closed skin. In other words, if the Jessner's peel did not frost, an occlusive agent such as Aquafor® need not be used. That said, sometimes the skin is very tight and dry. A thin layer of vaseline can help the skin from cracking and the patient from itching. The postcare will be better handled with a moisturizer. Specific moisturizers are available that are intended for postpeel use to ensure that the skin will be lubricated and hydrated; using one of these moisturizers is a better choice.

Irritation from the peel is also possible, which usually occurs when the patient returns to the therapeutic program too quickly. If the patient's skin is red and dry, additional peeling will usually follow. A topical 2% hydrocortisone will help with this problem.

Dry skin is common after peeling, especially around the mouth. Extra moisturizer will help. Additionally, giving the patient a facial is helpful. This hydrating process will alleviate the dry skin and exfoliate the loose skin.

Allergies to Jessner's solution are theoretic, and the clinician should be aware of a potential allergic reaction to the solution. An allergy would present itself in the same fashion as would any allergy: a rash, itching, and possible inflammation. Whether the allergy was caused by the solution or the products used would be difficult to know after the peel unless the allergy occurred immediately on application.

Infections rarely occur with Jessner's peels. If an infection occurs, it is usually in an area where the skin was compromised. If an infection occurs or you suspect an infection, you will need to have the patient see your clinic physician for treatment.

Herpes simplex (cold sores) can be precipitated by a Jessner's solution. Patients who are predisposed to herpes simplex should always have the antiviral, Valtrex®, on hand. For patients who are very sensitive, a wise course of action would be to have them begin Valtrex® 2 days before the peel and continue 3 days after the peel. Active herpes simplex virus, also called HSV-1, is the virus that causes cold sores. These viral infections appear as small clear blisters on the face, most commonly around the mouth or nose. After the lesion has healed, the virus will be dormant in the body, periodically reactivating. Herpes is contagious, and the patient should take care to avoid person-to-person contact while the lesion is open or weeping.

Acne breakouts can occur after a peel, which is usually isolated to individuals with oily, acne-prone skin. A topical antibiotic is helpful to control the breakouts, and, if necessary, an oral antibiotic can be used. Also useful for this patient is to be scheduled for a facial 1 week after the peel to avert an increase in breakouts (Table 8–2).

Table 8–2   Possible Complications of Jessner's Peels
Product sensitivity
Allergy
Irritation
HSV-1 breakout
Bacterial or viral infections

Combining Jessner's Peels with Other Treatments

Jessner's peeling is most appropriate to oily, acne-prone skin and hyper-pigmented skin. As such, this peel is generally not directed at the aging patient. Therefore combining this peel with common aging treatments is not applicable. However, any treatments such as facials that improve acne are highly recommended.

Other Peel Solutions

On occasion, the clinician may need to add a peel solution to Jessner's solution to enhance the result. An example of this instance would be the solar-damaged skin of a patient who has not properly used home-care products. Applying glycolic acid, perhaps 20%, may be useful to act as a keratolytic agent, loosing the stratum corneum, which will then allow the Jessner's to penetrate more effectively.

Neutralization of the glycolic peel comes into question in this procedure. Is it done before or after the application of the Jessner's solution? The safest approach is that the glycolic peel be neutralized before the application of the Jessner's solution. This action will ensure that the changes you see in the skin when you apply the Jessner's solution are related specifically to the Jessner's solution. Combining Jessner's solution with glycolic acid can be useful; just be sure to keep the glycolic acid at 20%.

5% 5-fluorouracil (5FU)

5FU is a chemotherapy agent that is used to treat actinic keratosis (AK). These AKs are not skin cancers but precursors to either squamous cell or sometimes basal cell skin cancers. 5FU cream can be prescribed by the physician and used at home. The usual protocol is a daily application until the areas blister, usually in approximately a week. The treatment is then discontinued. The process can be uncomfortable and unsightly. The loose AK material will usually blister off, and the skin will become smooth and free of potential skin cancers. 5FU is also used in the clinic in a solution form, combined with other peeling agents such as Jessner's, to attack and attach to the AKs. This treatment assists in removing AKs and is a gentler method of treatment compared with liquid nitrogen, surgery, or at home use of 5FU cream. This process is called **5FU pulse peeling** and can provide the same results without the discomfort and mess of cream application. The protocol calls for the patient to be peeled weekly with Jessner's solution followed by an application (in solution form) of the 5FU. The patient is instructed to avoid washing the treated area for 12 hours. The peel is not cooled in the clinic, with water or lotion of any kind. This approach is successful for the treatment of AKs and is frequently done for men, especially on the tops of their heads.

5FU pulse peeling
An alternative delivery to the daily fluorouracil cream. The treatment is done with weekly Jessner's peels and a fluorouracil solution.

Regimen of Clinical Treatments

Given that the Jessner's peel is meant as a component of the treatment regimen, a full program should be outlined for both the clinician and the patient. This care plan should reflect the different types of clinical treatments, the number of treatments, and the anticipated time required to achieve a result. When a treatment program is outlined and the anticipated results are discussed, the patient has direction (so does the clinician), which helps sustain realistic expectations. Remember that each patient is an individual and so is his or her skin; therefore create a program that is unique and customized to the patient's needs.

Number of Treatments

Initially, the best course of action is to see the patient every other week for a Jessner's peel. These peels should be moderate in depth, leaving the patient only 3 to 3.5 days of "shedding." This interval is the most effective for both oily, acne-prone skin and hyperpigmented skin. Once the treatment program has progressed through approximately four peels, then the time between appointments should be expanded to 3 weeks. Two to three more peels should be done after the 3-week interval. Finally, the patient should be placed on a monthly schedule. During this time, the clinician may skip a peel and do a facial instead. The skin may be too "peely" or sensitive to tolerate a peel. The clinician must have the experience and knowledge to assess the skin and know when a conservative approach is required.

Alternation with Other Treatments

Alternating the Jessner's peel with a facial or microdermabrasion commonly provides the best result. Obviously, this application depends on the problem that is being addressed. For example, when dealing with hyperpigmented skin, the clinician may find that the skin is dry or irritated and in need of a soothing treatment such as a facial. On the other hand, the skin may need additional stimulation to encourage faster cellular replacement. In this case, a microdermabrasion is the treatment to add. When acne-prone or oily skin is the problem, a facial is often necessary to help evacuate the pores and keep the skin free from debris. Once again, look at the skin, identify the problem, and then determine the treatment.

Facials

So many different types of facials are available on the market these days, and they are among the best treatment to alternate with Jessner's peels. A good facial, one that is medically directed, will provide the patient with several important treatment improvements, among them antibacterial effects, hydration, antioxidant effects, and exfoliation. Antibacterial facials are a good treatment for your patient with oily or acne-prone skin. This facial will help balance the oiliness of the skin, evacuate pores, and improve the overall appearance of the skin. A hydrating facial is always beneficial, and, in the case of Jessner's peels, it can improve the appearance of dehydrated and peeling skin. Antioxidant facials are good for all skin types, and candidates who are undergoing Jessner's peels are no exception. The benefits of antioxidants bring improvement to the skin that cannot be achieved by peeling alone. Finally, an exfoliating facial is a tremendous benefit, regardless of the skin condition. At least once every 6 weeks is recommended.

Microdermabrasion

Microdermabrasion can boost the results of Jessner's peels, which is especially true when the problem we are treating is hyperpigmentation. The idea of sanding the skin to improve its appearance is a long-standing technique that plastic surgeons and cosmetic dermatologists use. Whether the physician is using a small wire brush or pieces of actual sandpaper to abrade the skin in combination with chemical peeling, surgeons have had success "sanding" the skin to improve its appearance. Therefore a sensible step is to consider using microdermabrasion with Jessner's peels to improve the oily, acne-prone and hyperpigmented skin. Microdermabrasion should be done separately from the Jessner's peel to ensure that the skin is not overtreated.

■ WHEN TO CONSULT YOUR CLINIC PHYSICIAN

Several issues require a specific consultation with the physician before treating a patient with Jessner's solution. Those conditions include any suspicion of **body dysmorphic disorder (BDD)**, hepatitis C, acquired immune deficiency syndrome and human immunodeficiency virus (HIV/AIDS), lupus, any suspicious lesions, pregnancy and lactation, and complications. Each of these problems, though not necessarily contraindications, will need to be evaluated individually by the physician, or at the very least a standing order should be in place on the appropriate care of patients who fall into these categories (Table 8–3).

Body Dysmorphic Disorder

BDD is an emotional disease that causes individuals to be inappropriately concerned with their appearance. People with BDD are focused on

body dysmorphic disorder (BDD)
A psychosocial disease that causes individuals to be inappropriately concerned with their appearance. Persons affected with BDD are contraindicated for most aesthetic procedures.

Table 8–3   When to Consult Your Clinic Physician

Concern	Discuss with Physician
Truthfulness of a client	X
Ability to achieve desired results	X
Indications for a possible surgical procedure	X
Concerns about BDD	X
Efficacy of the care plan	X
Patient need for prescription medications	X
Clarification of medical conditions	X
Indications for chemical peel treatment	X
Possibility of an ongoing disease processes	X
Need for advanced acne treatment	X
Suspicious lesions	X

the appearance of their skin, hair, nose, or ears, in particular. They may have minor defects of the nose or small scars that they believe to be overwhelmingly obvious. Individuals with BDD also are concerned about their eyes and may believe that their eyes are too small or otherwise unattractive. Persons with BDD spend at least 1 hour a day thinking negative thoughts about their appearance.

Not surprisingly, patients with BDD have difficulty in their social life or work life, or both. They often have difficulty meeting new people or making and keeping friends because they are so self-conscious about their appearance. They often spend time alone in their home, often alienating family or people who care about them.

Clinicians in the world of cosmetic surgery and medical skin care find patients who are obviously afflicted and those who walk a gray zone between the well-adjusted and the afflicted.[2] Recognizing these clients will become a challenge for the skin-care professional. The skin-care clinician must be aware of patients who seem overly critical of their skin and appearance. Assuming that the patient is being treated by a psychiatrist, one of the easiest methods is to look at the medications that the client is taking. For persons under treatment, you will find a medication that is used to treat mood disorders. However, this circumstance can be easily misleading and does not always mean that all clients who are on medication for mood disorders have BDD. If BDD is suspected, the clinician should simply ask the patient if he or she is afflicted with the disorder.

Red flags for BDD include depression, anxiety, acute stress, and obsessive and compulsive behaviors.[3] Individuals with BDD will sometimes appear efficient and organized, but when the client is under stress, the previously subtle symptoms of BDD will become apparent. Clients with BDD have a high incidence of dissatisfaction with results, and any small complication can cause undue stress for both the clinician and the client.[4] The most important question the clinician should be asking in situations in which BDD is suspected is, "Can I satisfy this client?" If the clinician has a concern about his or her own ability to satisfy the patient, the client should be turned away or referred to the physician for further consultation.

Hepatitis C

Hepatitis is an inflammation of the liver caused by a number of viruses, including hepatitis A, B, and C. Hepatitis C is of greatest concern because of the chronic nature of the disease. Hepatitis C is transmitted through blood transfusion, unprotected sexual contact, shared needle use, and the mother-infant relationship. Health care workers are at great risk for hepatitis C. For those of us doing peels, coming in contact with blood should be rare.

Acquired Immune Deficiency Syndrome and Human Immunodeficiency Virus

HIV/AIDS is contracted through unprotected sexual contact, blood and blood product transfusions, shared needle use, and the mother-infant relationship. With the advanced treatments available today, finding people with the disease living longer and healthier lives is not uncommon. When a patient with HIV or AIDS seeks medical skin care and specifically peel treatments, understanding their health status is important. Therefore a consultation with the physician before beginning a program is important for both the clinician and the patient. Certain additional precautions may be necessary to protect the patient from infection. Similarly, the clinician must have a clear understanding and practice universal precautions. Patients with HIV/AIDS should be able to begin medical skin-care therapies as long as they are cleared by their physician.

Suspicious Lesions

Any lesion that worries you or looks unusual should be examined by the physician. The lesion may not be a skin cancer, but it might be a lesion of a different type that still requires attention before or concurrent with

---

Hepatitis C is on the rise and is the most likely virus to infect the clinician. Use universal precautions to ensure your safety at all times.

universal precautions
Preventative actions taken to prevent the transmission of infectious diseases; it involves the use of protective procedures and equipment, such as gloves and masks.

Individuals with HIV/AIDS are at greater risk for infection.

Suspicious lesions are all the lesions that worry you, regardless of the potential diagnosis. Do not be intimidated by the referral process to a proper physician. Think about what is in the best interest of your client.

the peel treatment. Additionally, your concern for lesions should not stop at the face, neck, and chest. Hands and arms are also at risk for suspicious lesions. Patients depend on you to look at lesions with and for them. Your motto should be "better safe than sorry" when it comes to having lesions examined by the physician.

Lupus

Lupus is a chronic autoimmune disease with no known cure. It is a familiar autoimmune disease for the clinician given that it is commonly associated with skin symptoms. Lupus is classified into two types: systemic lupus erythematosus (SLE) and discoid lupus erythematosus (DLE). SLE presents on the skin as a red rash on the face in the form of a butterfly. DLE, on the other hand, exhibits as round, red lesions over the skin. Lupus is much more prevalent in women than it is in men, making it a disease about which we tend to hear frequently. Lifestyle changes are necessary for the patient with lupus, including reducing sunlight exposure, getting regular exercise, avoiding stress, and getting immunizations to avoid disease. If the lesions of lupus (regardless of the origin of SLE or DLE) are active on the face, neck, or chest, the patient is not a candidate for peel treatment. Women with lupus may sometimes be treated with oral corticosteroids, making treatment with peels slightly more risky because of the potential delayed healing response of the skin.

> Lupus is a common autoimmune disease in women, with markings on the face, hands, neck, and chest.

Complications for the Physician

Several complications require assistance from the physician. When you determine that one of these problems exists, notify the physician and make sure that the patient is examined. Among the problems that should be seen by the physician are persistent erythema from a peel, herpes simplex breakout during the healing phase of the peel, infection, and an acne flare up that does not resolve quickly.

Persistent erythema is a redness that does not go away. This redness will sometimes be in one area, for example, where the peel went deeper; other times, the redness will be over the entire face, especially after the patient uses home-care products. This erythemic area will often thicken and become a scar if it is not properly addressed. The home-care program sometimes has to be adjusted; other times, the physician may recommend a topical steroid. In any case, this situation is one that you will want to refer to the physician.

Herpes simplex that breaks out during the healing phase of a peel can spread and be devastating. As the lesions heal, they will leave scars that will be difficult to minimize. If you suspect a herpes breakout, a physician must examine the patient immediately, and the protocol of oral medication should be adjusted.

Infections are just as problematic as is herpes. An infection can also leave scars on the face or area of treatment if it is not addressed quickly and efficiently. If you suspect an infection, be sure to have the patient examined right away.

Finally, acne that flares and does not resolve quickly will cause anguish for the patient and, in turn, for the clinician. If the acne is substantially worse after a peel, have the patient visit the physician. Patients will often scar themselves by picking at the acne, causing scabs and sores that are unnecessary. Addressing this problem head on will help keep the patient on the program and eliminate any emotional issues the patient might be having from the flare up.

TOP TEN TIPS TO TAKE TO THE CLINIC

1. Always keep a neat and clean treatment room.
2. Know where your supplies are at all times.
3. Make your client comfortable during and after the treatment.
4. Make sure you have signed a consent form with the patient.
5. Know how to apply a peel solution.
6. Create a peel treatment plan that includes microdermabrasion and facials.
7. Make sure the patient is on a viable home-care program.
8. Know when to contact the physician.
9. Select your candidates carefully.
10. Use the right peel solution.

CHAPTER REVIEW QUESTIONS

1. What is Jessner's solution?
2. How does Jessner's solution work to peel the skin?
3. What are the best indications for Jessner's solution peels?
4. How does Jessner's peels interface with other treatments?
5. What is the pretreatment protocol for Jessner's peels?
6. Describe the skin's normal response to Jessner's peels.
7. What are the objectives of Jessner's peels?
8. What are the potential complications of Jessner's peels?

CHAPTER REFERENCES

1. Obagi, Z. (2000). *Skin health restoration and rejuvenation.* New York: Springer-Verlag New York.
2. Leonardo, J. (2003, August). Negotiating the gray area of BDD, and the bottom line. *Plastic Surgery News*, 14(8), 24–25.
3. Leonardo, J. (2003, August). Negotiating the gray area of BDD, and the bottom line. *Plastic Surgery News*, 14(8), 24–25.
4. Wilhelm, S. (2004, January 14). *Body dysmorphic disorder clinic and research unit* [Online]. Available: http://www.mgh.harvard.edu

BIBLIOGRAPHY

911 Health Shop. (2005, May 16). *Ultimate H.A. (hyaluronic acid) formula by purity products* [Online]. Available: http://store.yahoo.com

Ancira, M. A. (1998). Chemical peels: An overview. *Plastic Surgical Nursing*, 19, 179.

Azer, M. (2002, March 1). *Salicylate toxicity* [Online]. Available: www.emedicine.com

Balin, A. K. (2002, February 27). *Seborrheic keratosis* [Online]. Available: www.emedicine.com

Blitzner, A., Binder, W. J., Boyd, J. B., & Carruthers, A. (Eds.). (2000). *Management of facial lines and wrinkles.* Philadelphia: Lippincott, Williams & Wilkins.

The Body Dysmorphic Clinic & Research Unit. (2004, January 14). [Online]. Available: http://www.mgh.harvard.edu

Breathnach, A. S. (1996, January). Melanin hyperpigmentation of skin: Melasma, topical treatment with azelaic acid, and other therapies. *Cutis.*, 57(Suppl 1), 36–45.

British Association of Cosmetic Doctors. (2004, April 20). *Chemical Peeling: What is chemical peeling?* [On line]. Available: http://www.cosmeticdoctors.co.uk

Brody, H. J. (1997). *Chemical peeling and resurfacing.* (2nd ed.) St. Louis: Mosby.

Coleman, W. P., & Lawrence, N., (Eds.). (1998). *Skin resurfacing.* Baltimore: Williams and Wilkins.

Deitz, S. (2004). *Milady's the clinical esthetician.* Clifton Park, NY: Thomson Delmar Learning.

Fagien, S., & Brandt, F. S. (2001). Primary and adjunctive use of botulinum toxin type A (Botox) in facial aesthetic surgery: Beyond the glabella. *Clinics in Plastic Surgery*, 28(1), 127–161.

Healthsquare.com. (2004, January 15). *Accutane* [Online]. Available: www.healthsquare.com

Kang, W. H., Chun, S. C., & Lee, S. (1998, September). Intermittent therapy for melasma in Asian patients with combined topical agents. *International Journal of Dermatology*, 25(9), 587–596.

Leffell, D. (2002, February). *New advances in treating actinic keratoses* [Online]. Available: www.skinandaging.com

Leonardo, J. (2003, August). Negotiating the gray area of BDD, and the bottom line. *Plastic Surgery News*, 14(8), 24–25.

Lim, J. T. (1999, April). Treatment of melasma using kojic acid in a gel containing hydroquinone and glycolic acid. *Journal of Dermatologic Surgery*, 25(4), 282.

MedicineNet.com. (2003, December 5). *Medical dictionary: Melanocyte* [Online]. Available: www.medterms.com

Merck Pharmaceuticals Company. (2005, May 16). *The Merck manual: Second home edition, section 211. Cellulitis.* [Online]. Available: http://www.merck.com

Obagi, Z. (2000). *Skin health restoration and rejuvenation.* New York: Springer-Verlag.

Palmer, G. D. (2001, October). Regarding the study on chemical peels on acne. *Journal of Dermatological Surgery*, 27(10), 914.

Perez-Bernal, A., Munoz-Perez, M. A., & Camacho, F. (2000, September-October). Management of facial hyperpigmentation. *American Journal of Clinical Dermatology*, 1(5), 261–268.

PlasticSurgery.com. (2004, May 13). *Chemical peel: How is a chemical peel performed?* [Online]. Available: www.plasticsurgery.com

Rubin, M. (1995). *Manual of chemical peels: Superficial and medium depth.* Philadelphia: Lippincott, Williams & Wilkins.

Thomas, C. L. (Ed.). (1997). *Taber's cyclopedic medical dictionary* (Vol. 18). Philadelphia: F. A. Davis.

U.S. Food and Drug Administration. (2003, December 12). FDA approves new product for facial wrinkles. *FDA Talk Paper* [Online]. Available: www.fda.gov/bbs/topics/answers/2003/ans01271.html

Venna, S. S., & Gilchrest, B. (2002, February). *Skin aging and photo-aging* [Online]. Available:www.skinandaging.com

Wilhelm, S. (2004, January 14). *Body dysmorphic disorder clinic and research unit* [Online]. Available: http://www.mgh.harvard.edu

Trichloroacetic Acid Peels

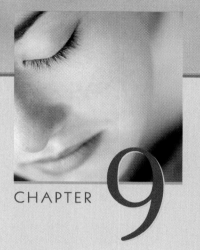

CHAPTER 9

LEARNING OBJECTIVES

After completing this chapter you should be able to:

1. Describe trichloroacetic acid solution.
2. List the indications and contraindications for trichloroacetic acid peeling.
3. List the anticipated results for trichloroacetic acid peeling.
4. Discuss the possible complications from trichloroacetic acid peeling.

223

INTRODUCTION

Trichloroacetic acid (TCA) has been a familiar peeling agent in the medical spa since the early 1980s.[1] Many physicians and clinicians believe that TCA is the gold standard of peeling agents. The product comes in varying strengths, beginning at 10% and moving up in 5% increments. TCA must be mixed in an aqueous solution to penetrate the skin.[2] Preparation of the peel solution and the subsequent analysis of percentage are complex and important components of the TCA peeling process. Done incorrectly, the percentage will not perform as predicted, creating either a peel that is too deep or one that is too light. Therefore the TCA product that you buy must come from a reputable source that is familiar with mixing and preparing peeling solutions. Commercial sources for TCA are available, but many clinics choose to use a local pharmacy to mix TCA products. This practice is fine as long as the pharmacist is familiar with the process and as long as the concentrations can be validated.

The mechanism of TCA injury is **protein coagulation** in the dermis and epidermis.[3] This mechanism is, of course, quite different than that of alpha hydroxy acid (AHA) or Jessner's solution. The benefits of TCA are many, but among the most notable is the ability to adjust the depth to fit the skin problem. For example, for patients who require only epidermal improvement, a single application of TCA peel of 10% to 15% will be effective. On the other hand, if the problems are in the papillary dermis, a stronger solution or more application passes can be applied. A word of caution should be noted at this time: *the number of coats or the volume of solution will increase the depth of the peel.* The percentage of solution you are using does not matter; the more coats you put on, the deeper the peel will be. Why? Remember the mechanism of action: TCA coagulates the dermal and epidermal proteins. Simply stated, the more solution that is applied, the deeper it will go looking for protein to neutralize itself (Figure 9–1). Other benefits that TCA brings include an improvement for all skin types (we will later discuss necessary safety measures for hyperpigmenting skin) and good results with a single application.

A discussion of TCA peeling would not be complete without acknowledgement and discussion of the **Obagi Blue® peel**. If asked, many physicians would agree that Dr. Zein Obagi is *the* expert on TCA peeling. Patients travel from around the globe to his office in Beverly Hills, California, for treatment. So what makes his treatment so different from yours? To start with, he is a physician with years of education and

protein coagulation
The point at which the peel solution reaches the protein of the skin.

Obagi Blue® peel
A simplified, uniform, user-friendly TCA peel solution indicated for all skin types, created by Dr. Zein Obagi.

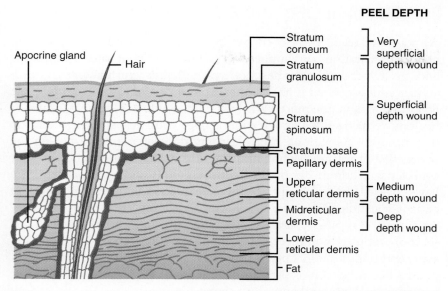

PEEL DEPTH

Apocrine gland — Hair — Stratum corneum — Very superficial depth wound — Stratum granulosum — Stratum spinosum — Superficial depth wound — Stratum basale — Papillary dermis — Upper reticular dermis — Medium depth wound — Midreticular dermis — Deep depth wound — Lower reticular dermis — Fat

Figure 9–1 TCA peels and Obagi Blue Peels® are medium-depth peels and can extend into the upper reticular dermis.

experience. He has spent his career focusing on TCA peeling, the benefits, the complications, the results, and the skin types of patients receiving the peels, a lot to learn. Many persons who are unfamiliar with TCA peeling immediately ask why the peel is blue, and this is a good question. According to Dr. Obagi, two misunderstandings about TCA are common: that the higher strengths of TCA penetrate faster and are more likely to scar and that conversely lower strengths penetrate slower and are less likely to scar. These statements are common misconceptions[4] that Dr. Obagi has attempted to eliminate by developing the Blue Peel™ and decreasing the variables that might otherwise exist. The variables that Dr. Obagi discusses include technique, patient pretreatment, patient skin type, ability to see the peel depth, variability of TCA strength, and the use of augmentation solutions. As we move through this chapter, we will address all of Dr. Obagi's concerns and discuss solutions (many recommended by him) to solve the problems (Figure 9–2).

As with all other peeling agents, TCA peels must be examined carefully. The process of patient consultation and selection, recognizing the proper indications and contraindications, the peeling process, and the aftercare all affect the patient's outcome. Given that TCA can dramatically affect the patient's appearance in one treatment, a lot of interest in the treatment can be found; so open your notebook, and let us talk about TCA peeling.

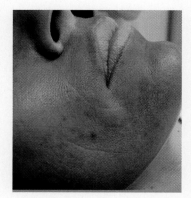

Figure 9–2 Very light Blue Peel™; little frosting is seen.

■ TRICHLOROACETIC ACID PEELS

As you have read, TCA peels can be variable, depending on strength, patient preparation, and application techniques. That said, TCA peels, once mastered, will be the best peel you will offer your patients. As with all procedures offered in the medical spa or plastic surgeon's office, the higher the risk is, the more likely you will be able to achieve a meaningful long-term result. The question is, can your nerves take it, and do they need to? As with all peels, learning the technique and having the knowledge of wound healing and the skin itself will give you the self-confidence to administer the procedure carefully and appropriately. We have covered the key points of the consultation and general points of patient selection. Before we discuss the important areas of patient pretreatment, clinical preparation, the consent, and choosing the TCA solution, let us talk in more detail about the appropriate skin types and skin conditions for TCA peels.

To begin, all skin types can benefit from TCA peeling. However, persons with postinflammatory hyperpigmentation require special attention. These patients will more than likely be patients in the Fitzpatrick IV, V, or VI skin types. Pretreating these patients with hydroquinone (at least 6% to 8%) twice a day for at least 4 weeks will significantly reduce the incidence of postinflammatory hyperpigmentation, but it will not eliminate it. (Remember a high SPF is also required.) Therefore the clinician has to be alert to the potential problems of postinflammatory hyperpigmentation. Once the skin has completely peeled, your clinic physician or medical spa clinician may have orders that allow the skin to be treated with a combination of topical steroids and hydroquinone. We will discuss this in detail later in the chapter.

The skin conditions that are appropriate for TCA peels are broad and include the following: hyperpigmentation, **rolling acne scars**, uneven texture, solar damage, and fine lines.

Given that one of our objectives for peels in general and TCA peels specifically is to avoid damaging the melanocytes, we must take into consideration the depth at which we will be peeling. Recommendations are that the clinician avoid using a solution stronger than 20%. In doing so, "... one coat will exfoliate the epidermis to the basal layer in medium-thick skin and may reach the papillary dermis in thin skin."[5] This amount is just perfect for our needs in the medical spa; a peel that penetrates any deeper will take us into territory in which we do not want to be, with potential problems that will require the assistance of your clinic physician.

rolling acne scars
Acne scars that appear in a wave pattern over the face.

Pretreatment Preparation

As with all peels, the pretreatment for a TCA or Blue Peel™ is important. However, as you may have gleaned, pretreatment is *really important* with TCA peels. The use of at-home therapeutic agents allows the
skin to exfoliate and flatten the stratum corneum. This process will permit an even and effective uptake of the peel solution, which will greatly
influence the result. Therefore what is this home-care program? Well, if
you plan to do an Obagi Blue® peel, a specific program is dictated by
the company, which highly recommends that the medical spa carry the
product line and follow the protocol accordingly. If, on the other hand,
a traditional TCA peel process is going to be done, the home-care
regime recommended by the spa needs to be in place. This home-care
program would include a morning routine of an acidic pH cleanser, a
12% to 18% glycolic acid treatment, 4% to 6% hydroquinone, vitamin C
serum, a multivitamin-antioxidant moisturizer, and a sunscreen. In the
evening, follow a similar course: an acidic pH cleanser, Retin A®
(usually 0.05%, but this varies, depending on the skin type), 4% to 6%
hydroquinone, a multivitamin serum, and a moisturizer. Be aware that
this program will cause the patient to peel and be erythemic, but this is
normal. You will need to support the patient or he or she will fall off the
program. The patient should be in the clinic for exfoliating facials or
product checks, or both, every week to 10 days. Performing lunchtime
peels on the skin is unwise. Given that the skin is peeling and exfoliating, a lunchtime peel may take up unevenly and cause a peel greater
than was anticipated. Encourage the patient to just let the home-care
program do its work, and make sure the patient has a facial and understands the importance of home exfoliation. The best home exfoliation is
one with papaya enzymes or **gommage** that will work without a lot of
scrubbing. One last word on pretreatment: before the patient starts on
the program, photographs should be taken. This precaution will be
important for a couple of reasons. First, photographs provide the visual
history that tells the story of the patient's face today, before treatment,
and they are used to compare the results of the treatment after the peel.
The skin changes slowly, and discerning a difference is sometimes difficult, but photographs never lie. Once the patient has been pretreated for
4 to 6 weeks, you are ready for the next step, the peel itself (Table 9–1).

gommage
An exfoliant without grains.

Clinical Preparation

As with any peel, make sure the room is properly set up and the supplies
are within reach. If you keep varying strengths of TCA peel solution,
these bottles need to be clearly marked. Remember, peel solutions with

Table 9–1 Pretreatment for TCA Peels

Morning routine	Acidic pH cleanser
	12%–18% glycolic acid
	4%–6% hydroquinone
	Vitamin C serum
	Multivitamin-antioxidant moisturizer
	Sunscreen
Evening routine	Acidic pH cleanser
	Multivitamin serum
	Retin A® (usually 0.05% but varied, depending on the skin type)
	4%–6% hydroquinone
	Moisturizer

Obagi Blue® peels have a specific pretreatment regime. For more information, refer to the manufacturer.

varying percentages should have the percentages marked on each bottle so that they are easy to identify. This precaution will help you avoid picking up the wrong bottle.

The supplies you will need for the TCA peel will be basically the same as those for other peels, except you will need either one big fan or a couple of small fans. Because this peel stings and burns more than other peels do, make sure you have fans that will keep the patient comfortable. Recommendations are that the patient hold onto one of the fans, which helps to take his or her mind off the stinging and focus on "fanning." On a disposable towel, set out all of your supplies, including a cleanser, Aquafor®, moisturizer, antiinflammatory gel, sunscreen, the peel solution, a medicine cup, soft and rough gauze, eyewash, cotton-tipped applicators, a bowl of cool water, and a bonnet or headband to protect the patient's hair. When you have all of your supplies organized, you can bring the patient into the treatment room.

Obtaining the Consent

Obtaining the consent for the TCA peel is not unlike that of any other peel. In fact, most of the education should have already taken place. However, some key points need to be made, among them are complications, potential results, and the aftercare. Obtaining another set of photographs before the peel is a good idea. This stage of the process is also an excellent time to check if the patient has been following

Consent forms are the tools that are used to inform the patient about the risks and complications of a peel procedure. This document also makes the clinician aware of the patient allergies, expectations (through discussions), and chronic medical problems. The clinician should make sure that a consent form accompanies each procedure performed.

the recommended pretreatment of Valtrex® and antibiotics, if recommended in your medical spa. If the patient has not followed the protocol deemed appropriate in your clinic, the procedure should be canceled and rescheduled to a time when all of the pretreatment protocol is in place.

The treatment can now begin. Have the patient change into a wrap or a traditional patient gown for the peel, which allows the peel to be done without worrying about the patient's clothing. Cover the patient with a blanket, and get him or her comfortable. Providing some soft music is a good idea to calm the patient. Additionally, a CD player with the patient's favorite CD is also a nice idea.

Choosing the Solution

Although choosing the percentage of glycolic acid for peeling can be as much an art as it is a science, choosing TCA is simply a science. You are choosing a solution that will penetrate well-prepared skin to a specific level for a specific reason. The percentages of the solutions, when applied appropriately, are usually predictable. If exfoliation of the upper epidermis is the objective of the peel treatment, use a 10%, 15%, or 20% TCA solution. As you know, when the epidermis is exfoliated (peeled) to the basal layer, significant improvement can be made. Among the possible changes are improvement in hyperpigmentation, fine lines, flat facial warts, actinic keratoses, and some skin laxity. The last of these improvements, however, should not be the reason for the peel. If a peel is focused on skin laxity, this level of peeling should be left to the physician.

10%, 15%, and 20%

As previously stated, the percentages of TCA recommended for the medical spa are 10%, 15%, and 20%. These percentages will give a nice epidermal peel. Remember the multiple considerations for the depth of the peel: skin preparation, number of coats, thickness (or "wetness") of the coats, and the clinician's technique. As the peel is being applied, it will begin to frost or turn white (or blue with the Obagi Blue® peel) once the solution has coagulated with the protein of the epidermis.

Obagi Blue® peel

The Obagi Blue® peel is a mixture of 30% TCA and the "blue mixture." Once diluted in the blue solution, the percentage is diluted to 15% or 20%. As previously stated, Dr. Obagi believes that this TCA mixture is controllable, providing consistent results for all skin types.

Peel Application

First, clean the skin with an acidic pH cleanser. If the patient arrived wearing makeup, be sure all of the debris is removed, especially around

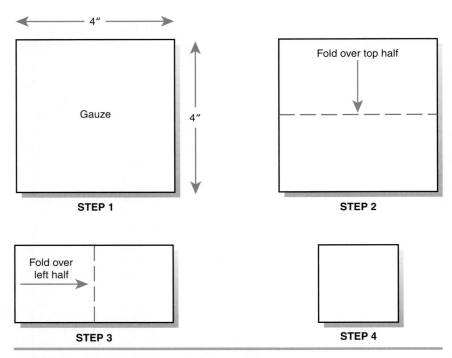

Figure 9–3 Fold the gauze precisely, and wring it out before applying solution to the face. Excess solution applied to the face will cause a deeper-than-anticipated peel.

the lower eyelid. Next, defat the skin. As we have previously discussed, the process of de-fatting can use any number of products; choose one and stick to it. The head of the table should be slightly elevated, which helps keep the peel solution from pooling. Elevating the head of the bed is also useful in keeping the patient comfortable.

The TCA peel application is simple, but it is technique sensitive. Use a folded gauze dipped into the medicine cup, saturate it with the TCA solution, then wring out the gauze (Figure 9–3). *Never* use dripping gauze on the face. The solution can run into the eyes or simply allow too much product to hit the skin at one time. The application needs to be *smooth* and *even*. Choose a place to begin and work methodically around the face (Figure 9–4). Some clinicians prefer to begin at the chin and work upward toward the forehead; others prefer to start on the forehead and work across the forehead and onto the face. Remember, find an approach that works for you (Figure 9–5). Some physicians like to do part of the face and watch for the frost; others like to complete the peel and watch the entire face for a frost. Either way is correct.

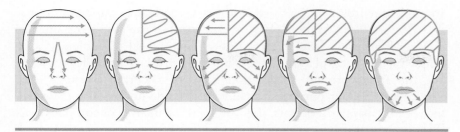

Figure 9–4 TCA and Blue Peels™ require a methodical peel application. Repeated overlapping will cause a deeper-than-anticipated peel.

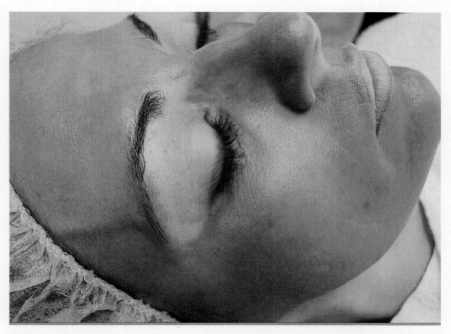

Figure 9–5 Blue Peel™ immediately after application of the solution, before the frost begins to show.

When peeling the area around the eyes, pull the skin tight so you can make the skin flat and therefore more evenly accept the peel solution by avoiding getting caught in a wrinkle. To keep a consistent peel, always peel the lower eyelids.

Skin's Response to Peel Solutions

The depth of the TCA peel is consistent with the frost achieved on the skin. That is to say, a light frost will equate to a light epidermal peel, and a deeper frost will produce a deeper epidermal or papillary dermal peel (Figure 9–6). Mark Rubin, MD, describes the skin's response to TCA at four levels: level 0, level 1, level 2, and level 3 (Table 9–2). To achieve a meaningful result, the skin must frost at some level; without the frost, protein coagulation has not occurred (Figure 9–7). Remember, for our purposes as clinicians, we do not want to penetrate through the papillary dermis; this will increase the risk of complications (Figure 9–8). When you have achieved the frost you are anticipating, rinse the patient's face with cool water. This action will do two things. First, any pooling of unnoticed peel solution will be rinsed away or diluted. Second, it helps the patient become more comfortable. Remember, TCA cannot be neutralized. After this step has been completed, either an ointment such as Aquafor® or a 2% hydrocortisone cream can be applied. A stronger topical cortisone is not recommended.

Use of occlusion

Some physicians recommend the use of ointment to drive the peel deeper when the peel itself has not reached optimal depths. Although some clinicians believe using an ointment is effective, others have discharged patients with and without occlusion and noted no specific results

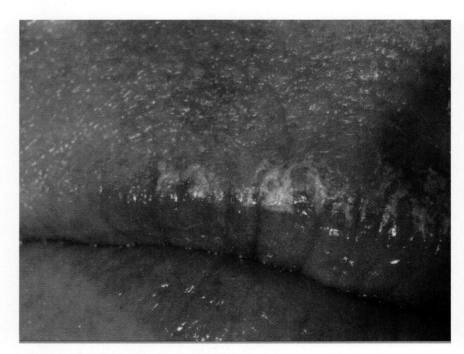

Figure 9–6 Deep lines will allow peel solution to creep into the fold, which can cause a deeper-than-anticipated peel in these areas.

Table 9–2 Frosting

Level 0	No frost	Skin appears shiny and slick, with minimal or no erythema.	Removes the stratum corneum.
Level 1	Irregular light frosting	Skin is shiny and slick, showing some erythema.	Depth extends into the superficial epidermis.
Level 2	White frost with pink showing through	The skin has a uniform white color, with noticeable pink background.	Depth extends into the full epidermis.
Level 3	Solid white frost	The skin has a uniform white color, with no pink showing through.	Depth extends into the papillary dermis.

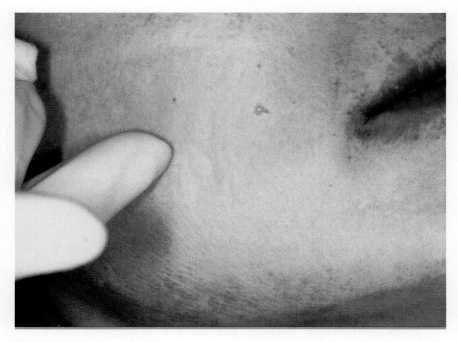

Figure 9–7 TCA frost.

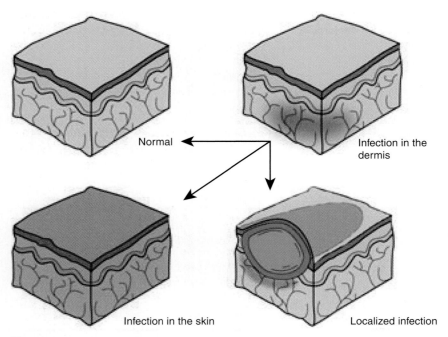

Normal

Infection in the dermis

Infection in the skin

Localized infection

Figure 9–8 Skin infections are a risk for deeper peels.

attributable to depth.[6] The right answer is to get the peel to the proper depth, rinse, and use the product of choice to moisturize or lubricate the skin before discharge.

Solid carbon dioxide

Harold Brody, MD, has spent time researching and working with solid carbon dioxide (dry ice) and TCA peeling. In Dr. Brody's approach, dry ice is applied to the skin for several seconds before the application of the TCA peel solution. The dry ice will cause a keratolytic effect. This process causes a deeper wound and, as a result, presumably a better outcome. This approach can be quite tricky and is not recommended for the inexperienced clinician.

Glycolic acid or Jessner's solution

Many physicians and clinicians prefer to prepare the skin with glycolic acid or Jessner's solution before applying the TCA solution. This approach causes a keratolytic effect that allows the TCA to penetrate quickly and perhaps more evenly. A few cautionary notes: if you use glycolic acid before TCA peels, be sure to avoid any areas of significant erythema, and always neutralize the face before applying the TCA. These two acids work differently. Glycolic acid requires neutralization to abbreviate its action, and TCA stops when the protein is coagulated. If you prepare with Jessner's solution and achieve a frost, be respectful of the injury you have caused. You may want to reconsider your TCA percentage or the number of coats you apply.

Patient's Response to Trichloroacetic Acid Peels

Most patients will tolerate TCA peels just fine, but they do hurt; there is no doubt about it. If the skin has been primed for 4 to 6 weeks as recommended, then the skin will already have a heightened level of sensitivity. When you apply the TCA, be prepared for the patient to tear and complain. You must keep the tears from falling onto the patient's face because this will dilute the peel and create streaking in the area where the tears fall. Having an assistant available during the peel is helpful in this instance. The assistant can blot the tears, hold an extra fan, and reassure the patient, all of which makes the treatment go a little faster. Some patients will have muscle quivering of the neck, representing the pain. Other patients may chill. All of these reactions are normal.

Talking the patient through the process is very important. Let the patient know what you are doing, what you are anticipating, and how much longer you believe the process to last. This communication seems to help the patient cope with the discomfort and focus on the endpoint of the peel. If you have a patient whom you believe will have a difficult time enduring the peel process, then talk with your physician about an oral sedative. If your patient is given an oral sedative, remember, they need someone to drive him or her to and from the clinic.

Posttreatment

Giving the patient an idea of how his or her skin will appear immediately after the peel and through the healing process is important. The change in the skin can be a little scary, and having a precise understanding of what is normal can be reassuring.

Once the frost has disappeared from the patient's face, the skin will be red and somewhat swollen. The patient sometimes wants to look in the mirror at the frost; this is just fine. Looking in the mirror can be a teaching tool to help patients understand what will happen to the skin next and where the deeper peeling (if applicable) will occur. The skin is going to feel tight and warm, similar to a sunburn immediately after the peel and through the next few days. This reaction is normal. Also common is for the skin to swell through the first night. Therefore when the patient wakes up the next morning, the face and eyes will be unusually puffy. This reaction is also normal. The swelling may continue through the peeling process, which is also fine. However, if the patient is complaining of a lot of swelling, then a physician should be consulted to evaluate the patient's status and consider an infection.

The posttreatment for TCA should be written down for the patient because the instructions can be easy to forget. The directions should take the patient day by day, beginning on the day of the peel. Generalized instructions include keeping the face lubricated and soft with Aquafor® for the first 3½ to 4 days, until it begins to peel. Letting the skin get dry will cause the process of peeling to take longer. The application of Aquafor® should be made at least four to six times a day in a thin, fine layer over the peel site. In the morning and in the evening, the skin should be cleansed with a mild cleanser appropriate for this skin condition followed by an application of lubricant (Aquafor®). Once the skin begins to peel, instruct the patient to avoid picking the skin or pulling loose pieces of skin off, which may cause scarring or at least put the areas at greater risk for longer healing (Figures 9–9 and 9–10). Once all of the necrosed skin has been sloughed, exfoliation can begin. The patient should be examined in the office before the exfoliation process. Make sure all of the skin is closed and that any areas of weeping or open sores are healed. If the skin looks good, then exfoliation can take place.

If possible, doing the first exfoliation in the office is a good idea to ensure that the skin is treated with care. Patients often rub too hard in an effort to remove the dead, dry skin and return their face to a more normal appearance. This action can sometimes cause the skin to bleed

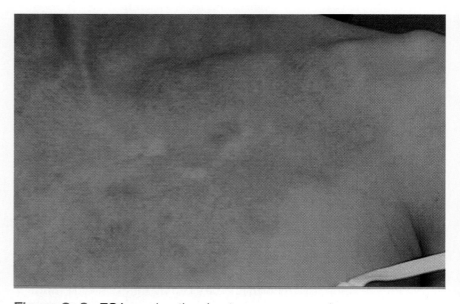

Figure 9–9   TCA used on the chest can cause scarring.

or become overly sensitive, which can be a setback in the healing process and a disappointment to both the patient and the clinician. A papaya enzyme mask is the best product to use because it will gently remove the loose skin without the rubbing that is required by grains. The patient should be instructed to wear a moisturizer and sunscreen (Figure 9–11). Approximately a week after the TCA peel, the skin may peel lightly again, somewhat similar to facial dandruff (Figure 9–12). This reaction is normal. A facial can be recommended to remedy this problem. When the skin can tolerate it, usually at approximately 2 weeks after the peel, a therapeutic home-care program should be started again, which would include the use of Retin A®, AHAs, vitamin C, and sunscreens (Table 9–3).

Anticipated Results

TCA peels are really the gold standard of peels, meaning that all of the other types of peels that are done are compared with the results of TCA peels. Although all skin types are candidates for TCA peels, those with *epidermal* lesions or pigment are going to respond better. These problems will have a superior outcome compared with dermal problems that require a deeper peel into the papillary dermis. Before peeling, consideration should be given to the potential result and the ability of

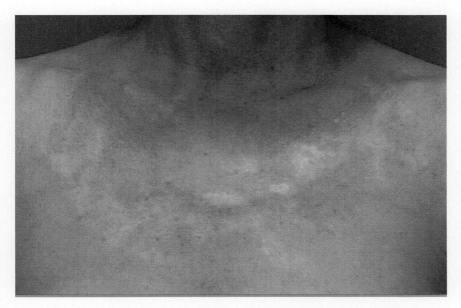

Figure 9–10   Chest scars 1 year later. Note the depigmentation that has occurred.

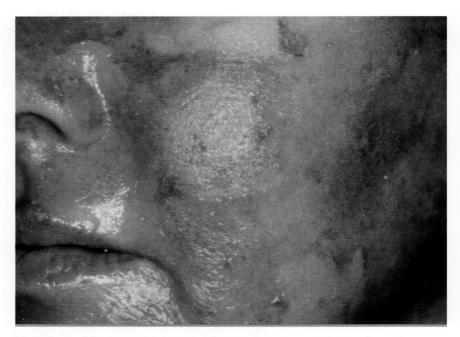

Figure 9–11   TCA peel 4 days after the treatment. This is normal.

Table 9–3   Posttreatment for TCA Peels

Aquafor®	The first 3 ½ or 4 days, four to six times a day, in a thin layer until it begins to peel
Mild cleanser	In the morning and in the evening
Papaya enzyme mask	After all of the necrosed skin has been sloughed
Moisturizer	Used daily, once the skin has peeled
Sunscreen	Used daily, once the skin has peeled
Therapeutic home-care program consisting of AHAs, vitamin C, Retin A®, and sunscreens	A week or more after the peel

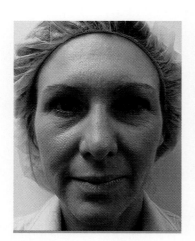

Figure 9–12   TCA peel 6 days after the treatment.

the peel to solve the problem and improve the skin's appearance (Figures 9–13 and 9–14).

A TCA peel can result in the reduction of fine lines, a slight tightening of the skin, and improving or clearing of hyperpigmentation.

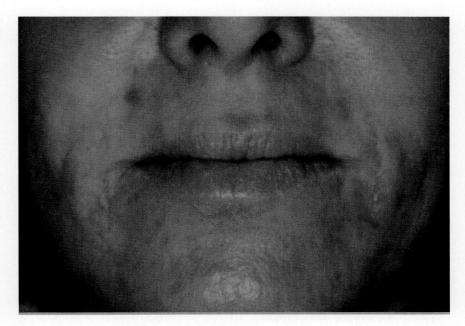

Figure 9–13   Patient before TCA peel.

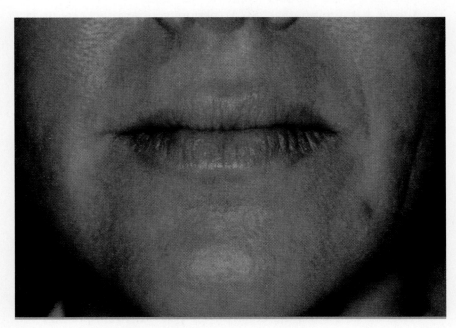

Figure 9–14   Patient after TCA peel.

Acne scars, depending on the type, will also be improved (with multiple TCA peels). Consideration should be given to the patient who has multiple actinic keratoses; this peel can work well to resolve these lesions. In general, TCA will provide the skin with an improvement in the quality, tone, and texture.

Solar-damaged skin in the Fitzpatrick types I, II, and III are great candidates for TCA peeling. These patients often have more lines, a sallow, gray color, and a pebbly appearance on the surface of the skin. These patients have usually had overexposure to sunlight, making them an appropriate choice for an aggressive preparation and a TCA peel to treat these problems. TCA will resolve most of the fine lines, improve the color, and help smooth the pebbly texture. Depending on the depth of the problem (epidermal versus dermal), the result will be significant.

For patients with hyperpigmentation, TCA peeling will be a viable option. The results of the peel are dramatic and generally require only one treatment to show improvement or complete resolution.

Skin tightening remains a controversial objective for TCA peeling, especially epidermal TCA peeling. Although the skin may be tighter initially, a long-term tightening effect cannot be expected from this treatment. Skin tightening from TCA peeling can be considered only a *side benefit* and should not be the primary reason for implementing a TCA peel.

Acne scars are another controversial topic for TCA peeling. Dr. Obagi has proven that TCA, performed properly, can in fact improve certain types of acne scarring.[7] TCA peels that treat acne scarring must be repetitive to be effective. The patient should be on the appropriate home-care program and be committed to the process of multiple peels. If the patient and clinician can coordinate, then positive results are achievable.

Complications

Given that TCA peeling reaches to the basal layer of the epidermis, and possibly into the upper papillary dermis, the risks increase over glycolic acid and Jessner's solution peeling. The clinician should be alert for several potential problems or complications when working with TCA. Among the problems associated with TCA peeling are a peel that is deeper than anticipated, infections (see Figure 9–5), herpes simplex breakout, acne and **milia**, premature separation of the skin, allergies to topical or oral products, irritations, scars, and changes in pigment (Table 9–4).

First, let us discuss the depth of the peel. If, while peeling, you notice the skin change from the normal white frost to a yellow, you have

milia
A small, white-headed cyst filled with keratin.

Table 9–4 Possible Complications after a Peel Procedure

Immediate (1-14 Days after Peel)		Recovery (2-6 Weeks after Peel)	Delayed (3-10 Weeks after Peel)
ANTICIPATED REACTIONS	UNANTICIPATED COMPLICATIONS	ANTICIPATED REACTIONS	UNANTICIPATED COMPLICATIONS
Edema	Herpes simplex virus eruption	Erythema	Hypertrophic reactions, keloids
Erythema	Infection	Postinflammatory hyperpigmentation	Scars
Darkening	Allergic reaction	Acne flare up	Hypopigmentation
Oozing	Irritation	Milia	Depigmentation
Scabbing	Premature skin separation	Demarcation lines, large pores, marbleization, persistent skin sensitivity	Ectropion

penetrated into the deeper dermis, and the potential for a problem looms. Getting the physician involved immediately will be important to avoid any potential scars or other types of problems.

Infections are always possible with any peel. Because of the slightly deeper depth of TCA peels, the chance of infection is slightly greater. Some physicians will have a protocol of using antibiotics before, during, and after the procedure to avoid a possible infection. Be sure to check with your clinic physician to determine if this course of action is appropriate. If an infection does occur, the patient will complain of tenderness and increased swelling, temperature, and oozing. Remember that patients can also have a fungal infection or a yeast infection. Therefore do not think only about bacterial infections. If an infection is suspected, a culture may be used to rule out fungal or yeast infections.

Herpes simplex is a big problem. Patients with a history of herpes simplex should be pretreated with Valtrex® or the antiviral of the physician's choice. The preferred protocol is 1 g the day before, 1 g the day of, and 1 g a day for 7 to 10 days after the peel. The clinician simply cannot be too careful in this situation. The eruption and spreading of the virus will cause scars and lengthen the healing time.

Acne breakouts and milia are not uncommon after a TCA peel. The treatment can be a little tricky though because the skin is sensitive and tender. Some physicians prefer a course of oral antibiotics, and others prefer facials and topical treatments. Whatever the recommended course your facility chooses, remember that picking at acne can cause scars; therefore try to keep the breakouts at a minimum.

A premature separation of the skin can occur when the patient has disregarded your instructions. The normal course of healing is a reepithelialization of the skin: sloughing of the injured tissue and replacement with newly formed skin. When the patient excessively sweats, picks, washes aggressively, or showers in a hot steamy shower for an extended period, the injured skin will lift, leaving the newly forming skin open to the environment. A premature separation can increase scarring, infection, and a lengthening of the recovery time. Once the tissue has lifted, the patient will have an increase in pain, and the new skin will require protection with a thick layer of Aquafor®.

Allergies and irritations can occur with any ointment you put on the skin. The patient should be alerted to the potential for rashes (especially from ointment products) and to call you if the problem occurs. Triple antibiotic ointment can cause allergies, just as oral antibiotics. For a patient to be allergic to one of the components in the product is common. Therefore, if the option is available, use Aquafor® or a bland ointment over one that is fortified with antibiotics. Patients will sometimes not realize they have an allergy until a situation such as a TCA peel takes place. Then, during the healing process, a nasty rash will develop. To avoid this potential, try to avoid using fortified products. Additionally, be alert to potential allergies to cleansers, moisturizers, and sunscreens. Remember, the skin will be sensitive and perhaps unable to tolerate the usual products. If such is the case, use products intended for sensitive skin. Finally, do not forget that patients can develop allergies to oral medications you might suggest or require. Keep your mind alert when problem solving a reaction with a patient. This circumstance provides a good opportunity to bring the physician into the picture to help you.

Scars are always a worry. If TCA is placed in the hands of an untrained clinician, a scar will probably occur (see Figure 9–9). Therefore bear in mind all that you know about wound healing and the skin as you embark on TCA peeling. Scars are rare, but they can and do occur. Scars usually occur when the peel is too deep or when the peel has been mismanaged. Scars can also occur after complications such as herpes simplex or infections. These complications usually create a full-thickness wound and, as such, create a scar. Once the wound is healed (with your clinic physician's help) the scar or scars can be addressed (see Figure 9–10).

The last important complication to discuss is a change in pigment, which can mean postinflammatory hyperpigmentation or hypopigmentation. Pigment, as you will recall, is related to the melanocytes and their ability to function.

Hypopigmentation is a loss of pigment and is directly related to the depth of the peel. The deeper the peel is, the greater the risk will be for hypopigmentation. For example, hypopigmentation is traditionally seen in phenol peels and is an accepted outcome. However, for TCA peels, hypopigmentation is not an accepted outcome. Certain skin types and conditions are more susceptible to hypopigmentation. Skin types that the clinician should suspect would include thin, fragile skin; skin that is previously treated with phenol, dermabrasion, or carbon dioxide (CO_2) laser; and skin that has had radiation for acne or other reasons.[8]

Hyperpigmentation or postinflammatory hyperpigmentation usually happens in Fitzpatrick skin types IV, V, and VI. The best course of action with these skin types is to assume that all will hyperpigment. In this fashion, you will not have a surprise and regret failing to be proactive. The best course is the following: Once the skin has sloughed, have the patient begin a course of a topical steroid, hydroquinone, and sunscreen. The topical steroid strength and hydroquinone strength should be at the discretion of your physician, but 4% to 6% hydroquinone twice a day mixed with a moderate-strength steroid such as **Cutivate**® will usually work great. Obviously, you know by now that sunscreen is a key in the treatment of postinflammatory hyperpigmentation and must be included to ensure the treatment success.

Cutivate®
A prescription steroidal cream.

Combining Trichloroacetic Acid Peels with Other Treatments

TCA can be combined with other clinical treatments to improve the final result. As with other peels, injectable dermal fillers and Botox® are a great augment with the TCA peel. These injectable products will help reduce the appearance of the moderate lines that did not have a great result with the TCA peel because of their dynamic nature. The patient should be prepared that some lines will not improve with TCA peeling and be made aware of the additional options available after healing. That said, some physicians prefer using Botox® in particular before the peel, which helps the area heal without movement, improving the result. Among the dermal fillers available are Restylane®, Hylaform®, and Radiesse®.

Dermal Fillers

A dermal filler is a substance used to fill lines or wrinkles on the face. Dermal fillers are also useful for filling shadows and areas of depression,

lipodystrophy
A disruption in fat metabolism.

such as **lipodystrophy**, that occur with certain medications. Dermal fillers are one of the best adjunct treatments to improve the results of TCA peels. These products allow the registered nurse or physician to target and treat specific lines, shadows, and depressions that cause the patient concern and that will not be helped by the TCA peel. Many dermal fillers are on the market today. The best dermal filler is really at the discretion of the injector together with the patient. Let us highlight the most familiar dermal fillers and the benefits they bring to the patient, especially after a TCA peel.

The oldest of the fillers is bovine collagen. Collagen® was approved for use in the early 1980s and began the stampede by women (and men) to the plastic surgeon's office. This product is placed in the papillary dermis and is an excellent choice for very fine lines, though its durability is not that long lasting. Bovine collagen was followed in early 2003 by human collagen products named Cosmoderm® and Cosmoplast®. The benefit of this product over traditional collagen is the decrease in allergies or sensitivities and a greater durability than the original Collagen®. Once again, Cosmoderm® or Cosmoplast® is injected into the upper dermis. Following Cosmoderm® in U.S. Food and Drug Administration (FDA) approval were Restylane® and Hylaform®, both hyaluronic acid injectables. Hyaluronic acids fillers are currently extremely popular. The benefits of hyaluronic acid fillers are (1) they are hypoallergenic, (2) their ease of injection, and (3) their durability over bovine or human collagen. These fillers are the most popular, but many others in various stages of clinical trial are being developed, awaiting FDA approval.

Botox®

Botox® is one of the fastest-growing and most popular tools in the non-surgical armamentarium. Each vial of Botox® has 100 units of *Clostridium botulinum* type A. When reconstituted and injected into the muscle, this product causes paralysis of the muscle groups and, in doing so, relaxes the overlaying skin and lines. Unlike dermal fillers, the purpose of Botox® is not to fill the lines with a product, but rather relax the lines through paralysis. Botox® is a popular product for treating lines and wrinkles, especially those of the crow's feet and forehead. This treatment before a TCA peel can be quite helpful. In cases in which the crow's feet and forehead lines move aggressively, the lines will continue to progress and will be minimally affected by the peel. However, when the muscles have been paralyzed, Botox® helps the healing progress and the appearance of the lines.

Facials

Facials are highly recommended in concert with TCA peels, especially before the peel when the patient may be experiencing a good deal of peeling and flaking from the use of the home-care products. A facial can be relaxing, exfoliate the skin, and help the patient "bond to" the clinic before the peel. A facial should not be done within 4 days of the peel itself. After the peel, the patient must go through the "peel and heal" phase of approximately 7 to 10 days before a facial. A facial must be avoided if persistent erythema or complications of any kind are present. Approximately 1 month after the peel, the patient can usually plan to have a facial.

Microdermabrasion

Microdermabrasion is a great treatment to sustain the results of a TCA peel. However, the patient should wait at least 4 to 6 weeks before considering such a treatment. The microdermabrasion treatment should be a monthly treatment and will best serve the patient if it is combined with a facial or a light peel.

Repeating the Trichloroacetic Acid Peel

TCA peels need to be repeated. Depending on how you are using the TCA, the peel can be done quarterly as a "freshener peel." This peel would be very light, with only light flecks of white frost appearing at the time of the peel and with minimal recovery time. On the other hand, if the peel is aggressive, intended to solve significant problems, it may need to be repeated two to three times over a 6- to 8-month period to achieve acceptable results. If you are going to set in place an aggressive plan of action for your patient, be sure you give the skin adequate time to heal before insulting the already vulnerable surface a second time. TCA has flexibility and reliability on its side and can be used to achieve most reasonable results.

■ WHEN TO CONSULT YOUR CLINIC PHYSICIAN

Remember that your clinic physician is available to help you. You should be capable of managing this peel without his or her assistance, but you must know when to ask for help. Knowing when to ask questions is in large part a function of the detailed policy and procedure manual. However, knowing when to ask for help is also part of the relationship that the clinician and physician create (Table 9–5).

Questions before and after the procedure are always appropriate. As a clinician, anticipating problems is important by taking an in-depth patient history, evaluating past treatments, and understanding from the patient the desired results.

Table 9–5   When to Consult the Physician

Body dysmorphic disorder is suspected.

Patient has sensitive or thin skin.

Patient is a "sun worshipper."

Patient has chronic herpes simplex breakouts.

Patient is pregnant or lactating.

Patient has suspicious lesions.

The peel goes deeper than you anticipate.

Peeling a nonfacial area.

A TCA peel is a safe but sometimes tricky treatment. Although we rarely think about the idea of *precautions*, all treatments have them, and TCA is no exception. Body dysmorphic disorder, sensitive or thin skin, the "sun worshipper," the patient with chronic herpes simplex breakouts, the pregnant or lactating patient, and patients with suspicious lesions are instances that warrant a discussion with the physician before peeling.

TCA is safe on areas of the body other than the face. However, the clinician must recall the anatomy and physiology of the skin and its variations from location to location over the body. Before peeling a nonfacial area, an important precaution would be for the physician to examine the patient to make comments and suggestions about the treatment.

Finally, if you are involved with a TCA peel that goes deeper than you anticipate, giving the skin a yellow tinge during the peel, the physician must be contacted right away. This proactive approach will help the progress of the patient's healing. The clinician must also create a team approach to dealing with patient problems. Two brains dealing with a problem is always better than just one.

▶ ▷ ▷ TOP TEN TIPS TO TAKE TO THE CLINIC

1. The volume of TCA solution applied to the skin will determine the depth of the peel. Therefore, if you get too much solution in an area, blot it off to prevent a deeper than desired peel.
2. Peeling the neck and chest is possible with TCA but should be applied lighter in these areas.

3. The intensity of the frost is an indication of the depth of the peel.
4. Patient selection is important. Persons who continue to avoid using sunscreen and worship the sun are not good candidates for this peel.
5. TCA can be used on all skin types, but attention and care must be given for those who have a tendency to hyperpigment.
6. Pretreat patients who get cold sores with Valtrex®.
7. The Obagi Blue® peel is a TCA peel.
8. Using Botox® to paralyze active areas such as the crow's feet will provide a better result.
9. TCA is the gold standard for peeling.
10. Aggressively watch for complications and treat accordingly.

CHAPTER REVIEW QUESTIONS

1. What is TCA?
2. How does TCA work to peel the skin?
3. What are the best indications for TCA?
4. How does TCA interface with other treatments?
5. How do you choose the strength of TCA?
6. What is the pretreatment protocol for TCA?
7. What are the skin's normal responses to TCA?
8. What are the objectives of TCA?
9. What are the potential complications of TCA?
10. Is TCA neutralized or diluted?

CHAPTER REFERENCES

1. Obagi, Z. (2000). *Skin health restoration and rejuvenation*. New York: Springer-Verlag New York.
2. Brody, H. J. (1997). *Chemical peeling and resurfacing* (2nd ed.). St. Louis: Mosby.
3. Obagi, Z. (2000). *Skin health restoration and rejuvenation*. New York: Springer-Verlag New York.
4. Obagi, Z. (2000). *Skin health restoration and rejuvenation*. New York: Springer-Verlag New York.
5. Obagi, Z. (2000). *Skin health restoration and rejuvenation*. New York: Springer-Verlag New York.
6. Rubin, M. (1995). *Manual of chemical peels: Superficial and medium depth*. Philadelphia: Lippincott, Williams & Wilkins.
7. Obagi, Z. (2000). *Skin health restoration and rejuvenation*. New York: Springer-Verlag New York.

8. Obagi, Z. (2000). *Skin health restoration and rejuvenation.* New York: Springer-Verlag New York.

BIBLIOGRAPHY

Bioform Medical. (2004, April 11). *Product characteristics: Radiesse* [Online]. Available: www.bioforminc.com

Brody, H. J. (1997). *Chemical peeling and resurfacing* (2nd ed.). St. Louis: Mosby.

Coleman, W. P., & Lawrence, N. (Eds.). (1998). *Skin resurfacing.* Baltimore: Williams and Wilkins.

Daresbury Imaging Group. (2005, May). *Collagen* [Online]. Available at: http://detserv1.dl.ac.uk

Fagien, S., & Brandt, F. S. (2001). Primary and adjunctive use of botulinum toxin type A (Botox) in facial aesthetic surgery: Beyond the glabella. *Clinics in Plastic Surgery, 28*(1), 127–161.

Nassif, P. S. (2004, April). Radiesse: An injectable calcium hydroxylapatite. *Plastic Surgery.com* [Online]. Available: www.plasticsurgery.com

Obagi, Z. (2000). *Skin health restoration and rejuvenation.* New York: Springer-Verlag New York.

Rubin, M. (1995). *Manual of chemical peels: Superficial and medium depth.* Philadelphia: Lippincott, Williams & Wilkins.

Samalonis, L. B. (2004, January-February). Restylane: Approval spurs analysis of new treatments. *Cosmetic Surgery Times* [Online]. Available: www.findarticles.com

Sengelmann, R. T., & Tull, S. (2004, May 14). Dermal fillers [excerpt]. *eMedicine Specialties: Dermatology* [Online]. Available: http://www.emedicine.com

Salicylic Acid and Designer Peels

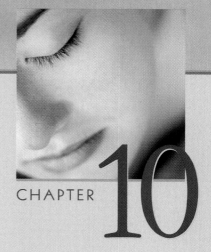

CHAPTER 10

LEARNING OBJECTIVES

After completing this chapter you should be able to:

1. Discuss the indications and contraindications for salicylic acid peeling.
2. List the potential complications of salicylic acid peeling.
3. List the anticipated results from salicylic acid peeling.
4. Define a designer peel.
5. State the common ingredients in designer peels.

■ SALICYLIC ACID PEELS

beta hydroxy acid
An isometrically distinct relative of alpha hydroxy acids.

beta peel
A 20% or 30% salicylic acid peel solution.

Salicylic acid was originally extracted from the willow bark,[1] and is still found in homeopathic remedies and skin-care products as willow bark today. Salicylic acid is a **beta hydroxy acid**, which is different from glycolic acid (an alpha hydroxy acid). The difference in the chemical structure exists specifically in the position of the hydroxy group. Although this subject is fascinating to persons interested in chemistry, other specifics about salicylic acid might prove more important to the clinician. For example, the clinician may want to know that salicylic acid is antibacterial and antiinflammatory and, as a result, works well for acne. Salicylic acid also has the ability to reduce the spots and bumps associated with acne. Finally, a combination program (at home) of salicylic acid and a retinoid of some type (perhaps Differin®) can be an effective program for the patient with grade 2 or possibly grade 3 acne. As a peeling solution, salicylic acid has gained popularity in the modern medical spa for the treatment of acne. It is often referred to as a **beta peel** and is found in solutions of 20% and 30%. In the dermatology practice, salicylic acid has been in and out of favor. It is usually found as a 50% paste used to treat lentigines, pigmented keratoses, and actinically damaged hands and forearms.[2]

Salicylic acid has sometimes been overlooked for the more trendy agents such as glycolic acid. However, this mild beta hydroxy acid is a good tool for the clinician to have on the back bar as a peeling agent for acne or for the patient with oily and acne-prone skin. Let us learn more about salicylic acid, how it is used, and why we would choose it over other peeling agents.

Salicylic is oil soluble[3] and is therefore used to penetrate pores and digest the debris that accumulates and causes pimples. The peels are recommended every 2 weeks if the acne is grade 2 and every 3 weeks if the acne is grade 1. Remember that some patients are candidates for more aggressive treatments such as Accutane® or oral antibiotics. If your patient is a candidate for aggressive treatments such as Accutane®, he or she will not be a candidate for salicylic acid peels or peels of any kind for that matter. If the patient is taking oral antibiotics, check to see if the specific medication causes the skin to be solar sensitive. If it does cause skin sensitivities, the peel may react differently on the skin than is anticipated. This situation does not preclude your patient from having light salicylic acid peels; it simply means you should be more cautious.

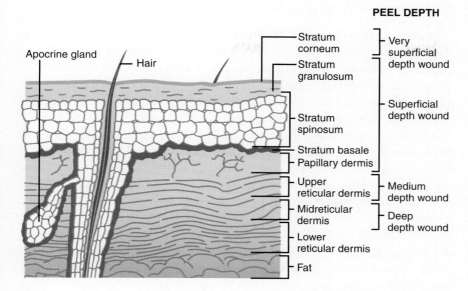

Figure 10–1 The depth of home-care peels is very superficial as defined by this illustration.

Pretreatment Preparation

As with all superficial peeling, home-care programs are extraordinarily important (Figure 10–1). Because the primary indication for salicylic acid peeling is skin that is acne prone or has active acne, the home-care program should also be based on these conditions. The best clinical home care for patients who are acne prone includes home-care products such as salicylic acid, benzol peroxide, Retin A® or Differin®, and hydroquinone if indicated. Topical vitamins, especially vitamin C, can be helpful with acne conditions.

Patients with acne are usually difficult to manage. They are, understandably, very self-conscience and fastidious regarding their appearance. Once a home-care program has been established, examining the patient at the 1-week mark is a good idea to ensure that the program is going well and to answer any patient questions. Moreover, patients who begin new home-care programs often have episodes of breakout or irritation, which can be upsetting to the patient and, in some cases, can cause the patient to discontinue the program. Patients with acne require attention and nurturing to ensure their success. Facials, in combination with peels, for patients with acne help ensure a good relationship and a greater opportunity for success.

Clinical Preparation

Salicylic acid peels usually come in a boxed kit. On the outside of the box, the strength of the peel is marked. These kits have all of the necessary products—cleanser, preparation and peel solution—to provide the peel. As with any other treatment, all supplies should be placed on the counter for immediate use. Included in these supplies are application supplies (gauze, brushes, cotton-tipped applicators, and a small medicine cup), a bowl of water, eyewash, two types of cleansers, two types of moisturizers, neutralizing solutions, and two types of sunscreens. Also necessary is a small motorized fan to help cool the patient's skin during the treatment. Lastly, a bonnet or headband to protect the patient's hair is needed. Once you have all the supplies at hand, you are ready to begin the treatment.

Obtaining the Consent

As with all treatments, the salicylic acid peel requires consent for treatment. The clinician should review the consent in detail, highlighting the specific information of which the patient should be aware. These highlights should include the specific language regarding risks, complications, and anticipated results. Patients with acne or acne-prone skin will be sensitive to the complications, especially potential breakouts. Be clear with these patients.

> Consent forms are tools that are used to inform the patient about the risks and complications of a peel procedure. This document also makes the clinician aware of the patient allergies, expectations (through discussions), and chronic medical problems. The clinician should ensure that a consent form accompanies each procedure performed.

Peel Application

As with all of the peels previously discussed, the key to a successful peel is the peel application. This process includes how the skin is prepared (at home and in the clinic), the choice of the application device, the gauze or sponge that is used to clean the skin, how the solution itself is applied, and the method of neutralization.

Many different application devices can be used: a brush, gauze, or a cotton-tipped applicator. The best results come from using folded gauze or a soft sponge. Folded gauze also works well to neutralize the peel, although cotton balls can also be used.

Before you bring the patient into the room, double-check that all the supplies you will need are on the counter. Make sure you have a bonnet, the gauzes, the solution, and the fan. Make your back bar professional and organized, which will help you eliminate mistakes and perform as the professional that you are.

Now that your treatment room is organized and stocked, you are ready to begin. Bring the patient into the treatment room, and have him or her review and sign the consent form. Once this duty is accomplished and the patient's questions are answered, you are ready to begin the treatment. Make the patient comfortable on the bed, protect the hair, and drape the chest with a towel. If you are going to be peeling the chest or the back, the patient should change into a wrap or patient gown. Using a mild cleanser on soft gauze or a soft sponge, clean the face until all of the makeup and debris has been removed. This process may take two applications of cleanser. Next, de-fat the skin with alcohol or acetone; choose one, not both. This process will take away most of the oils on the skin, allowing the peel solution to penetrate evenly and effectively. When the process of de-fatting the skin is done well, the peel solution will not get hung up on oily patches of the skin (usually on the T-zone). Next, dip the folded gauze or sponge into the peel solution. Squeeze out any extra solution against the side of your medicine cup; your gauze should not be dripping. Salicylic acid solution is applied in the same methodical process as other peel treatments, ensuring that the entire face is covered with solution for the best result.

Skin's Response to Salicylic Acid Peels

The skin will be red and sometimes have a veil of **salicylate** on the surface, not unlike the Jessner's peel. This appearance may resemble a frost; but unlike a frost, it can actually be moved, whereas a true frost cannot. This reaction is normal. In some cases, the skin will have a temporary anesthesia effect. In other words, the skin will be numb from the peel. The skin will usually peel in sheets or big "chunks" with this solution, beginning, of course, around the mouth.

Solid carbon dioxide

"The use of solid carbon dioxide (dry ice) is a physical modality for peeling and not a true peeling agent."[4] Solid carbon dioxide is commonly used to treat patients with active acne and works well as an adjunct to salicylic acid peels. Once the peel is complete, the dry ice is lightly applied to the peeled area. Remember, the skin has already been injured; therefore if you linger in any one place, you will cause a burn on the skin. This process should be done quickly and lightly with attention to the active breakouts. The dry ice is wrapped in gauze and lightly touched to acetone to activate the process. Acetone has two functions under these circumstances. First, it changes the dry ice from a solid into a liquid. Second, the acetone dissolves any stubborn **sebum** in the pores. The dry ice will not last long under these circumstances, so move quickly. Additionally, be careful on the bony prominences of the face; the skin is thin and at a greater risk for injury. After this step of the peel is complete, apply the sunscreen or moisturizing sunscreen before discharging the patient.

salicylates
The salt of salicylic acid.

sebum
The semifluid secretion of the sebaceous glands consisting chiefly of fat, keratin, and cellular material.

After the Peel

The posttreatment for the salicylic acid peel is simple (Table 10–1). Use an antiinflammatory gel product to reduce the stinging and burning, if any exists. Many postpeel agents are on the market, some of them using healing agents such as sea whip or other antiinflammatory agents. Such agents should be used for the first 12 hours after the peel. After the first 12 hours, the skin should be kept soft with a moisturizer that is specifically designed for postpeeling. Any "hot spots" or "rug burns" need to be kept soft with Aquafor®. At the third day, the skin should be exfoliated. Once again, stick to an enzyme mask to exfoliate; it is gentler compared with a mask with grains and does not subject the skin to potential scratches.

On the day of the peel and the day after the peel, the patient should avoid therapeutic home-care products such as salicylic acid or Retin A®. These products may be too irritating and may cause the skin to become erythemic and sensitive. The best approach is to place the patient on a "peel kit," which includes a gentle cleanser, an emollient moisturizer, a sunscreen, and an exfoliant. The usual protocol is to begin the normal home-care program the second day after the peel.

Probable Results

Salicylic acid peels are generally effective at reducing the quantity and quality of acne lesions. The skin will be less oily and clearer after this peel. The skin will also take on a glow as a result of the exfoliation that is accomplished through the peeling process.

Possible Complications

The patient with active acne or acne-prone skin may break out after peeling; this is understandably the patient's biggest worry. Acne breakout is a common event and should not be met with horror or surprise.

Table 10–1 Posttreatment for Salicylic Acid Peels	
Antiinflammatory gel	Reduces the stinging and burning during the first 12 hours after the peel
Aquafor®	Used to treat any "hot spots" or "rug burns"
Enzyme mask exfoliate	Used on the third day following a peel
"Peel kit" (gentle cleanser, emollient moisturizer, sunscreen, and exfoliant)	The usual home-care program on the second day after the peel.

A matter-of-fact attitude on the part of the clinician is required to sustain the patient relationship. Treatment options for acne breakouts after peeling include a short course of oral antibiotics, topical antibiotics, a facial, or a change in the home-care program. The patient should always be examined in the office to evaluate the situation. Remember to listen to the patient's concerns and understand that the patient may believe the situation is worse than it actually is. If you believe that additional therapies are recommended, you will need to follow the protocol set forth in your spa or clinic. If on the other hand, if you believe the situation can be improved by a facial or a change in the home-care program, you should follow the protocol recommended in the policy and procedures of the clinic. The clinician should be alert to the amount of stimulation that the peel provides. If the skin is getting too irritated by the peel, decrease the percentage; irritation can be the potential cause of a breakout. Other complications for salicylic acid peels are minor and include minor abrasions and a failure to peel (Table 10–2).

Combining Salicylic Acid Peels with Other Treatments

Although many physicians use this peel to decrease pigment associated with solar damage, doing so typically requires high percentages of salicylic acid. In the hands of an aesthetician, salicylic acid peels have a specific target audience: patients with acne-prone and active-acne skin. Therefore recommendations are that the programs be directed primarily at this problem and not for an improvement of solar-damaged skin. Improvement in solar-damaged skin may be seen, but this should be considered only as a bonus for you and your patient. Salicylic acid peels are often combined with other peeling modalities (as previously discussed) and with other clinical treatments such as facials and microdermabrasions. These treatments will provide a boost to the salicylic acid peel itself. Facials and

Table 10–2 Possible Complications for Salicylic Acid Peels	
Possible breakout for acne-prone skin	Patient should be examined and treated accordingly; decrease the percentage.
Minor abrasions	Treat accordingly with Aquafor®.
Failure to peel	Increase the percentage; make sure the patient is adhering to the home-care program.
Irritation	Decrease the percentage.

salicylic acid peels, when done concurrently, can provide the patient with one of the best acne treatments available today, which is especially true if the treatment is concluded with a brush of dry ice. The clinician must talk with the patient, develop a customized protocol, and evaluate the skin at each visit to determine the success of the program. Microdermabrasions can also be a successful adjunct to the salicylic acid peel.

Facials

The combination of facials and beta peels can be the most effective clinical treatment for acne. The facial should be the first step, followed by the salicylic acid peel. To cool off the peel, rinse and apply a mask. The treatments are generally done every 2 to 3 weeks, depending on the status of the skin. However, more frequent treatments are acceptable.

Regimen of Clinical Treatments

Beta peels are usually performed every other week in the beginning then reduced to once a month as the skin improves. Obviously, much of this process involves the skin's response to the peel and the patient's ability to keep appointments. No limit exists as to the number of peels that the patient can receive; however, the clinician must be mindful to avoid overtreating the skin.

■ DESIGNER PEELS

designer peel
Custom-made combinations of herbal and prescription ingredients.

The newest peel therapy on the market is the **designer peel**: a combination of herbal and prescription ingredients compounded together to create a peel for a specific problem or concern. Designer peels are typically found in the medical or luxury spa to treat dyschromia, dry skin, and aging skin. In the medical spa, designer peels are used before or after microdermabrasions or with facials to enhance the overall results. Designer peels are pricey for the patient, not because of the result per se, but more because of the price of the peel solution. Therefore understanding the properties of the peel solutions and the intended outcome is important to ensure that the peel you are using will provide the best result for the patient's concerns. The clinician may be unfamiliar with many of the herbal ingredients. Although venturing out into new territory may be exciting, you may be surprised about the nature of some of these ingredients and the possible results and complications. The purpose of these designer peels remains controversial, especially in the face of the tried-and-true peeling agents that show remarkable results. Nevertheless, these peel solutions are becoming popular; thus being aware of all of the properties of these solutions is important.

Designer peels claim to decrease the appearance of fine lines, improve pigment, or simply tighten the skin. The solutions usually have familiar peeling agents or prescriptions as the base of the product, such as lactic acid, trichloroacetic acid (TCA), glycolic acid, azelaic acid, or even hydroquinone, which is combined with the herbal component. One of the challenges for the clinician who uses a designer peel will be "what solution" and "what reason."

The first step in using a designer peeling agent is to understand the herbal ingredients and their potential for results. Understanding the impact of mixing these ingredients together and the problems they may create on the skin is also important. These peeling solutions are generally benign, with little if any problems. However, this feature does not allow the clinician an excuse of ignorance.

Solution Choice

These herbal solutions are generally mild and intended for combination with other treatments. Additionally, the products are recommended when the patient has sensitive skin or is concerned about a lengthy downtime. These reasons are excellent in selecting a designer peel.

In most cases, you will be using these peeling agents as an adjunct to another procedure, for example, with microdermabrasion or after a facial. Naturally, you must first understand the patient's skin concerns before choosing the peeling solution and treatment regime. The home-care program and the clinical program must work in tandem to ensure a positive result. Let us take the example of dyschromia, a common problem. The discoloration may respond to designer peels but only if the home-care program is complete with hydroquinone and sunscreen, as well as other agents, to attack the dyschromia. Additionally, this peel solution is going to perform better if the skin is exfoliated through a process such as microdermabrasion. Logically, if the stratum corneum is polished and thinned through microdermabrasion, the peel solution will penetrate more effectively. In this case, you would want to use the peel solution with ingredients most likely to improve the dyschromia, perhaps azelaic acid, bearberry, or kojic acid. Another important consideration is the frequency of treatments. Light peels such as designer peels can be performed more frequently compared with other more aggressive treatments, and as such, the clinician may choose to treat the patient more often in the clinic in an attempt to improve and accelerate the outcome.

Azelaic acid

Azelaic acid or Azelex® (the trade name) is commonly a 20% prescription cream or gel and is used to treat acne. It is usually part of the home-care program used in the evening. However, azelaic acid is also known to

> Using a designer peeling agent requires that the clinician have an understanding of herbal ingredients and how they affect the skin.

improve discoloration. Savvy clinicians know that the home use of azelaic acid in combination with hydroquinone for stubborn dyschromias will dramatically improve the patient's result in a short period.

Azelaic acid is also used in designer peels to treat discoloration. Given that azelaic acid is a prescription medication, manufacturers that do not have prescription privileges will not be able to prepare this peel solution. Azelaic acid is found in wheat, rye, and barley.[5] Therefore you may be able to use a solution with these precursors to azelaic acid. When used as a peeling agent, azelaic acid can be irritating and, as such, penetrate slightly better compared with home-care preparations. When azelaic acid is used as a peeling agent, it is primarily directed at discolorations rather than acne.

Lactic acid

Lactic acid is an alpha hydroxy acid. Lactic acid comes from milk (you remember the story about Cleopatra). However, as with glycolic acid, lactic acid is now synthetically manufactured. Remember, the molecules of lactic acid are slightly larger than those of glycolic acid, making it less penetrable and generally a milder peeling agent. Lactic acid is also a humectant and part of the natural moisturizing factor of the stratum corneum. For this reason, lactic acid can be among the base acid of designer peels. Lactic acid will, however, exfoliate the skin just as does glycolic acid by breaking apart the cellular glue. In doing so, the herbal ingredients are allowed to penetrate more effectively.

Kojic acid

Kojic acid comes from fermented Japanese mushrooms. It can also be derived in the manufacture of sake. Kojic acid has been studied both **in vitro** and **in vivo**, with convincing results. Kojic acid chelates copper, which is required by tyrosine to produce melanin.[6] This product is used not only as a home-care product, but also increasingly as an ingredient in designer peeling solutions. The storage and stability of kojic acid seems to be the main problems regarding its efficacy. Kojic acid is an unstable formulation in higher percentages and oxidizes when exposed to air.

Mulberry root

Mulberry root has a high content of **arbutin**, which is a hydroquinone derivative.[7] Arbutin is also isolated from the bearberry shrub, cranberry, blueberry, and most pears.[8] Although the research on arbutin and, as such, mulberry root has been performed mainly on animals and in vitro,[9] evidence suggests that it has efficacy in the treatment of dyschromias. The recommended percentages for mulberry have not yet been established.

in vitro
Not on a living subject.

in vivo
On a living subject.

mulberry root
The precursor to hydroquinone.

arbutin
A glycoside found in the bearberry and related plants; hydroquinone derivative.

Bearberry

Bearberry also contains high concentrations of arbutin and is therefore effective as an herbal ingredient to treat dyschromias. Bearberry must be in higher percentages (though exactly what that means remains unclear) to provide an effective result. The reality is that bearberry, although it appears in cosmetic products today, has not been tested for cosmetic use on the skin. The potential results are only speculative at this time.

Licorice

Licorice (*Glycyrrhiza glabra*) contains **glycyrrhetic acid** and is used for its antiinflammatory properties. In home-care products, you may find this ingredient appropriate for treating acne and rosacea or as an afterpeel ingredient. Licorice is sometimes found in designer peels. As a peel ingredient, the purpose of its use is not clear because inflammation of the skin is, in part, the purpose of a peel.

Echinacea

Echinacea was originally used by Native Americans. A derivative of the purple coneflower, Echinacea is best known as an herbal medicine to assist the immune system. As a modern society, we used Echinacea to treat colds and influenza. However, Echinacea has also found a place in designer peel preparations. Used in peel solutions, mainly as an antibacterial, Echinacea has been shown to be effective in treating mild acne. It is also an antiinflammatory agent. Only Echinacea purpurea and Echinacea pallida have been shown to have effectiveness.[10]

Green tea

Tea and its benefits, topical and oral, are of great interest to researchers at this time because of its strong antioxidant properties. Research has confirmed these antioxidant benefits, as well as anticarcinogenetic properties[11] of black, green, and white teas. Although this information is abundant for the oral consumption of tea, research for tea applied topically is minimal. However, as studies are being conducted, the research is beginning to confirm that the antioxidant, antiinflammatory, and anticarcinogenetic qualities of these ingredients can improve the skin when applied topically.[12] As a peeling agent, green tea brings all of the antioxidant, antiinflammatory, and anticarcinogenetic qualities of regular topical use.

Kola nut

Kola nut is native to Nigeria and was originally used as currency and traded for goods and services. Kola nut has high quantities of caffeine and will therefore be addictive to persons who consume large quantities of the nut. Kola nuts also are thought to contain amine, which may form nitrosamines

bearberry
A botanical used in skin-care products and peeling agents to treat hyperpigmentation.

licorice
A dried root that contains glycyrrhetic acid, a known antiinflammatory.

glycyrrhetic acid
A bioactive natural glycoside known for its antiinflammatory qualities.

Echinacea
A purple coneflower native to western United States and known to be an antibacterial and antiinflammatory herb.

kola nut
An African nut tree commonly used for strong medicinal qualities. Kola nut also contains high levels of caffeine.

(potential carcinogens).[13] As a peeling agent, kola nut is probably a skin irritant, but the exact reason for its use as a peeling agent is unknown.

Lavender

Lavender is typically used as a fragrance and as a calming agent in aromatherapy. However, no research has been conducted as to its effect on the skin as a peeling agent. Potential actions of lavender on the skin are irritation and a remote possibility of antibacterial actions.

Vitamin C

Vitamin C is a well-known and very powerful antioxidant. Used as both an oral and topical component, the benefits of vitamin C are well recognized and well documented. As a peeling agent, vitamin C will assist in stimulating collagen and reduce the signs of solar damage.

Skin's Response to Designer Peels

Having realistic expectations is important while using any designer peel solution. Even if the patient is using topical prescription creams such as Retin A®, a designer peel will not render a similar result as, for example, TCA. Both the clinician and the patient should understand this property. The skin will have a mild response to designer peels, especially if used independently of adjunct treatments such as microdermabrasion. The skin will not likely burn, sting, or show any signs of erythema with the use of these ingredients. Remember, erythema is a benchmark in the peel process to evaluate the outcome of the treatment. However, skin can still derive a benefit from a designer peel treatment. With the proper combination of herbal ingredients, the skin should show moderate improvement in dyschromias, mild acne, and mild photoaging.

Posttreatment

The postcare treatment will, more than likely, be dictated by the adjunct treatment. For example, if the peel is done in conjunction with microdermabrasion, the postcare of microdermabrasion may be directed by the clinician. These peels are generally so mild that the patient is advised to wear the peel home and wash it off several hours later. As with all treatments in the clinic, a specific protocol should be written and followed by the clinician. This precaution is important for the safety of both the patient and the clinician.

Anticipated Results

Although the results of designer peels cannot be described as significant, they are still a valid and legitimate choice for the clinician. The anticipated mild improvements for the skin are predictable and provide an effective adjunct to other treatment modalities. For patients who

---

lavender
A plant used primarily as a fragrance and thought to have antibacterial qualities.

are seeking a gentler approach to treatment, designer peels are an appropriate option. With the use of designer peels, the patient's skin can look refreshed, evenly colored, and hydrated.

Complications

Although the common complications known to other peel solutions are highly unlikely with the light designer peels, the clinician should still be alert for complications. The most likely complication to afflict the patient would be an allergic response to the peel solution, which would present itself as a rash or erythema unassociated with a traditional peel result. However, these situations are rare, and even if the protocol is to send the patient home with the product on his or her face for 24 hours, reports of significant complications, if any, are rare.

Combining Designer Peels with Other Treatments

As previously discussed, the best approach with herbal designer peels is to combine them with other clinical treatments. The combination approach allows the other clinical treatment to do the "heavy lifting," allowing the peel solution to penetrate into the skin evenly and more effectively. Some of the best treatments to combine with designer peels are microdermabrasion, facials, and dermaplaning.

When using microdermabrasion, the concept of implementing a physical polishing process before the application of the peel solution makes sense. A debate is underway at this time about the timing of the peel application. Many clinicians prefer to apply the solution before the microdermabrasion. In the case of keratolytic peeling agents, this course of action is correct. However, when the objective is to allow a deeper penetration of the peeling agent, application after microdermabrasion is the correct order. In the case of a designer peel, the product would not likely have a keratolytic effect; therefore the solution should be applied after the microdermabrasion treatment.

Using a designer peel after a facial is a good idea, especially when treating acne or dry skin. Because the skin is soft from the heat, it will be ready to accept the peel solution. In this case, a facial will allow penetration and greater efficacy. Apply the designer peel in the final steps of the facial, and follow the peel with a cooling mask.

This stage brings us to the treatment called dermaplaning. Dermaplaning is a great treatment to combine with a designer peel application. The treatment was made famous by BioMedic®, a medical skin-care company. The procedure uses a straight-edge blade, usually a surgical #10 blade at a 45-degree angle. Special blades are now made by La Roche/BioMedic® used specifically for this purpose. The entire face is "bladed," removing the hair and loose stratum corneum. Following the dermaplaning, the peel solution can be applied. The solution can deeply penetrate and can sometimes result in an uneven penetration if the dermaplaning technique has been applied heavier in a particular area. However, this treatment generally gives a great result, and patients love it!

Regimen of Clinical Treatments

Obviously, the number of treatments is directly related to the problem you are trying to solve. If the patient can tolerate a weekly or bi-weekly microdermabrasion treatment with a peel application, the results will be achieved more quickly. On the other hand, if the patient has only a mild problem and the peel is used as an adjunct treatment to a facial, for example, monthly may be suitable. The decision will be up to you, the clinician, to determine how often the patient should be seen.

TOP TEN TIPS TO TAKE TO THE CLINIC

1. Know what the herbal ingredients do before choosing a solution.
2. If you do not know the ingredients, look them up.
3. Antioxidants are popular ingredients for designer peels.
4. The best results with designer peels will be achieved in conjunction with microdermabrasions, facials, and dermaplaning.
5. Complications with designer peels are rare; the complications will usually come with the adjunct treatment, such as microdermabrasion.
6. Designer peels can be a good choice for sensitive skin.
7. Designer peel solutions can be expensive; therefore make sure you develop a meaningful treatment for the patient.
8. Salicylic acid peels or beta peels are best used for acne treatments.
9. Patients with acne will respond best if a home-care treatment is followed in coordination with the clinical treatment.
10. Salicylic acid can cause rug burns in areas of irritation or open skin.

CHAPTER REVIEW QUESTIONS

1. What is salicylic acid?
2. How does salicylic acid work to peel the skin?
3. What are the best indications for salicylic acid peels?
4. How does salicylic acid peeling interface with other treatments?

5. How do you choose the strength of the peel solution?
6. What is the pretreatment protocol for salicylic acid peeling?
7. What are the skin's normal responses to salicylic acid peels?
8. What are the objectives of salicylic acid peels?
9. What are the potential complications of salicylic acid peels?
10. What is a designer peel?
11. How does the designer peel work on the skin?
12. What are the best indications for designer peels?
13. How does designer peeling interface with other treatments?
14. How do you choose the solution for a designer peel?
15. What is the pretreatment protocol for designer peeling?
16. What are the skin's normal responses to designer peels?
17. What are the objectives of designer peels?
18. What are the potential complications of designer peels?

CHAPTER REFERENCES

1. Lowe, N., & Sellar, P. (1999). *Skin secrets: The medical facts versus the beauty fiction.* New York: Collins & Brown.
2. Brody, H. J. (1997). *Chemical peeling and resurfacing* (2nd ed.). St. Louis: Mosby.
3. American Academy of Dermatology. (2004, May 13). *Public resources: Combination therapies offer new management options for acne and rosacea* [Online]. Available: http://www.aad.org
4. Brody, H. J. (1997). *Chemical peeling and resurfacing* (2nd ed.). St. Louis: Mosby.
5. Begoun, P. (2004, June 7). *Cosmetic dictionary: L* [Online]. Available: www.cosmeticshop.com
6. Centurion, S. A. (2004, February 4). *Cosmeceuticals. eMedicine. com* [Online]. Available: www.emedicine.com
7. Begoun, P. (2004, June 7). *Cosmetic Dictionary: L* [Online]. Available: www.cosmeticshop.com
8. Begoun, P. (2004, June 7). *Cosmetic dictionary: L* [Online]. Available: www.cosmeticshop.com
9. Begoun, P. (2004, June 7). *Cosmetic Dictionary: L* [Online]. Available: www.cosmeticshop.com
10. Begoun, P. (2004, June 7). *Cosmetic dictionary: L* [Online]. Available: www.cosmeticshop.com
11. Begoun, P. (2004, June 7). *Cosmetic dictionary: L* [Online]. Available: www.cosmeticshop.com
12. Begoun, P. (2004, June 7). *Cosmetic dictionary: L* [Online]. Available: www.cosmeticshop.com

13. Begoun, P. (2004, June 7). *Cosmetic dictionary: L* [Online]. Available: www.cosmeticshop.com

BIBLIOGRAPHY

1911 Edition Encyclopedia. (2004). [Online]. Available: http://encyclopedia.org

American Academy of Dermatology. (2004, May 13). *Public resources: Combination therapies offer new management options for acne and rosacea* [Online]. Available: http://www.aad.org

American Society for Dermatologic Surgery. (2004, May 13). *Chemical peel: Patient fact sheet* [Online]. Available: http://asds-net.org

Azer, M. (2002, March 1). *Salicylate toxicity* [Online]. Available: www.emedicine.com

Begoun, P. (2004, June 7). *Cosmetic dictionary: L* [Online]. Available: www.cosmeticshop.com

Brody, H. J. (1997). *Chemical peeling and resurfacing* (2nd ed.). St. Louis: Mosby.

Centurion, S. A. (2004, February 4). Cosmeceuticals. *eMedicine.com* [Online]. Available: www.emedicine.com

Grieve, M. (2004, June 8). *Kola nut: A modern herbal* [Online]. Available: www.botanical.com

Kunin, A. (2003, November 12). Chemical peels. *Dermadoctor.com Newsletter* [Online]. Available: www.dermadoctor.com

Latona, V. (2000, August). Saving face: Adult acne. *Vegetarian Times* [Online]. Available: www.findarticles.com

Lee, H., & Kim, I. (2003, December). Salicylic acid peels for the treatment of acne vulgaris in Asian patients. *Journal of Dermatologic Surgery*, 29(12), 1196–9.

Leigh, E. (2004, June 8). Herb information: Echinacea. *The Herb Research Foundation* [Online]. Available: www.herbs.org

Lowe, N., & Sellar, P. (1999). *Skin secrets: The medical facts versus the beauty fiction*. New York: Collins & Brown.

Tabibian, M. (2001, November 5). Skin lightening/depigmentation agents. *eMedicine.com* [Online]. Available: www.emedicine.com

Peels in Your Practice

CHAPTER 11

KEY TERMS

annual business plan
competition
cost to acquire
cross selling
database
demographics
economy pricing
goals
indicator hot sheet

indicators
inventory
marketing strategies
marketplace
penetration pricing
"powering" the patient
   database
premium pricing
pricing strategies

product bundling pricing
referral programs
revenue goals
revenue strategy
standard pricing policy
understanding your client
understanding your
   competition
yearly business objectives

LEARNING OBJECTIVES

After completing this chapter you should be able to:

1. Discuss the development of a "peel practice."
2. Describe marketing concepts available to build a peel practice.
3. Discuss how the current patient base can be used to build a peel practice.
4. Describe practice indicators.
5. Discuss the use of practice indicators.

INTRODUCTION

Chemical peels are an essential component of many individual medical skin-care programs and, from a business perspective, an essential service of medical spas. They often create the need for repeat clinic visits, an important piece of the business of providing skin care. Yet the financial success of the *business* of providing the peel service depends on understanding and analyzing several crucial but basic business concepts, beginning with the development plan.

Writing a development plan looks simple, but it will be wrought with details you usually do not consider. This is the beauty of a development plan: it makes you *think* and *plan*. In the process of thinking about how you will develop your peel business, you will have to answer questions and solve initial problems. This process helps make your development plan solid and void of potential holes that can later cause problems. For our purpose, the development plan has two simple components: getting your business started and keeping your business moving.

CREATING A PEEL BUSINESS

Introducing chemical peels into a business can be both exciting and challenging. The sophisticated nature of these businesses can elevate your spa to the next level. The startup process involves evaluating the practice landscape, which includes an understanding of demographics, current patient base, competition, pricing strategies, and marketing. This understanding will encompass creating **marketing strategies** to bring the clients through the door. Adding a service to your menu will be hard work that you want to bear fruit as soon as possible. The best way to accomplish this task is through a strict and methodical process. A development plan is the launch pad for the success you will later enjoy; so read carefully, and take notes. There is a lot to learn.

Practice Landscape

For your new chemical peel service to thrive, you will need to keep up with the trends, regulations, and **competition** associated with your new service, or even the spa industry at large. These aspects are collectively referred to as your business landscape. The business landscape will be the deciding factor in many areas, most notably, marketing your program accurately and effectively.

marketing strategies
The planned use of marketing elements and media pathways to create a strategy to introduce new clients or reactivate former clients.

competition
Businesses in your region that offer comparable services.

Three deeply intertwined aspects of evaluating your practice landscape are the marketplace, clients, and competition. Independently and consequentially, these three components are in a state of constant change. By identifying the present conditions of each category, you have defined the current landscape. The **marketplace** is different in every city, and it is sometimes even more localized than your city; it may be your local community. Therefore, to have a firm grasp on the marketplace, you must understand your city and local community.

With a comprehensive understanding of local dynamics, narrowing the general population down to your business's demographic and client base is the second and most misunderstood component of the practice landscape. **Understanding your client** will have a domino effect on marketing, pricing, and many other components that are critical to the success of your business.

Next, although knowing your marketplace and your clients will have a significant role in your daily operations, **understanding your competition** does not. Therefore this aspect should not have an equal share of consideration. Worrying about your competition can become a distraction (or an obsession) that will only harm your practice. You should limit your understanding of competition to the few bits of information you really need to compile about your competition (prices, menu, and advertising promotions).

In addition to keeping current with your practice landscape, maximizing your peel service, and understanding business risks, establishing indicators and goals can play a pivotal role. In the following sections, we discuss the issues of your practice landscape in more detail.

Current Patient Base

An analysis of the existing client base will give you a composite sketch of your target demographic. The information you should seek includes service preferences, price sensitivity, age, household income, knowledge of the industry, referral source, and preconceived notions of the facility and services.

Take note of the existing clients in the current **database** who might be interested in a chemical peel treatment based on your composite sketch criteria. This task can be done two ways: through a survey or by a mathematical analysis based on growth. If you use a survey, the process is simple. Create a survey that clients can fill out while waiting for their treatment. Filling out the questionnaire can include a treatment offer at an "introductory promotional price." Persons who are not in the clinic during the time you are doing the survey can be contacted by telephone or e-mail for the survey.

marketplace
Any environment in which two or more people buy or sell a product or service.

understanding your client
A component of the business landscape during which a business evaluates and acquaints itself with its target demographics.

understanding your competition
A component of the business landscape during which a business evaluates its competition in terms of pricing, procedures, demographics, and advertising promotions.

database
An electronic compilation of extensive categorical information relevant to business processes, such as marketing, inventory, or customer names.

Using the mathematical approach is a stab in the dark, but it is still useful and effective. Knowing the number of clients you currently have in your database, realistically project the potential number of clients that will cross over. Keep the number low, for example 2% to 5% of the database.

With this information in hand, create an in-house campaign to capture these patients. Current clients will be the first to experience the treatment and enjoy your peel treatment. To further improve the number of chemical peel clients, create a referral offer for those who experience the treatment and refer a friend.

However, to maximize the potential of your new service, you will need to bring in new clients. Not all existing clients will be interested in the new service. Similarly, an entire pool of prospective clients remains who have yet to be reached. Given that most of this pool of potential clients will not seek you out, you will need to use demographics as the most effective tools of contacting them by means of marketing materials.

Demographics

demographics
General statistical data used to define consumer markets.

Understanding your **demographics**, or general statistical data used to define consumer markets, is helpful when designing your marketing plan. Most marketing principles are general and are considered "the norm" because they have proven to change or modify consumer behavior. However, with a well-considered interpretation of your potential clients, you will be able to tailor your campaign to your client base, as opposed to broader populations. Enhanced collection and analysis will help you refine your campaign from conception to implementation.

Competition

Your competition is everywhere, across town or across the hallway, and they can be distracting. Like it or not, the ideal is the marker against which the commonplace is compared. Your waiting area will be compared with the most exquisite furnishing fit for royalty. Your customer service will be held up to virtually unattainable standards; and yes, your treatment programs will be expected to surpass the abilities of the leading plastic surgeons. This view is just the way the customer or client thinks and does not suggest that your business must settle for mediocrity. Rather, it should ground you against putting undeserving emphasis on "keeping up with Joneses" or overreaching your own business goals. Your business success will be served best by an internal motivation to satisfy your own client. Other clinics across town and the *Fortune 500* conglomerates across the globe are all your competition, but you must shrink your description of the competition down to a bulleted list of information, which can facilitate your individual business goals.

You want to know what your competitors are doing: who their patients are, what their treatments are, and so forth. The few key points that you should know about your competitors are their pricing, common procedures, demographic target, and advertising promotions. Once you know these things or have an idea of the direction of their business, stay informed, but leave it alone. Use your time efficiently by growing your own business, not paying attention to someone else's.

Competition across the country is important because it gives you an idea of the direction of the industry. Look for a few progressive businesses on each coast and in the middle of the country. Stay on top of what they are doing, including their pricing, procedures, promotions, literature, and written materials and web site promotions. This knowledge will help you keep up with the trends and fads that are developing in the industry and adjust your business, if you wish.

Pricing Strategies

Pricing strategies may sometimes seem as though they are part of the marketing plan. However, pricing is quite different and should be evaluated independently of marketing. The theories and implementation of pricing strategies can be sophisticated. For our purposes, we will focus on four distinct pricing strategies: price and costs, price and competitors, price and customers, and price and business objectives. These pricing strategies will drive your business objectives, unlike promotional pricing, which is an occasional *price break* that may be used, for example, to move overstocked **inventory**.

In retail business, the common thinking holds that the price of an item is the price the customer will pay,[1] meaning that the price of a product is consumer driven. This theory is no less true in the spa and medical spa business. An important first step in setting your peel prices is understanding your customer. Because peels can be competitive, your customers may already be receiving the treatment at another clinic. This area is one of the few instances when a customer survey is recommended. However, elaborate data collection is not necessary. Pricing surveys should be focused on price sensitivities about procedures and products, as well as value. In our environment, perceived value tracks closely with the price the client will pay.

Surveys can be tricky to put together. Preparing the questions in a manner that does not influence the answer can sometimes be difficult. Therefore surveys that affect significant decisions, such as pricing, should be prepared by a professional. Otherwise, the information you get will be exactly what you thought it would be because you asked the question to get the predicted answer.

pricing strategies
A process by which a business determines the best way to price its product or service to entice customers while allowing for profit.

inventory
An itemized list of merchandise or supplies on hand.

Some simple survey questions might include:

- ► Have you ever had a chemical peel?
- ► If not, would you consider having the treatment?
- ► How much do you think is reasonable to pay for a peel?

Making a profit is the number one reason for being in business. Otherwise, you are a nonprofit organization or out of business. Figuring out how to hold down costs, meet goals, pay bills, keep employees happy, and provide outstanding customer service can sometimes feel overwhelming. One particular strategy ranks on top to keep a business moving forward, and that is a revenue strategy, or *how you price*. Understanding pricing strategies, how the competition prices, and what the market will bear in your patient demographic require insight, skill, and intuition.

Pricing peel treatments to facilitate your business's growth and profitability is a smart business tactic. When companies drastically cut prices in an effort to attract customers, the end result can be disastrous. To avoid using desperate, last-option pricing decisions (and suffering the subsequent consequences on your bottom line), consider implementing a **standard pricing policy**. A standard pricing policy is a document that is controlled by the clinic manager or spa director and is a list of all the prices. The initial prices are calculated through a mathematical formula based on cost and a specific markup percentage. When prices are increased, a standard price increase formula is used. This method is far more effective than saying, "What is spa ABC charging? Oh, let's charge 50 cents less."

Standard pricing policies help the company meet its **yearly business objectives**. The yearly objectives are part of the **annual business plan**, which is a complex document that includes a budget, a marketing plan, and a growth plan, and which includes isolated development plans for specific services. The annual business plan gives focus and depth to the business growth.

When a spa adds a service, creating an isolated development plan for the growth of the procedure within the clinic is insurance for success. When you use a model such as the one depicted here, you will want to make the information detailed and appropriate to your individual situation.

A business that offers chemical peels has to ensure that the revenue it generates will cover the costs and yield a profit. Several different pricing tactics cover costs and should be evaluated based on different business models. In the medical spa and day spa sector, one usually thinks first of **premium pricing**. This pricing strategy uses high prices to communicate the uniqueness of the product or service.

The next type of price strategy that might be used in the medical spa area is **penetration pricing**. In penetration pricing, the price is set low to allow access into the market by gaining market share. The costs in this strategy are at break-even or loss levels.

Next is **economy pricing**. Economy pricing keeps all costs low to provide the lowest cost to the customer. This strategy has been made famous by Wal-Mart.

Product bundling pricing is a tactic that is commonly used in the day spa and is finding its way into the medical spa. This concept involves *packages*, but product bundling is more sophisticated than packages. This type of pricing combines multiple services (e.g., facials, peels) sold together. For product bundling, you look at the costs and determine how much discount can be taken in exchange for collecting the fee in advance. Product bundling can also help the clinic become efficient at scheduling and increase clinic utilization by knowing the number of clients who have packages and predicting the number of patients that should be scheduling. Although many other different types of pricings have been developed, these four are the most familiar and most commonly used in our industry.

Evaluate your business objectives for the year before choosing a pricing strategy. Your objectives might include maximizing profits, attracting new clients, achieving a **revenue goal**, preventing further competition, and maintaining your market share. A business might use each of these pricing models at different times in the year to execute its plan.

Marketing

Creating marketing strategies and watching them *bring in the clients* can be rewarding at times, and equally disconcerting other times. Business growth followed by success is dependent on innovative and effective marketing. The marketing plan you create should use as many tactics as possible because each of them will have a different reach, appeal, and anticipated impact on the practice. These tactics should include direct mail, e-mail, newspaper, radio, in-house strategies, and literature, to mention a few.

Marketing strategies. Direct mail is a commonly used tactic to introduce new services. The clinic or spa usually sends out a card or letter with an offer attached. Direct mail has a success rate of 1.5% or less. The average clinic may believe this tactic to be a terrific way to introduce a service or product, but it can be expensive. Let us take a look.

If you send out a 1000 cards, you will get, at best, 15 clients through the door. If the direct mail piece cost $2.00 per card plus postage, the total per card is $2.37. The total cost for the mailer will be $2370.00, meaning that each of the 15 patients that come through the door must spend $158.00 to cover just the cost of the mailer. This amount is calculated before you begin to cover the overhead or make any money. An unexpectedly low yield may end up being costly. Although direct mail can be successful, with this and all strategies, do the math to make sure the ends justify the means. Bearing in mind that direct mailings are a crap shoot, consider taking proactive steps to decrease the risk by trimming the fat from your mailing pool. Send direct mail pieces only to clients who have responded positively to an in-house survey or who have been in the clinic in the last 6 months. A well-conceived database should be able to do as much with little time. Additionally, consider a "cross-selling" direct-mail campaign that combines one treatment, for

premium pricing
A pricing strategy in which the price is set high to compensate for a high-quality product, usually with a high production cost as well.

penetration pricing
A pricing strategy in which the price is set low to allow for introduction into an existing market.

economy pricing
The low pricing of a product or service as a means to entice customers to buy.

product bundling pricing
A pricing strategy in which one or more products or services are offered at a discount.

revenue goal
The process used to define the monetary objectives of a business.

example, Restylane® or Botox®, with a promotional treatment. Because of the unpredictable nature of direct mailings, mail the offer to a select number of more qualified patients rather than your entire database.

Making it easy and rewarding for your existing clients to volunteer their e-mail addresses for in-house marketing and promotional use is to your advantage. By far, e-mail is the most cost-effective means of communicating with your clients. You can develop regular e-mail specials and introduce new offerings with little effort and surprising results. When you put promotional signs in your office that say, "Ask about our e-mail-only specials" you will be surprised by how many people will give you their e-mail addresses because no one wants to be left out when a special becomes available (Table 11–1).

Newspaper advertising is tried and true. In most cities, every weekend, literally hundreds of ads can be found for plastic surgery, spas, and medical skin care. Is your ad special, or is it just one in the maze of many? Are you participating in "advertorials?" What is the competition doing right next to you? Newspaper advertising can be an expensive tactic to acquire new patients. The question that must be answered when it comes to newspaper advertising (as with all tactics) is the **cost to acquire**. In other words, how much money must be spent to get one new patient to walk through the door? Taken one step further, how many appointments were needed for the patient to spend enough money to cover the cost of the newspaper ad and begin to produce a profit for your clinic? Add into the financial mix the variable costs of ad design and any additional marketing and you may find that newspaper ads are

cost to acquire
The average cost per new customer of any one marketing strategy.

Table 11–1   Marketing Strategies

Marketing Strategy	Breadth of Market Reach	Cost	Cost to Acquire Risk
Direct mail	Low	High	High
E-mail	Low	Low	Low
Newspaper	Moderate	High	High
Billboard	Moderate	Moderate	Moderate
Radio commercial	Moderate	Low	Low
Regional magazine	High	High	Moderate
Local affiliate television commercials	High	High	Moderate

rather expensive unless you can really attract a large number of patients. Radio advertising is a viable option for smaller markets. In larger metropolitan areas such as Los Angeles or New York, the reach of the radio station may be too great to merit radio advertising. In other words, a large percentage of potential clients are simply too far away to consider driving to your clinic. Even under this condition, radio will provide great name recognition and tremendous branding, but the important question to ask is, "What is the objective of radio advertising?" If the purpose is to attract clients, the larger the size of the metropolis, the greater the risk is of unsatisfactory new client yield. Having said that, in smaller communities, radio may work well, especially if a drive-time slot is open and an announcer is available who will broadcast a live advertisement or, better yet, a testimonial.

In-house strategies are among the most effective and low-cost means of attracting new patients and increasing revenue. By implementing cross selling, **"powering" the patient database**, and **referral programs**, you can create a sophisticated, layered initiative to generate additional revenue, as well as flex your know-how.

First, learn and implement **cross selling**. This tactic is one that will begin to build your practice today. Cross selling is the technique of using an active client in one category and moving him or her into other categories. For example, an injection client, one who is in the clinic only for Botox® or dermal fillers, may be open to the opportunity of experiencing something new. In fact, the client may be receiving services at another clinic or spa. Cross sales can be made in a couple of ways. First, offer a gift certificate, followed by a discount on a package sale. Cross selling can also happen subtly when you combine procedures in a package. For example, when a client buys a microdermabrasion package, include a couple of facial treatments. Almost everyone can benefit from this strategy, so it is really a win-win proposition for everyone.

Powering the database uses your existing database to uncover potential candidates for new treatments. This strategy requires investigative work on the part of the staff, but it is worth it. Gaining a new client can cost 10 times more money than keeping an old client,[2] so get to work on clients you already have in your database. Look through the database and find out who has not been in the clinic for a while. Evaluate the number of "lost clients," and create a cross-selling campaign to get them back into your clinic.

Creating new clients from your current database may seem redundant, but a referral program will do a great job of creating new clients. Most clinics experience at least a 30% referral rate. In other words, each month, 30% of your new clients come from the referral of happy clients. Do you reward these clients that send you business? If not,

"powering" the patient database
An in-house marketing strategy that involves innovative and detailed use of information already contained in a business database to increase traffic.

referral programs
An in-house marketing strategy that rewards an existing client for referring a new one.

cross selling
The process of selling related, peripheral items to a customer.

why not? This person is the easiest new patient you will encounter, and he or she is already sold because a friend told this new potential client that your clinic was the best. Create a referral program for your established clients. Use gift certificates or cash rewards. Everybody wins.

Having literature available for the procedures you offer is an essential part of the in-house marketing campaign. Original literature specific to your practice can be informational, educational, and identifiable. If you do not print original literature, then be sure to have literature that is supplied by the manufacturer. If the manufacturer does not supply literature or brochures, several vendors create "boilerplate" literature that will work just fine. The important part is that the literature is accurate and available. Included in the literature category should be *posttreatment* instructions. Even if these items are copied on your copy machine, you can still customize and dress up the presentation. However, the content is the important part, and function should take obvious precedence over form. Written posttreatment instructions are important to ensure that the patient follows your instructions and that any misunderstandings will be minimal.

> The best and worst forms of advertising are word of mouth or experienced based. These ways of spreading the word are reliable, affordable, achievable, and manageable. Try to make each client satisfied enough to want to tell at least one other person. Just think of the profound effect this will have on your business success.

Setting Up Goals and Indicators

Company history speaks not only to the traditional history, such as "this is where we came from and this is what we look like now," but also, and more importantly, about the comparatives of **indicators** and goals. Although these categories may initially seem financial in nature, the reality is that indicators and goals really speak to history and the ability to exceed against the historic goals.

indicators
A key value used to measure performance over time as it relates to an organization's goal progress.

goals
General statements of anticipated business outcomes resulting from well-stated objectives.

Creating Goals

Setting **goals** for both the clinic and the clinician is appropriate. The goals should reflect the number of patient calls, the number of patients scheduled, the number of patients treated, the referral patterns, and other important indicators for the clinic. These goals should translate directly into the revenue goal for the clinic.

The goals you set up should be attainable otherwise everyone gets discouraged. Failure is a bad feeling and one that you do not want in your clinic. If the peel procedure is being brought into an already established practice, the goals can be a little more aggressive because you have an already established patient base. If, on the other hand, your clinic is a startup, then conservative numbers are in order. The goals should be set for 6 months and evaluated monthly. This way, you can determine how successful the process is and if you need to add additional advertising or marketing to stimulate the number of visits.

Set your goals and let the front desk and clinician know the goal. Some managers like goal setting to be a collaborative process. This process works only if you, as the manager, stretch your employees to accept goals that seem out of reach. Employees are somewhat more conservative than managers are; so do not be surprised if you find that your goals are a little higher in comparison to your employees' goals. Your goals might initially be broken down by (a) how many clients are scheduled and (b) how many clients are treated. Once you get these numbers, you can extrapolate the revenue. For example, if the goal is 50 clients and the price for the peel is $125.00, then your revenue goal is $6250.00 per month. This goal is just a treatment goal. The product goal also exists. For example, does every ticket need a product sale of at least $25.00? We know this will not happen, but the average product sales on peel tickets may be $25.00, and this is what you are looking to accomplish: a focus on additional sales.

Creating Indicators

Indicators track the progress of business goals. Daily or, at the longest interval, weekly review of each clinician's **indicator hot sheet** will provide you with daily (or weekly) goal progress reports.

Without a weekly or daily hot sheet, you do not have the opportunity for improvement. A hot sheet for chemical peels may include number of clients scheduled, number of clients seen, number of clients rebooked, average ticket revenue, and the breakdown between product and service revenue. You also might be interested in the referral pattern. The indicator hot sheet should be the tool to evaluate, redirect, and grow the business. Over time, the information will be the comparative you use to measure your progress. Indicator sheets are simple in form; they need only the information you are wanting and should not be cumbersome (Table 11–2).

indicator hot sheet
A daily or weekly progress report that measures and provides daily insight into a business or employees' performance.

Initially, you may find that a daily review of indicators is not necessary. In this event, a weekly sheet will do. However, do not extend this period past a week. Forgetting about the growth process is too easy. At the end of the month, you will get the numbers, and they can be disappointing, and by this point, nothing can be done to improve the numbers for the month.

	Week One	Week Two	Week Three	Week Four	Actual	Goal
Number of new clients booked						
Number of clients seen						
Number of clients rebooked (after treatment)						
Number of packages sold						
Revenue per ticket						
Service revenue per ticket						
Product revenue per ticket						

Table 11–2 Indicator Sheet: Chemical Peels

Conclusion

Starting a new business or adding to your existing business can be exhilarating and full of challenges, but doing so is never as easy as it seems. Successful people follow the intricate steps of business development, analysis, and the daily monitoring of progress. A chemical peel is a worthwhile procedure, one that will bring improvement to the client's skin and an expansion of the menu offerings. A well-conceived and carefully implemented plan will make a business more competitive and certainly more successful.

▶ ›› TOP TEN TIPS TO TAKE TO THE CLINIC

1. Chemical peels are an essential offering for a medical spa.
2. Become an expert at understanding your client.
3. Develop a feature/benefit communication style to increase sales.
4. Understand possible marketing opportunities.
5. Identify the benefits of marketing opportunity before executing it.
6. Use goals to achieve success.

7. Use indicators to measure success.
8. Keep organized business records.
9. Learn to read financial statements.
10. Be organized, methodical, and focused.

CHAPTER REVIEW QUESTIONS

1. What are indicators?
2. How do you identify the indicators for peel treatments?
3. What are the four pricing strategies?
4. Why is marketing an indirect cost of chemical peeling?
5. What are the other indirect costs of chemical peeling?
6. What are income statements?
7. How do you keep money from slipping through your fingers?
8. What are indirect costs?
9. What are direct costs?
10. Discuss writing a business plan to implement chemical peeling.

CHAPTER REFERENCES

1. Canada Business Service Centre. (February 15, 2004, February 15). *Setting the right price* [Online]. Available: www.cbsc.org
2. Keller, K. L., Sternthal, B., & Tybout, A. (2002). Three questions you need to ask about your brand. *Harvard Business Review*, 80(9).

BIBLIOGRAPHY

American Management Association. (2004, February 15). *A baker's dozen pricing strategies* [Online]. Available: www.amanet.org

Beer, K. (2003, September). *The cosmetic clinic: Six secrets to success* [Online]. Available: www.skinandaging.com

Bennis, W. G., & Thomas, R. J. (2002). The crucibles of leadership. *Harvard Business Review*, 80(9), 257–267.

Canada Business Service Centre. (2004, February 15). *Setting the right price* [Online]. Available: www.cbsc.org

Entrepreneur.com. (2001, October 02). *Avoid these "destroy your business" pitfalls* [On line]. Available: www.entrepreneur.com

Gail, S. (2003, July 1). *Mirror, mirror on the wall, are men so vain afterall* [Online]. Available: www.cosmeticsurgerytimes.com

Grima, D. (2004, February 15). *Keeping tabs on your competition* [Online]. Available: www.santuccibrown.com

Keller, K. L., Sternthal, B., & Tybout, A. (2002). Three questions you need to ask about your brand. *Harvard Business Review*, 80(9).

Khurana, R. (2002). The curse of the superstar CEO. *Harvard Business Review*, 80(9).

MarketingTeacher.com. (2004, February 13). *Pricing strategies lesson* [Online]. Available: www.marketingteacher.com

Matarasso, S. L., Glogau, R. G., & Markley, A. C. (1994, June). Wood's lamp for superficial chemical peels. *Journal of American Academic Dermatology*, 30(6), 988–992.

Millenium Research Group. (2002, July). *US market 2002* [Online]. Available: www.mindbranch.com

Nemko, M. (2000, March). *Perfecting your pricing strategies* [Online]. Available: www.entrepreneur.com

Parisian Peel Medical. (2000, October 10). *Aesthetic buyers guide: Market study defines industry leaders and market size* [Online]. Available: www.parisianpeel.com

Parisian Peel Medical. (2004, March 10). *Skin renewal market study confirms growth, cites "second generation technology"* [Online]. Available: www.parisianpeel.com

Smith-Isroelit, B. (2004, January 21). *Spa finder's 2004 trends and predictions* [Online]. Available: www.spatrade.com

Spatrade. (2004, February 5). *Spas leading outlets for professional skin care brands* [Online]. Available:www.spatrade.com

Troy, B. (2003, October 1). *Patient experience makes your bottom line* [Online]. Available: www.cosmeticsurgerytimes.com

Tutor2u.com. (2004, February 13). *Pricing* [Online]. Available: www.tutor2u.net

Urbany, J. (2003). *Getting the price right: What gets in the way* [Online]. Available: www.nd.edu

Glossary

5-flourouracil (5-FU) A chemotherapy agent that is given as a treatment for some types of cancer. Used as a topical peeling agent. Also known as Efudex® when used on the skin.

5FU pulse peeling An alternative delivery to the daily fluorouracil cream. The treatment is done with weekly Jessner's peels and a fluorouracil solution.

A

acetic acid A mild organic acid derived from vinegar.

acetylcholine An enzyme found in various tissues and organs, associated with muscle movement.

acid mantel A thin coating on the stratum corneum that is intended to protect the skin from infection. It has a pH of 4.0 to 6.5.

acidic Any substance that has a pH less than 7.0.

actinic keratoses Precancerous lesions of the skin, generally from sunlight exposure.

acute Having a rapid onset with a short but severe course.

adipose cells Fat cells.

aging The universal experience of change associated with the passage of time.

aging analysis An assessment that examines how aging physically presents itself in the skin, particularly, what sorts of damaging conditions to which the skin has been exposed in the past and what the results of that damage are. Aging analysis considers both intrinsic and extrinsic aging modalities.

albinism Inherited skin dyschromia characterized by a lack of pigment.

alkaline Any substance that has a pH greater than 7.0.

alpha hydroxy acids Mild organic acids used in cosmeceutical products. AHAs "unglue" cells in the epidermis, allowing keratinocytes to be shed at the stratum granulosum, providing skin with a healthier texture.

anagen The growth phase of the hair follicle.

anatomy The study of the body and how its structures work in relation to one another.

annual business plan A growth plan that outlines business objectives, marketing plans, and budgets for the period of 1 fiscal year.

anthranilates Weak UVB filters. They absorb mainly in the near UVA portion of the spectrum.

antimicrobials An agent that halts or prevents the development of microorganisms.

apocrine sweat glands The larger of the two sweat glands that are housed in axillary (under the arm), pubic, and perianal areas.

appendages Any anatomic structure that is associated with a larger structure. For the skin, its appendages include hair follicles, sweat glands, and nails.

arbutin   A glycoside found in the bearberry and related plants; hydroquinone derivative.

arrector pili muscle   Located at the hair follicle, the arrector pili muscle contracts when we are cold and creates piloerection (goose bumps).

ascorbyl palmitate   A fat-soluble form of ascorbic acid.

atopic dermatitis   A skin irritation or rash of unknown origin.

atrophic   To undergo deterioration.

atrophic scars   Flat, small, round, and generally inverted scars; usually seen in acne or chicken-pox scarring.

avascular   Lacking in blood vessels and thus having a poor blood supply.

Ayurveda   Indian theory, dating back to 2500 B.C., known as the science of living. Ayurveda defines the essentials that were perceived as being necessary to health.

azelaic acid   An antibacterial agent that is usually used for acne treatment. It also has shown promise in minimizing dyschromias.

B

Baker-Gordon solution   A phenol deep-peel solution.

basal cell carcinoma (BCC)   A slow-growing tumor that generally does not metastasize. It is the most common form of skin cancer, which usually occurs in regions of repeated sunburn.

basophils   A type of white blood cell.

bearberry   A botanical used in skin-care products and peeling agents to treat hyperpigmentation.

benzophenone   A chemical absorber that responds to UV light by generating a free radical capable of rapid polymerization.

beta hydroxy acid   An isometrically distinct relative of alpha hydroxy acids.

beta peel   A 20% or 30% salicylic acid peel solution.

bicarbonate solution   Any salt containing bicarbonate anion; pH above 7.

blanch   A rapid loss of coloration.

Blue Peel®   TCA peel solution that is combined with blue color and acid penetration–slowing or modifying agents.

body dysmorphic disorder (BDD)   A psychosocial disease that causes individuals to be inappropriately concerned with their appearance. Persons affected with BDD are contraindicated for most aesthetic procedures.

body surface area (BSA)   A term used to represent an amount when calculating the percentage of the body burn.

burns   Thermal or electrical injuries that wound the skin.

C

camphors   Used topically as an antiitching agent. Derived as a gum from evergreens native to China and Japan.

carbohydrates   One of a group of chemical substances (including sugars) that contain only carbon, hydrogen, and oxygen. Common in fruits, grains, and nuts, carbohydrates are thought to be the most common chemical compounds on earth.

carbolic acid   *See* phenol.

carbon dioxide (CO_2) laser   Aggressive type of laser used for skin resurfacing, which vaporizes skin and causes thermal injury, allowing for improved collagen production.

career plan   Action taken by an individual to set goals and actions taken to ensure that these goals are realized.

catagen   The transitional phase of the hair follicle.

cautery   Tissue destruction, usually done using electricity.

cellulitis   A potentially serious infection of the skin.

ceramides   A class of lipids that do not contain glycerol cholesterol.

chemical peeling   The use of chemical agents to destroy layers of skin.

chemoexfoliants The use of chemical agents to exfoliate the stratum corneum.

Chi (or Qi) Concept originally theorized by the Yellow Emperor of China's Han Dynasty. According to Chi, nature has a delicate balance and describes nature as an imbalance.

cholesterol A precursor to most steroid hormones; a single molecule is called alcohol.

chronic A disease or occurrence showing little or no change over a long period.

cinnamates A derivative of cinnaminic acid, useful for protection against low levels of UVB rays. Also makes sunscreens waterproof.

citric acid An AHA derived from citrus fruit (oranges, grapefruit, and so forth).

clinic protocols Any set of rules or guidelines established by a clinic to ensure safe practice. These guidelines will vary by location yet are expected to be observed by clinicians working within the individual clinic.

Clostridium botulinum The bacteria derived for Botox®.

cocamidopropyl betaine A foaming agent used in shampoos and cleansers.

collagen An insoluble protein found in connective tissues. Particularly, type I collagen forms a network in the epidermis, and it is credited with providing skin with its tensile strength and firmness.

Collagen® A dermal filler and the trade name for injectable bovine collagen.

competition Businesses in your region that offer comparable services.

consent form Required clinical documentation in which associated risks, complications, and presumable outcomes are outlined in association with a given procedure. This document gives permission by the patient to the clinician to provide the procedure.

consultation The initial visit with a professional during which both the client and the professional investigate whether a specific treatment or service is warranted or achievable.

continuing education units (CEUs) Any certified training or event that is intended to build or add skills.

cornified Hardening or thickening of the skin.

cosmeceutical Products that do more than decorate or camouflage but less than prescription drugs would do. The term was originally coined by Dr. Albert Kligman.

cost to acquire The average cost per new customer of any one marketing strategy.

cross selling The process of selling related, peripheral items to a customer.

croton oil A fixed oil extracted from the croton plant (castor oil).

Cutivate® A prescription steroidal cream.

D

***d*-alpha tocopherol** *See* vitamin E.

database An electronic compilation of extensive categorical information relevant to business processes, such as marketing, inventory, or customer names.

deep epidermal wounding Injury that reaches deep into the epidermis, as with peeling solutions.

deep peels A peel depth extending into the papillary dermis or upper reticular dermis. Most notable of deep peels are phenol.

defatted The use of isopropyl alcohol or acetone to remove all oils from the skin, which will allow peel solutions to work evenly.

demographics General statistical data used to define consumer markets.

dermal-epidermal junction The superficial side of the dermis, connected to the epidermis.

dermaplaning The use of a sharp surgical blade to exfoliate the stratum corneum.

dermis The second layer of skin, which is responsible for attaching the skin to the body.

designer peel Custom-made combinations of herbal and prescription ingredients.

desmosomes   Small hairlike structures in the spiny layer of the epidermis.

detergents   A synthetic cleansing agent that acts as a wetting agent and emulsifier.

diabetes   Many different types; the most familiar is that which is associated the rise and fall of blood sugars and the associated complications therein.

dibenzoylmethanes   A UVA ray absorber.

diethanolamine (DEA)   An emulsifier or foaming agent.

discoid lupus   Cyclic breakouts and remissions of a scaly red rash.

drug-induced lupus   Growing old; aging eccrine glands.

dynamic rhytids   Wrinkling that occurs as a result of facial movement.

dyschromias   Discoloration of the skin.

epithelialization   The growth of new skin over a wound.

epithelium   Membranous tissue covering internal organs and lining skin appendages.

erbium laser   Less-aggressive type of laser that causes less thermal injury while still causing epidermal and papillary dermal injuries.

erythema   A spot on the skin showing diffused redness caused by capillary congestion and dilation.

ester   A fragrant water- and fat-soluble compound formed by the combination of an organic acid and alcohol, removing the water from the compound.

etiology   The cause of a disease.

extrinsic aging   Changes that are brought on by the effects of the environment and our choices relating to them, specifically sunlight exposure.

E

eccrine sweat glands   The smaller of the two sweat glands that reside all over the body.

Echinacea   A purple coneflower native to western United States and known to be an antiviral and intiinflammatory herb.

economy pricing   The low pricing of a product or service as a means to entice customers to buy.

elastin   Connective tissue proteins.

Eldopaque®   A 4% concentration of hydroquinone.

emollients   A product that has a softening or soothing effect on the skin.

eosinophils   Granulocyte blood cell characterized by multiple-shaped nuclei, present in full-thickness wounds.

epidermal cells   Cells found in the outermost layer of skin.

epidermis   Outermost, avascular, protective layer of skin.

epidermolysis   Separating of the epidermal cells.

F

fatty acids   One of many molecules that are long chains of lipid-carboxylic acid found in fats and oils.

filaggrin   Synthesizes lipids (fats) that are thought to serve as "intercellular cement," an important component of NMF.

Fitzpatrick skin typing   A method of skin typing that considers skin's complexion, hair color, eye color, ethnicity, and the individual's reaction to unprotected sunlight exposure.

flash injuries   A tissue injury caused by a sudden and rapid exposure to electricity, heat, cold, or chemicals.

folliculitis   An infection of the hair follicle, such as "in-grown hairs."

four humors   Early medical concept originally documented by Hippocrates that states that the character of a man was determined by the specific balance of the four fluids (as he perceived as) running through the body: black bile, yellow bile, blood, and phlegm.

free radicals Molecules lacking an even number of electrons. Free radicals play an important role in tissue ischemia, injury, and aging.

frost Coagulation of protein in the skin that turns the skin a white color.

full-thickness wounds Wounds that penetrate to a specific depth in the papillary dermis or upper reticular dermis. These wounds are associated with slower healing, and scarring will usually develop.

fungal infection Any infection caused by the kingdom of organisms, which includes yeasts and molds.

G

gel solution Semisolid material that is easily absorbed in the skin without the irritation associated with other cream-based solutions.

generalized posttraumatic dyschromias A hyperpigmentation caused by an insult.

glabella The area between the eyebrows.

Glogau classification of aging analysis A system of aging analysis that calculates the degree of aging-related damage and assigning a numeric typing. The Glogau classification considers both intrinsic and extrinsic aging.

glycolic acid Alpha hydroxy acid derived from sugar cane. It has a small molecular size that allows for easier penetration into the skin.

glycosaminoglycans (GAGs) Polysaccharide chains, most prominent in the dermis that bind with water, smoothing and softening the surface from below.

glycyrrhetic acid A bioactive natural glycoside known for its antiinflammatory qualities.

goals General statements of anticipated business outcomes resulting from well-stated objectives.

gommage An exfoliant without grains.

granulocytes White blood cells involved in immune response; these include neutrophils, eosinophils, and basophils.

ground substance Consists mainly of glycosaminoglycans (hyaluronic acid, chondroitin sulfate, and dermatan sulfate); involved in maintenance and repair of dermis.

H

health history sheet A document used by medical professionals to gather information on past and present health conditions, as well as likelihood for future conditions. This information includes allergies, medical conditions, and prescription information.

Health Insurance Portability and Accountability Act (HIPAA) A federal regulation that dictates procedural protocols to protect patient privacy.

Help Us Understand You sheet A document that should be used by skin-care professionals to gauge a client's knowledge, expectations, and concerns so that the treatment will be mutually advantageous. It is also used to differentiate the business and identify with the client.

hemochromatosis Dyschromia characterized by a buildup of pigments; known as hemosiderosis.

hepatitis A condition caused from multiple viruses defined as hepatitis A, B, or C; it is a contagious inflammation of the liver, with possible chronic consequences, particularly with hepatitis C.

herpes simplex An infectious disease caused by herpes simplex virus (HSV)-1, characterized by thin-walled vesicles that tend to occur repeatedly in the same place on the skin's surface.

Hippocrates Greek physician and "father of medicine" who theorized the Hippocratic oath and the four humors.

Hippocratic oath Oath taken by all physicians relative to the practice of medicine and created by Hippocrates.

hormone replacement therapy A therapeutic replacement of natural and synthetic hormones as a means to counter the side effects of their absence, usually given to postmenopausal patients.

human immunodeficiency virus/acquired immunodeficiency syndrome (HIV/AIDS) Opportunistic infections that are associated with a compromised immune system.

humectants Moisturizing agents.

hydroquinone A safe, topical bleaching agent that inhibits the production of tyrosine within melanocytes.

Hylaform® An injectable hyaluronic acid manufactured from rooster combs.

hyperpigmentation The overproduction of melanin.

hypertrophic scars Overly developed scar tissue that rises above the skin level, often overfed by an abundance of capillaries. These scars usually regress over time.

hypodermis A layer of subcutaneous fat and connective tissue lying beneath the epidermis.

hypopigmentation The lack of melanin production.

I

image business The type of business in which the way the public views the company is based largely on how things look—or how they are perceived—more than actual performance.

impetigo A skin infection from staphylococcal or streptococcal bacteria.

impression A lasting opinion or judgment of something.

in vitro Not on a living subject.

in vivo On a living subject.

indicator hot sheet A daily or weekly progress report that measures and provides daily insight into a business or employees' performance.

indicators A key value used to measure performance over time as it relates to an organization's goal progress.

inflammatory phase The early wound-healing phase during which blood and fluid collect and substances begin to fight infection and promote healing.

insult An injury or a trauma that causes an inconsistency in tissue.

integumentary system The skin and its appendages (nails, hair, sweat glands, and oil glands).

intrinsic aging Changes that would occur over time without the effects of any environmental factors.

inventory An itemized list of merchandise or supplies on hand.

ischemia A localized restriction of blood flow usually caused by an obstruction of normal circulation.

isohexadecane A highly emollient cleansing agent.

J

Jessner's solution Peel solution for the skin that is 14% resorcinol, 14% salicylic acid, and 14% lactic acid in ethanol.

K

keloid scars Scar formation in which tissue response is excessive in relation to normal tissue repair.

keratinization The process keratin cells go through as they move up to the stratum corneum layer.

keratinocyte Any cell in the skin, hair, or nails that produces keratin.

keratolysis Separation of the skin cells in the epidermis.

keratoses Horny growths on the skin.

kojic acid A bleaching agent derived from bacteria on a Japanese mushroom, usually used in conjunction with hydroquinone.

kola nut An African nut tree commonly used for strong medicinal qualities. Kola nut also contains high levels of caffeine.

L

lactic acid An AHA derived from milk.

lamellar granules Control lipids that produce NMF.

lamellar ichthyosis An inherited skin disorder with scaly, dry patches of skin; also known as fish scale disease.

Langerhans cells Cells that are intimately involved in the immune response of skin.

l-ascorbic acid Topical vitamin C that is both water and fat soluble.

lavender A plant used primarily as a fragrance and thought to have antibacterial qualities.

lentigines Flat brown spots appearing on aged or sunlight-exposed skin. Commonly called liver spots, they are not related to any liver disease.

leukocytes White blood cells without granules involved in immune response; these include lymphocytes and monocytes.

lichen simplex chronicus Itching papules; also known as Vidal's disease.

licorice A dried root that contains glycyrrhetic acid, a known antiinflammatory.

lipids Fat or fatlike substances that are descriptive, not chemical.

lipodystrophy A disruption in fat metabolism.

lupus An autoimmune disease that is a chronic, progressive, ulcerating skin disease.

lymphatic drainage Drainage of lymphatic fluids.

lymphocytes White blood cells involved in the body's immune system; their numbers increase in the presence of infection.

M

macrophages Part of the immune system in the skin; these cells are scavengers that clear debris in tissue injury.

magnesium ascorbyl phosphate An ester that converts to vitamin C on the skin

malic acid An AHA derived from apples.

malignant Cancerous or harmful to one's health.

malnutrition The result of any condition that causes a lack of nutritional substances for the body to use and distribute.

marketing strategies The planned use of marketing elements and media pathways to create a strategy to introduce new clients or reactivate former clients.

marketplace Any environment in which two or more people buy or sell a product or service.

melanin The cells that produce color in the skin.

melanocytes A group of cells (in the epidermis) that produces the pigment melanin.

melanoma The most serious form of skin cancer.

Melaquin® A 3% concentration of hydroquinone.

melasma An overproduction of melanin.

melasma gravidarum An increase in melanin production caused by pregnancy, also known as the mask of pregnancy.

milia A small, white-headed cyst filled with keratin.

mission statement A written statement of a business's individual philosophy.

moderate peels A peel depth extending into the papillary dermis.

moisturizers An agent that replenishes moisture to the skin.

mulberry root The precursor to hydroquinone.

N

naso-labial folds   The area of skin connected to the nose and lip.

natural moisturizing factor (NMF)   A compound found only in the top layer of skin that gives cells their ability to bind with water.

necrosis   Death of cells, when tissue is deprived of blood supply.

neutral   A pH of 7.0.

neutralization   A process by which active agents lose their potency, either with the addition of another agent or the loss of time.

neutrophils   The most common type of white blood cells that kill bacteria and discourage infection.

nicotinamide   A member of the vitamin B complex that has been shown to decrease TEWL.

nonsurgical aesthetic skin care   Any non-invasive procedure that is intended to improve overall skin health and appearance.

normal aging   Intrinsic aging.

O

Obagi Blue® peel   A simplified, uniform, user-friendly TCA peel solution indicated for all skin types, created by Dr. Zein Obagi.

occlusion   The state of being closed.

organelles   A specific location within the cell.

P

papillae   Projections of any kind; in the skin, papillae hold the dermis and the epidermis together.

papillary dermal wounding   Any injury to the skin that is sufficient to cause bleeding.

para-aminobenzoic acid (PABA)   A cousin of the vitamin B complex found in animals other than humans, the most common use of which is that of an effective sunscreen.

Parsol 1789®   Preferred sunscreen ingredient that protects against photodamage and premature aging of the skin from exposure to UVA light.

partial-thickness injury   A wound that penetrates only the epidermis or the upper layer of the papillary dermis. These wounds tend to heal more quickly and with less risk of scarring.

patient information sheet (PI)   A document used by medical professionals to gather social, personal, and demographic information.

peel depth   The depth of skin injury by chemical peeling agents.

peel percentage   The amount of bioavailability of the active ingredient, not to be confused with pH.

penetration pricing   A pricing strategy in which the price is set low to allow for introduction into an existing market.

perception   A process by which individuals use their senses to make decisions or gather information.

pH (potential of hydrogen)   The scale by which a material is characterized as being acidic (pH less than 7.0), alkaline (greater than 7.0), or neutral (7.0).

phenol (carbolic acid)   Highly corrosive acid used in peel solutions that dissolves cells to make room for newer and healthier ones.

photodamage   Damage caused by repeated and unprotected sunlight exposure over time, also called *solar damage*.

photographs   The reproduction of an image on film. A necessary component of skin-care treatment program that accurately documents the original skin condition so as to prove or disclaim treatment results.

physiology   The study of body functions.

pilosebaceous unit   Hair follicle and accompanying sebaceous glands and arrector pili muscle.

postinflammatory hyperpigmentation   Pigment that occurs in response to skin injury.

postmitotic cells   Cells that have completed mitotic division.

poultices   An herb or other substance made into a paste, used to relieve congestion or pain on the skin.

"powering" the patient database   An in-house marketing strategy that involves innovative and detailed use of information already contained in a business database to increase traffic.

predisposed   Possessing attributes that increase the likelihood of an event taking place.

premium pricing   A pricing strategy in which the price is set high to compensate for a high-quality product, usually with a high production cost as well.

preservatives   An agent used to prevent spoilage.

pricing strategies   A process by which a business determines the best way to price its product or service to entice customers while allowing for profit.

product bundling pricing   A pricing strategy in which one or more products or services are offered at a discount.

professional ethics   A set of guidelines that should set a framework for professional behavior and responsibilities.

progressive improvement plan (PIP)   Administrative document intended to record a problem and the actions taken to correct the problem and prevent its reoccurrence.

proliferative phase   The phase of wound healing during which replacement of protective epithelial tissue occurs over the old wound site.

protein   A class of complex compounds that are synthesized by all living creatures. Proteins are broken down into amino acids for use, including the rebuilding of tissue.

protein coagulation   The point at which the peel solution reaches the protein of the skin.

pseudofolliculitis barbae   In-grown hairs.

pyruvic acid   An alpha keto acid that has properties of acids and ketones. Pyruvic acid is a powerful peeling agent.

R

Radiesse®   Calcium hydroxylapatite (a dermal filler).

radio frequency   Frequency used with the newest technology for promoting collagen growth.

Raynaud's phenomenon   A chronic peripheral vascular disease.

reepithelialization   The replacement of protective epithelial tissue.

referral programs   An in-house marketing strategy that rewards an existing client for referring a new one.

reflexology   A system of massage in which certain body parts are massaged in specific areas to influence other body functions favorably.

remodeling phase   Phase of wound healing during which collagen is assembled to replace skin.

Renova®   A tretinoin that is meant specifically for aging and is recommended for patients with drier-than-normal skin.

resorcinol   Equal parts of hydroquinone and catechol, a peeling agent with similarities to phenol.

Restylane®   Trade name for the first FDA approved hyaluronic acid for dermal filling.

rete-pegs   Anatomic features that hold the dermis and epidermis together.

reticula   A netlike formation or structure; a network.

reticular dermis   The sublayer of the dermis that connects the dermis to the epidermis and is home to the skin's appendages (nails, hair, and glands).

Retin A®   Topical vitamin A, also known as tretinoin.

retinol   A vitamin-A derivative that must first convert to retinoic acid before it can be useful to the skin.

retinyl palmitate   A vitamin-A derivative that must first convert to retinoic acid before it can be useful to the skin. It is also thought to be useful for collagen synthesis.

revenue goals   The process used to define the monetary objectives of a business.

revenue strategy   A pricing plan to keep the business moving forward.

rhytids   The clinical name for wrinkles.

ringworm   A popular term for dermatomycosis caused by a species of fungi from the Microsporum family.

rolling acne scars   Acne scars that appear in a wave pattern over the face.

Rubin classification of aging analysis   A system of aging analysis that calculates the degree of photodamage and assigns a numerical level. The Rubin classification considers only extrinsic aging.

S

salicylate toxicity   Absorption of too much salicylic acid, resulting in ear ringing, dehydration, and possible convulsions.

salicylates   The salt of salicylic acid.

salicylic acid   Beta-hydroxy acid, a peeling agent usually reserved for acne treatment.

scar   A mark left in the skin or on an internal organ that is the result of deep tissue trauma. Scars are a result of injury, disease, or medical procedures.

sebaceous glands   Small glands, usually located next to hair follicles in the dermis that release fatty liquids onto the hair follicle to soften hair and skin.

seborrheic keratoses   A benign skin tumor common in older adults, thought to develop from prolific epidermal cells.

sebum   The semifluid secretion of the sebaceous glands consisting chiefly of fat, keratin, and cellular material.

secondary intention   The process of healing that includes coagulation and inflammation, reepithelialization, granulation tissue formation, angiogenesis, and collagen remodeling.

selenium   A chemical agent resembling sulfur that helps protect the skin from solar-induced skin cancers.

senescence   Growing old; aging.

Septisol   An antibacterial cleansing agent.

skin condition   A fundamental skin classification in which an individual's skin is grouped according to the degree of moisture retention or its reaction to products and environment, or both.

skin history sheet   A document used by skin-care professionals to provide information on a client's past and present skin health, including past treatment, sunburns, and conditions that are necessary for treatment.

skin turgor   The flexibility of the skin.

skin typing   A more detailed skin classification that gives indications as to how a certain skin type will react to various treatment conditions.

sodium lauryl isethionate   Similar to sodium lauryl sulfate but not as irritating. Additionally, it is less effective as an emulsifier.

sodium lauryl sulfate   A common ingredient in household detergents and soaps most commonly used as an emulsifier.

solid carbon dioxide   The clinical name for dry ice.

squamous cell carcinoma (SCC)   A malignant cancer of the epithelial cells.

standard pricing policy   A business document that outlines the specific price range of a given product or service, preferred pricing strategy, and circumstances during which each might change.

static rhytids   Wrinkles that show without reference to movement.

stem cells   Unspecialized cells that give rise to specific specialized cells.

stratum basale   The lowest layer of the epidermis. The stratum basale (basal layer) houses germinal cells and regenerating cells for all layers of the epidermis.

stratum corneum   The superficial sublayer the epidermis; this layer varies in thickness over the body.

subcutaneous   Beneath the skin.

sun protection factor (SPF)   The amount of time you can be exposed to sunlight before you burn.

sunscreens   Any agent that protects the skin from harmful ultraviolet A and B (UVA, UVB) light. In turn, sunscreen helps protect skin from photodamage, including skin cancers, dyschromias, and so forth. Sunscreens block rays by either physical or chemical means.

superficial peels   A peel depth that extends into the stratum granulosum.

surfactants   A surface-active agent that lowers surface tension.

systemic lupus   Chronic disease of connective tissue, which results in injury to various affected tissue, identified by butterfly mask over the nose.

T

tartaric acid   An AHA derived from grapes.

technique sensitive   Results of a treatment that depend on the clinician's ability to administer consistent results.

telangiectasia   Dilation of a group of small blood vessels.

telogen   The resting phase of the hair follicle.

tinea corporis   Body ringworm.

tinnitus   Ringing in the ears.

titanium dioxide   Physical sunscreen that scatters light rather than absorbing or filtering it.

transepidermal water loss (TEWL)   The process by which our bodies constantly lose water via evaporation.

trichloroacetic acid   Chemical used in peel solutions that dissolve aging and abnormal cells to make room for newer and healthier ones.

tyrosine   An enzyme that produces melanin in melanocytes. Overproduction of melanin is associated with hyperpigmentation.

U

ubiquinone   Lipid soluble cellular antioxidant present in virtually all cells.

understanding your client   A component of the business landscape during which a business evaluates and acquaints itself with its target demographics.

understanding your competition   A component of the business landscape during which a business evaluates its competition in terms of pricing, procedures, demographics, and advertising promotions.

universal precautions   Preventative actions taken to prevent the transmission of infectious diseases; it involves the use of protective procedures and equipment, such as gloves and masks.

V

Valtrex®   An antiviral treatment for herpes simplex.

vasoconstriction   Narrowing of the blood vessels.

very superficial peels   A peel depth that does not achieve erythema or flaking and thus is ineffective.

vesiculation   The process of forming blisters.

vitamin B   *See* nicotinamide.

vitamin C   An antioxidant that is a necessary factor for the formation of collagen in connective tissue and maintenance of integrity of intercellular cement.

vitamin E   An antioxidant that has been shown to inactivate free radicals. However, the exact mechanism of function is unknown.

vitiligo   Smooth depigmented white spots on the skin.

W

Wood's lamp   A device that uses UV rays to detect fluorescent material in the skin, which are indicative of certain diseases or conditions.

wound   A disruption of normal tissue that results from pathologic processes, beginning internally or externally to the involved organ.

wound healing   The restoration of tissue continuity following injury or trauma.

Y

yearly business objectives   A part of the annual business plan that identifies the goals a business would like to attain during a given fiscal year.

yeast infections   A viral infection caused by several unicellular organisms that reproduce by budding. Oral yeast infections are common in persons with compromised immune systems.

yin and yang   Concept, originally devised by Fu Xi, that describes the harmony between nature and its daily phenomenon.

Z

zinc oxide   Physical sunscreen that scatters light rather than absorbing or filtering it.

Index

291